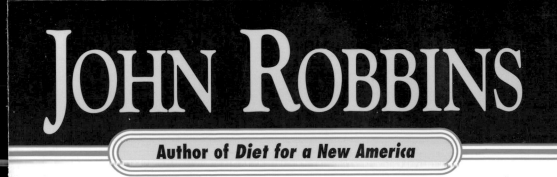

JOHN ROBBINS

Author of *Diet for a New America*

RECLAIMING OUR HEALTH

Exploding the Medical M
and Embracing the
Source of True Heali

WHAT OTHER PEOPLE ARE SAYING ABOUT
RECLAIMING OUR HEALTH

"In this wonderful new book, John Robbins meticulously documents how and why the factors associated with true healing are often missing from the so-called health-care systems of our country, and then gives us some very up lifting and practical solutions to this dilemma. But to understand the importance of these solutions, you have to first understand what created the situation we've inherited today. Robbins explains the history of our health-care system in a highly entertaining, personal, and accurate fashion. For instance, though I've long been familiar with many of the forces that have kept drugs and surgery in the forefront of the medical armamentarium, often at the expense of other solutions, and though I know well the mindset that perpetuates this, I was completely shocked to learn about the disgraceful relationship between conventional organized medicine and the tobacco industry. This riveting story and the many others that are equally compelling now need to reach the widest possible audience if Americans are to awaken from the trance that is holding the state of their health hostage. Frankly, I'd make this book required reading for everyone in the country who has any decision-making power whatsoever about health. It's time that everyone in this country knew the truth about health and healing that is presented so eloquently and convincingly in *Reclaiming Our Health*."
> —Christiane Northrup, M.D., Assistant Clinical Professor of
> Obstetrics and Gynecology, University of Vermont College
> of Medicine, Past President of American Holistic Medical
> Association, Author of *Women's Bodies, Women's Wisdom*

"What Rachel Carson's *Silent Spring* did for the environmental movement, John Robbins's *Reclaiming Our Health* does for health care."
> —Dana Ullman, M.P.H., Author of
> *The Consumer's Guide to Homeopathy*

"John Robbins has done it again! The author of *Diet for a New America* has courageously taken on the medical establishment. The section on cancer treatment is particularly excellent. Robbins shows in vivid detail how often the 'proven' methods do not work while alternative treatments are given short shrift. Robbins's book provides a sober yet highly encouraging look at the most promising alternative treatments. No one can come away from this book without realizing that major reforms are necessary in the way we as a society deal with the cancer problem."
> —Ralph Moss, Ph.D., Author of *The Cancer Industry*
> and *Questioning Chemotherapy*

"*Reclaiming Our Health* is one of the most profound books I have ever read. It will not only change medical practice; it will change the world."
— Howard Lyman, Director,
Humane Society of the United States

"John Robbins's new book tears the mask off Medicine in America. It is a shocking exposé of what is wrong, yet a beautifully optimistic view of what can be very right when we change from a disease-centered culture to a health-centered one. John Robbins is a true visionary, and his latest work is powerful and compelling."
— Neal D. Barnard, M.D., President,
Physicians Committee for Responsible Medicine

"*Reclaiming Our Health* is excellent. It is beautifully written, and an out-standing example of patient empowerment."
— Bernie Siegel, M.D., Author of *Love, Medicine, and Miracles*

"Modern medicine can be life-saving and compassionate, but also lethal, un-caring, and self-serving. *Reclaiming Our Health* is a bombshell of a book that takes an unflinching look at the dark side of our current medical system, and points the way toward a more effective, humane, and life-affirming health-care system."
— Larry Dossey, M.D., Author of *Healing Words*

"As a physician reading John Robbins's *Reclaiming Our Health,* I was moved by this powerful indictment of physician arrogance and the institutional in-sensitivity that often passed for today's medical care. Written with compassion and the sincere intent to heal the situation, Robbins's words ring with legiti-macy and had me thinking again and again: You know, he's right."
— Michael Klaper, M.D., Director,
Institute for Nutrition Education and Research

"Wow! Even though I've been studying and researching the politics and eco-nomics of health care for over 25 years, I was stunned by the data John Rob-bins has unearthed for *Reclaiming Our Health.* The work is so well researched and presented that it just can't be ignored or discredited. A must-read."
— Joseph Pizzorno, M.D., President, Bastyr University

Reclaiming
Our
Health

Exploding the Medical Myth
and Embracing the
Source of True Healing

John Robbins

H J KRAMER
TIBURON, CALIFORNIA

H J Kramer Inc
P.O. Box 1082
Tiburon, CA 94920

Editor: Nancy Grimley Carleton
Editorial Assistant: Claudette Charbonneau
Cover Design: Jim Marin/Marin Graphic Services
Book Design and Composition: Classic Typography
Book Production: Schuettge & Carleton
Manufactured in the United States of America.
10 9 8 7 6 5 4 3 2 1

The Library of Congress has catalogued
the hard-cover edition as follows:

Library of Congress Cataloging-in-Publication Data

Robbins, John.
    Reclaiming our health : exploding the medical myth and embracing
the source of true healing / by John Robbins.
        p.   cm.
    Includes index.
    ISBN 0-915811-69-3 (hardcover)
    1. Medical care—United States.   2. Holistic medicine.
3. Alternative medicine.   4. Medical care—Philosophy.   I. Title.
RA395.A3R623   1996
362.1'0973—dc20   96-19149
                                                              CIP

Contents

Part Five

Foreword

IN SEVERAL AREAS of our collective existence, the status quo guards crumbling mansions, and nowhere are the cracks more evident than in Western medicine. While modern Americans have acquiesced almost hypnotically to the prejudices of our medical establishment, the suppression of free thinking has never been, and never will be, a permanent thing. In medicine, as elsewhere, a renaissance in higher consciousness is beginning to take hold in America. It awakens us from our collective enslavement to an overly materialistic bias, and herein lies our greatest hope for the healing and renewal of the Western world.

I am honored to preface the following material with the acknowledgment that John Robbins is one of the foremost evocateurs of the new American renaissance. In *Reclaiming Our Health*, he guides our understanding of a natural modality for health and healing, an area of intimate concern for each and every one of us, for our families, and for our future. As a woman, I am particularly grateful to him for restoring to our awareness the unique function of women's minds and bodies in a healed and whole society.

A time of whole-systems transition is upon us, replete with crumbling mansions and coalescing castles of light. New force fields of awareness are pushing up from the bottom of things, and from this pressure shall come a quantum leap forward in human possibility. In *Reclaiming Our Health*, John Robbins helps us clear a path of illumination through a medical fog which has lasted for decades. Let's not be angry at the people and institutions who so clearly have deceived us, but let us be full of hope that on the path ahead, we will be far too sophisticated in our understanding to ever let ourselves be so deceived again.

—Marianne Williamson
Author of *A Return to Love* and *A Woman's Worth*
Spring 1996

Acknowledgments

The creation of *Reclaiming Our Health* has truly been a partnership effort. There is no way I can adequately express my gratitude for the tremendous support given by my partner and wife, Deo; my son and dear friend, Ocean; and his fiancee and my spirit daughter, Michele. Their contributions, both directly to the book and to my life, have been more important than words can say.

I also want to express my deepest thanks to Hal and Linda Kramer, who have been far more than publishers for this book. In their vision for the book and in their faith in me, they have been midwives to its birth, and coparents in its life.

Marianne Williamson and Riane Eisler have honored *Reclaiming Our Health* by contributing their splendid Foreword and Introduction. I am forever grateful to each of them, not only for blessing this book, but also for the strength and direction their work has given to our generation.

My deepest thanks and appreciation also goes to Christiane Northrup, M.D., Andrew Weil, M.D., Ralph Moss, Ph.D., and all of the other health professionals and activists who have helped inspire this book, and who are working to bring healing to our medical system and our lives.

Among my dear friends whose support has been especially meaningful to this work, I want to particularly acknowledge Joyce Vissell, R.N., and Barry Vissell, M.D.

I am also grateful for the assistance of Patricia Carney, Shams Kairys, Steve Lustgarden, Richard Glantz, Eleanor Wasson, Howard Lyman, Amy Bacheller, Earle Harris, Ian and Terry Thiermann, Sheila Hoffman, and my many other friends and colleagues on the EarthSave board and staff.

There are so many people who have all in their different ways provided crucial support for me and the book: Nancy Grimley Carleton, Salima Cobb, R.N., Michael Klaper, M.D., Raven Lang, Lois Berry, Glenn Warner, M.D., Michelle Winkler, Barbara Harper, John Lee, M.D.,

Bob Kradjian, M.D., Anna Keck, R.N., Ken Ausebel, Dana Ullman, Katchie Shakti Egger, Keith Block, M.D., Phil Kline, Jim Marin, Steve Roth. . . . I cannot name them all, but I am eternally grateful for the community of beings whose work and love have enabled me to write *Reclaiming Our Health*.

—John Robbins
Spring 1996

Introduction

SOMETIMES A BOOK COMES ALONG at precisely the right moment in history. This is such a book. America's health-care system is in crisis, and *Reclaiming Our Health* points the way toward *real* health-care reform.

Reclaiming Our Health is not only an extremely timely, urgently needed book; it is a landmark book that, like John Robbins's earlier *Diet for a New America,* helps us look at ourselves and our world with fresh eyes.

In *Reclaiming Our Health,* Robbins makes another major contribution to the health of our nation and our world. Like his *Diet for a New America,* this book is an impeccably researched work in the honorable tradition of such "muckraking" classics as Rachel Carson's and Upton Sinclair's earlier exposes of harmful and unethical practices. And like *Diet for a New America,* this book charts a new course that is both healthier and more cost-effective.

These are some of the reasons I was delighted, and honored, when John asked me to write the Introduction to this book. But there are also some more personal reasons. One is my affection and admiration for this remarkable man, whose passion for justice, gentle humor, and dedication to human welfare imbue every page of *Reclaiming Our Health.* The other is that in *Reclaiming Our Health* John brilliantly applies what I have identified as the dominator and partnership models to health care, showing how the dominator perspective has led to many of our health-care difficulties and using the partnership model as a prescription for healing and a guide for action.

Reclaiming Our Health shows how the dominator model—for example, the view that our bodies have to be controlled through drastic interventions and the notion that all will be well if we simply follow "doctor's orders"—has distorted health care, and with it, our lives. It shows how the dominator gender stereotypes—for example, the notion that men must control both women and nature—lie behind many of the inadequacies and failures of our health-care system. More important, it shows how a partnership model of health care, melding the most ancient wisdom with the newest scientific insights, can help us fully use our own extraordinary healing powers.

Unlike many of the orthodox approaches to health-care reform, *Reclaiming Our Health* is not about limiting conventional medicine by cutting funds for social programs, such as Medicare. It is not about herding health-care providers into HMOs, where they, and we, are restricted by considerations of short-term financial profit, which in the long term results in huge economic and human costs. Rather, it is about how we can care for ourselves and one another in more appropriate and affordable ways, through both time-honored and innovative approaches.

In the process, *Reclaiming Our Health* offers a rich storehouse of information and tells many fascinating stories. It explores the lost spiritual dimensions of health and healing that women and men all over the world are today struggling to reclaim. It takes us way back, to ancient traditions that we lost during the prehistoric shift from a time when humans lived more in partnership with one another, our bodies, and the rest of nature, to a time when conquest and domination became the norm. It looks at the resurging profession of midwifery—and with this, childbirth at home, often in a sacred space—and how today's persecution of midwives is a milder replay of the witch burning of the Middle Ages, when untold numbers of women were hunted down, tortured, and burned alive by "men of God" for the crime of healing through herbal and other natural means. But it also recognizes that modern medicine has made, and can continue to make, important contributions—if these are contextualized in a health-care system guided by a partnership ethos free from the conventional biases against women, nature, and spirituality.

In short, this is a book that can profoundly change not only health care, but our lives. I hope it is read by our policy makers—and by everyone who wants to play an active and informed part in moving us toward the better future we want for our children and future generations.

> —Riane Eisler
> Author of *The Chalice and the Blade*
> and *Sacred Pleasure*
> April 1996

1

Reclaiming Our Health

ONCE UPON A TIME there was a large and rich country where people kept falling over a steep cliff. They'd fall to the bottom and be injured, sometimes quite seriously, and many of them died. The nation's medical establishment responded to the situation by positioning, at the base of the cliff, the most sophisticated and expensive ambulance fleet ever developed, which would immediately rush those who had fallen to modern hospitals that were equipped with the latest technological wizardry. No expense was too great, they said, when people's health was at stake.

Now it happened that it occurred to certain people that another possibility would be to erect a fence at the top of the cliff. When they voiced the idea, however, they found themselves ignored. The ambulance drivers were not particularly keen on the idea, nor were the people who manufactured the ambulances, nor those who made their living and enjoyed prestige in the hospital industry. The medical authorities explained patiently that the problem was far more complex than people realized, that while building a fence might seem like an interesting idea it was actually far from practical, and that health was too important to be left in the hands of people who were not experts. Leave it to us, they said, for with enough money we will soon be able to genetically engineer people who do not bruise or become injured from such falls.

So no fences were built, and as time passed this nation found itself spending an ever-increasing amount of its financial resources on hospitals and high-tech medical equipment. In fact, it came to spend far more money on medical services than any nation had ever done in the history of the world. Money that could have gone to community services, decent housing, education, and good food was not available to the people, for it was being spent on ambulances and hospitals. As the costs of treating people kept rising, growing numbers of people could not afford medical care.

There were increasing numbers of homeless, and ever more hungry people and families torn apart by the stress. As a result of these and similar mis-allocations of national energy and resources, violence, gangs, and inner-city riots welled up as outlets for the frustration and despair people felt.

The more people kept falling off the cliff, the more a sense of urgency and tension developed, and the more of the country's money was poured into the heroic search for a drug that could be given to those who had fallen to cure their injuries. When some people pointed out how fruitless the search had been thus far, and questioned whether a cure would ever be found, the research industry answered with massive public relations campaigns showing men in white coats holding the broken bodies of children who had fallen, pleading, "Don't quit on us now, we're almost there."

When a few families who had lost loved ones tried to erect warning signs at the top of the cliff, they were arrested for trespassing. When some of the more enlightened physicians began to say that the medical authorities should publicly warn people that falling off the cliff was dangerous, representatives from powerful industries denounced them as "health police." A fierce battle ensued, and finally, after many compromises, the medical establishment did issue warnings. Anyone, they said, who had already broken both arms and both legs in previous falls should exercise utmost caution when falling.

Of course, this is just a fable.

AWAKENING FROM THE MEDICAL MYTH

Like most people in our society, I grew up believing in the medical myth. I grew up believing that health comes from the doctor, the drugstore, and the hospital.

I never suspected that illness might be a messenger, or that our experience of our bodies, whether well or ill, could provide us with self-understanding. I did not know that I could create a lifestyle that would support the radiant health of my body, mind, and spirit. I did not understand that the choices I made and the way I lived could make a tremendous difference to the quality of life I experienced. I never imagined that the source of true healing lay within each of us.

But over the years I have come to realize that while doctors and medical technology have an important role to play in health care, they do not hold the ultimate secrets to health. Taken together, factors such as the food we eat, whether and how we exercise, the way we give voice to our feelings, the attitudes we hold, and the quality of the environment in which we live are far more important to the quality of health we experience than even the most sophisticated medical technologies. It has been liberating to see that health comes from learning to live in vibrant harmony with ourselves, with the natural world, and with one another.

In our society, the medical myth has led to an emphasis on intervention instead of prevention that has generated a crisis in health care of epic proportions. The current level of dissatisfaction and frustration with the U.S. medical system is enormous. Corporate health-care expenditures now exceed corporate profits. Doctors and patients alike feel depersonalized and used. Year after year, the difference between our system and that of other nations becomes more embarrassing and disturbing. We spend far more money for health care than any other country in the world, and yet we are the only nation in the industrialized world that does not guarantee minimum health care to every single citizen. Increasing numbers of Americans—42 million at last count—have no health coverage. We lead the world in malpractice suits, but continue to fall further behind in infant mortality rates, life expectancy, and the other indicators used to measure the health of a people.

In New York City, 10.8 infants out of 1,000 die before their first birthday, while in Shanghai, China, the rate is only 9.9. Life expectancy at birth in Shanghai is now 75.5 years, compared to a life expectancy in New York City of 73 years for whites and 70 years for people of color.[1] Shanghai is an extremely overcrowded and polluted Third World city in a country with a per capita income of only $350. Shanghai spends just $38 per person annually on medical care, compared to New York City's $3,000, yet generates a better health record because it channels what funds it has toward prevention and basic care, because its elders are respected and revered, and because only very recently have its people begun to fall prey to the high-fat, meat-based American diet.[2]

Our medical establishment's fixation on drugs, surgery, and other high-tech interventions at the expense of low-cost preventive approaches is perhaps most evident in its failure to fully appreciate the important role of nutrition in health. A board member of the Ohio Dietetic Association recently said, "A hospital is one of the few places in the U.S. where a person can starve to death unnoticed."[3] The average U.S. physician, in four years of medical school, gets only two hours of course work in nutrition.

Only 25 percent of the accredited medical schools in the country have a single required course in nutrition.[4] Meanwhile, McDonald's is opening up franchises in hospitals!

A HEALING CRISIS

We all know that the American medical system is in the throes of a horrendous crisis, and many of us feel overwhelmed and desperate in the face of it all. The question I seek to answer is whether it might be possible for this chaos, upheaval, and dysfunction to serve a healing purpose. Could the very intensity of our medical crisis somehow represent a potential turning point, an unprecedented opportunity for fundamental personal and social change? Is it possible that the breakdown of our medical system could lead to a greater healing, both in our society and in many of our lives?

Increasing numbers of us are seeing that we cannot remain passive bystanders to our own health, and then expect the medical system to rescue us. We're seeing how false and destructive is the belief that the more money we spend and the more technology we have, the healthier we will be. We're seeing how alienating and harmful it can be to think that experts always know more than we do about our bodies and our lives.

The current medical crisis is serving to challenge the assumptions many of us have held, and in the process leading us to become aware of more satisfying and fulfilling ways to live. We're seeing that there may not be a technological or pharmaceutical answer to all our ills, and that consuming drugs that have been prescribed by a physician may not always be the best way to alleviate our difficulties. We're seeing that if we don't want to be dependent on a system that is increasingly expensive and dehumanizing, we need to find other approaches on which we can reliably depend. Increasingly, we are utilizing alternative forms of medicine that rely on the natural healing wisdom our bodies possess, and selecting foods and making other personal choices based on what we believe will produce the healthiest outcomes.

By disrupting our blind faith in the medical system, the current crisis is throwing us back on ourselves, and compelling us to ask such questions as: What can I do to optimize my health and healing? How must I live in order to attain and preserve well-being? For which conditions is orthodox medicine of value, and for which conditions are alternative approaches more appropriate? How can I become less dependent on an impersonal system, and more connected to and trusting of the sources of true healing within me?

Many of us are turning our attention toward what we can do for ourselves on an ongoing basis, building and nurturing our health, rather than ignoring our bodies' needs and then automatically taking ourselves to the doctor to be fixed when illness strikes. We are learning that our health is intimately interwoven with our mental outlook, emotional tone, and spiritual well-being, and coming to understand that taking responsibility for our health means more than simply lowering our cholesterol or blood pressure. It means learning to tap the powerful regenerative forces that dwell within our own beings. It means opening our lives to the joy of awakening and the gift of peace.

FROM DISEASE CARE TO HEALTH CARE

I sometimes think we don't really have a "health-care" system; we have a "disease-care" system. For our medical establishment does not teach us how to live so that we can achieve the maximum health and highest quality of life of which we are capable. Instead, it teaches us to manipulate ourselves from the outside, a process that has left many of us numb to the signals our bodies constantly send. Some of us have become so out of touch with our bodies that we may fail to register when we need to exercise, stop eating, open a window, change body positions, take a deep breath, tell others we love them, or rest. We may not know when we need caring or nurturing, or when we need to express ourselves. We may ignore fatigue, hunger, and discomfort to the point of doing real harm to ourselves. We may find ourselves continuing in jobs, relationships, and lifestyles that are killing us, yet close our ears even as our bodies scream out to us in distress.

Many of us do not really know how to take care of ourselves, nor what choices we can make to keep ourselves well. When I was growing up, I believed that eating a balanced diet meant enjoying a wide variety of the 31 flavors my family's business made available to the world. As far as I was concerned, the basic four food groups were Chocolate, Vanilla, Strawberry, and Jamoca Almond Fudge. I had no idea that the standard American diet, based as it is on high-fat meat and dairy products, and deriving nearly 40 percent of its calories from sugar, creates problems that even the most expensive medical technology can't repair.[5]

Because our dominant medical system has focused on intervention instead of prevention, growing numbers of people are beset by a host of physical problems and difficulties. Most adults, and even many children, suffer from allergies, headaches, back pain, lack of energy, stiff joints, digestive and respiratory disorders, and problematic emotional states, including periodic depression and anxiety. Most of us don't often feel all that wonderful, yet consider ourselves "normal" because most of the people we know are equally lacking in vitality. Meanwhile, there are massive industries profiting enormously from our overreliance on drugs, and from our following unhealthy lifestyles that lead to an ever-increasing demand for their services and products.

Although there is much in modern medicine that is of great value, we need to pick and choose very carefully from among its offerings. Many of its prescriptions and practices, while carrying numerous troubling side effects, merely suppress symptoms, sometimes even causing the disease process to take new and more virulent forms. Some of these treatments are no more truly healing than turning off a fire alarm without attending to the fire.

When we are taught to repress symptoms with no attempt to understand the needs they represent, our experience of ourselves becomes distant. We sense our bodies not as sources of self-awareness and guides to our healing needs, but as enigmas that must be analyzed and explained to us by experts. We easily become bewildered and lose trust in ourselves. If we become ill, we slip all too often into passivity and helplessness, believing ourselves dependent on the doctor to make us well, acting like bystanders to our own healing process, disconnected from the incredible creative powers that always lie within us.

After years of assisting people with cancer, the noted surgeon and author Bernie Siegel, M.D., remarked that the people who survive the disease are typically those who don't submit passively to the patient role. He said that he could tell that a patient was going to do well when nurses told him, "Your patient is a real problem; he won't take his clothes off; I can never find him in his room, and he keeps questioning every blood test."[6]

In studies done at Yale, Bernie Siegel says, "It got to be a joke. There was a 100 percent correlation between the head nurse's opinion of the patient and the long-term survival rates. If the head nurse said, 'He's a real s.o.b. and won't let you draw the blood for the test,' they would find no trouble with the immune system. If he was a submissive, gentle patient who would not question anything, and would always let the nurses draw his blood, he was in trouble."[7]

If you want to be well, Bernie Siegel concludes, the key is to stand up for yourself and make your needs known. People who give their power away to their doctors and to the hospital staff not only feel helpless—they die sooner. And yet this is exactly what most of us have been trained to do—subjugate our command over ourselves to anyone wearing a white coat and a stethoscope.

Some people wonder how I can presume to write with authority about these subjects, when I am not a doctor. Many of us have been taught that doctors, by virtue of their medical training, constitute a special class of human being, almost a priesthood. The truth is that if I had been trained as they have been, and if I were subject to the same financial pressures they are, I might be preoccupied with technology and drugs, oblivious to their drawbacks and risks, and dismissive of alternative approaches, just as many physicians today are. If I had spent six or eight years of my life being trained to practice orthodox medicine, and had sacrificed greatly in order to do this, as most of our doctors have, I would hardly be in a position to consider the subject without personal bias. It is precisely because I am not a doctor that I can more easily stand outside the fray, and hopefully bring a measure of objectivity to the discussion.

We struggle today, as a culture, to get over the idea that M.D. stands for "Medical Deity." It wouldn't hurt us to remember that in Israel in 1973, doctors went on strike for a month, and the death rate dropped 50 percent. There had not been a month with so few deaths since the previous doctors' strike, 20 years before. A few years later, in Bogota, Colombia, a two-month-long physician strike resulted in a 35 percent drop in the death rate. And when Los Angeles county doctors went on a work slowdown to protest soaring malpractice insurance premiums, the death rate dropped 18 percent. But when the slowdown ended, and the medical industry got back in gear, the death rate jumped right back up to where it had been before.[8]

THERE ARE ALTERNATIVES

I once believed that the medical establishment was unbiased and open-minded in its search for healing. I thought that the only people who would fall into disfavor with organized medicine would be charlatans and quacks who posed a danger to the public. But I have come, none too happily, to see otherwise. In fact, one of the reasons that so many other nations have better health outcomes while spending far less money than we do is that they are far more open to what we call preventive or alternative medicine. In no other nation are legitimate holistic alternatives to the pharmaceutical orientation marginalized and discredited the way they are in the United States.

Unlike much of orthodox medicine, alternative approaches to healing typically honor the wisdom and capability of the human body. Their goal is often to support and strengthen the powerful healing forces already at work within us. There are, of course, alternative methods that have no merit, and some that make fraudulent claims. But there are others that have been of great value to countless numbers of people. The sadness is that very few have been given the opportunity to be tested or appraised impartially. It is hard to overestimate the human suffering that continues to occur because these approaches are being condemned without a fair trial. An integration of orthodox and alternative medicine, a *partnership* approach to healing, would allow patients access to the best ideas and practices available, regardless of whose economic interest is served in the process.

When holistic and preventive methods of health care are dismissed as quackery without being given fair consideration, people are not only deprived of the health benefits these approaches can bring, but of the values and the relationship to life that they represent. To allow acupuncture, chiropractic, naturopathy, midwifery, homeopathy, herbs, massage therapy, and many of the other valid alternative methods fully into the medical picture would not only make medicine more effective, it would also incorporate a more compassionate perspective into medicine, for these approaches have in common that they nurture the inherent healing forces and potentials of the body, something orthodox medicine often neglects to do.

The medical myth casts an intimidating shadow. Many of us continue to believe that when we fall ill, there is nothing we can do but turn for deliverance to orthodox medical authorities. We expect our doctors to know what is best for us, and assume that if natural approaches and remedies worked, our doctors would tell us so. But the unfortunate truth is that American physicians have been trained in a system that has been closed historically to natural and alternative approaches, and is only now barely beginning to open.

This is why the American Medical Association (AMA) continues to attack acupuncture, biofeedback, homeopathy, and naturopathy as "unproven, disproven, controversial, fraudulent, and/or otherwise questionable."[9] This is why the AMA *Journal* hasn't written anything positive about acupuncture since Nixon went to China. And why the American Cancer Society continues to denounce unconventional approaches to cancer that show great healing promise and that have never been properly tested or impartially evaluated, even while chemotherapy is useful in only a very small percentage of cancers and is often horrendously toxic. Many people today who use alternative treatments do so without telling their medical doctors, for fear of being ridiculed. A prominent spokesperson for the AMA point of view who was evidently not terribly impressed with the value of alternative medicine recently took it upon himself to announce: "Freedom of choice in health care is a euphemism for freedom to defraud. What they want is the freedom to lie."[10]

AN ENTRY POINT FOR TRANSFORMATION

I have been asked what has motivated me to take on the medical establishment, to challenge its biases, and to expose its abuses of power. My answer is that I see how much needless harm is being done, and how much better things could be. I see how much healthier and happier people can be when they are educated and able to act wisely and make their own choices regarding their bodies. Freedom of choice is essential to the American way of life, and I believe that people ought to have a right to do with their bodies what they want to do, as long as they aren't hurting anyone else. There are many conditions that can best be treated by standard medicine, including trauma, medical and surgical emergencies, bacterial infections, and certain mechanical difficulties. But there are many other conditions, including most forms of cancer, viral infections, allergic and autoimmune disorders, and most chronic degenerative diseases, that are more effectively handled with alternative approaches. To my eyes, the monopolization of health care by the medical-pharmaceutical complex not only violates our rights to health freedom. It drains us of our potential for wholeness and healing by slighting the power of the human body to restore itself, and by rejecting the value of natural medicine.

I believe it is possible that the current medical crisis, as dire as it is, can be an entry point for transformation. The situation holds vast opportunity as well as danger. The movement to reclaim our bodies and our lives may in fact represent the most powerful grassroots movement that has yet emerged to challenge the underlying paradigm of our society, the basic philosophical assumptions that have us marching, in the name of progress and control, toward ecological disaster and social chaos.[11]

I believe it possible that the current medical crisis can yet become a healing crisis, one that could usher in greatly needed change. Alternative therapies that help us contact the regenerative powers that lie within us, that help us take care of ourselves and prevent disease, and that give us greater control over our lives have a major role to play in the future of health care, and in the healing of our society.

It is important to add that it has never been my intention to add further rage to an already highly inflamed situation. My purpose in exposing the darker side of the AMA and others in the medical establishment is to help make possible genuine health-care reform. I do not wish to condemn those whose actions are hurtful, but to lift the veil of ignorance and fear that cloaks us all. I do not wish to be inflammatory, but truthful. I bring the darker side of the medical establishment to light because I want to see people have access to legitimate alternatives, because I want no one to be left out, and because people deserve support in reclaiming power over their own bodies and lives.

Physicians in our society are granted special status, and given tremendous authority. They have in their arsenal enormously potent drugs and procedures, and they deal with people in their times of greatest vulnerability. They are the ones in whose hands we have placed our trust and our lives, and with that trust comes a responsibility to put their own self-interest aside in order to serve those in their care. Though there are many fine physicians, the medical system as it exists today frequently does not support them in fulfilling this sacred trust.

I write to show a way out of this predicament. I write to restore our faith in our bodies, in ourselves, and in those activities that truly generate and protect health.

WOMEN'S HEALTH ISSUES

Women are the world's mothers, and they carry within themselves the nurturing and compassionate instinct that Western technological medicine is in so much danger of losing. They are the ones whose voices are most needed today, and yet they are the ones who are least heard.

The subjugation of women deprives us all. When I focus on women's health issues, as I do in the first portion of this book, I do so on behalf of both women and men. For each of us, whether we are male or female, was born of a woman's body, and was nurtured, from our tiniest beginnings, in the body of a woman. Our primary sense of who we are and of the relationship we have with life was formed through the most intimate possible relationship with a woman. Regardless of our gender, the female body was our gateway to life.

If we are to bring healing to ourselves, to our society, and to our world, we must regain respect for our bodies, and particularly for women's bodies, for it is women who are most devalued, and it is women in whose wombs and hearts future generations are shaped. The way we are each treated by our mothers and what they pass on to us is largely a product of the messages they have internalized. In a world where women are demeaned, all children inherit a legacy of alienation and dishonor.

Unfortunately, our medical system has come to maintain a patriarchal attitude toward women, to possess what Riane Eisler has called a dominator rather than a partnership perspective. By medicalizing natural life events such as childbirth and menopause, and viewing women's bodies as inherently prone to malfunction, the medical establishment today perpetuates a disrespect for women that has plagued us for centuries.

Awakening from patriarchal, dominator medicine will not only help women to take charge of their health. It will also help all of us, both male and female, to regain our balance and recover our reverence for the feminine perspective and wisdom. It will help our medicine become more humane, more holistic, and more effective. It will help us become a society which, instead of revering the power to control and dominate, will truly honor the power, on the part of both men and women, to give, nurture, and illuminate life.

RECLAIMING OUR SELVES

I write to help all of us, male and female, doctors and patients, take authority over our lives into our own hands, and to take back our power from institutions, groups, and individuals who have lost sight of their mandate to serve. My urge is to help all of us take greater responsibility for every aspect of our lives—including our deaths. When we fail to do this, when we leave matters in the hands of a medical system that has grown increasingly impersonal, the results can be heartbreaking.

Sandra Bertman, director of the Program in Medical Humanities at the University of Massachusetts Medical Center, tells the all-too-common story of a 78-year-old man in another hospital who witnessed the intubation and unsuccessful resuscitation attempt on a fellow patient. Afterwards, he begged to be left alone.

"Listen, doctor. I don't want to die with tubes sticking out all over me. I don't want that my children should remember their father that way. All my life I tried to be a mensch, you understand? All my life, I tried to live so I could hold my head up. Rich I wasn't, but I managed to put my sons through college. I wanted to be able to hold my head up, to have dignity, even though I didn't have much money and didn't speak good English. Now I'm dying. Okay. I'm not complaining, I'm old and tired and have seen enough of life, believe me. But I still want to be a man, not a vegetable that someone comes and waters every day—not like him."[12]

Although this man was a competent adult, and made his wishes clear, they were not honored. He was "coded," tagged by hospital personnel to be resuscitated at all costs. Eventually, he managed to disconnect himself from the machinery, leaving a handwritten note to his physician: "Death is not the enemy, Doctor. Inhumanity is."[13]

My work is to bring compassion back into medicine, and to help all of us take possession of our lives. I write to help all of us find within ourselves, through the natural transitions, cycles, and rhythms that are ours to experience, something to be honored and kept sacred. My goal is to help heal how we relate to our bodies, to doctors, and to health, and to help us discover sources of true healing in the wisdom of our bodies.

Our life stories begin with birth—a natural process of immense power and extraordinary significance—and it is to this topic that we now turn. Here, as elsewhere, when we uncover the darkness in our medical system, it is always in order to more fully reveal the light in the human heart.

Part One

2

The Goddess in Stirrups

Jane English, a biologist from Soquel, California, became involved in the childbirth controversy when, after she had labored for 24 hours while awaiting her first child, her hospital's doctors insisted she have a cesarean section. When her objections were disregarded and nurses began restraining her, she fled to a hospital bathroom, where she easily and successfully gave birth on the floor while her friends and relatives fended off the staff.

IN THE MIDDLE OF THE 19TH CENTURY, a young Hungarian-born obstetrician by the name of Ignaz Philipp Semmelweis was delivering babies in a famous Viennese hospital. Women coming to give birth here were sent to one of the hospital's two sections—the First Clinic, where obstetricians prevailed and medical students received training, or the Second Clinic, staffed entirely by midwives. Noticing that women were literally begging to be admitted to the Second Clinic, Semmelweis began to look carefully at the autopsy records from the two sections. His investigation was to lead to one of the most remarkable advances in medical history. What he discovered was that the death rate from puerperal (childbed) fever for women in the doctors' wards was more than four times higher than for women under the midwives' jurisdiction.

Semmelweis, like the other doctors of his time, had no idea that germs could cause disease. This was some 20 years before Joseph Lister would advance the use of antiseptics in surgery. But in a moment of inspiration he decreed that the medical students handling deliveries on his ward should wash their hands in a chlorine solution after dissecting corpses, and after each examination of a woman in the ward. To this end, he arranged for washbasins to be placed strategically between the rows of beds.

The results were outstanding. Before the hand washing, one out of every eight women giving birth in the First Clinic had died of puerperal fever. But now the death rate dropped almost immediately to less than 1 in 100.

What do you think the reaction was when Semmelweis published the records of this spectacular success? Was he heralded and applauded, and his ideas immediately put into practice in all obstetrical clinics?

Not quite. Orthodox obstetricians virtually declared war on the poor man, battering and insulting him at every opportunity. He was hounded from Vienna, and eventually driven insane by the relentless attacks. He died without ever knowing that his views would eventually triumph, and that thanks to his discoveries, puerperal fever would nearly disappear. Humanity owes a great debt of gratitude to this courageous pioneer.

Why were such spectacular results dismissed by the medical establishment of the day? Part of the answer is that the finger was being pointed at obstetricians, who found it inconceivable that their own hands might be spreading the fatal infection. Members of the medical establishment were at that time implacably resistant to any insinuation that their own practices were harming women.

In the United States, the chief advocate of Semmelweis's ideas was the illustrious Oliver Wendell Holmes, M.D. In April 1843, Holmes published an article titled "The Contagiousness of Puerperal Fever" in what was then known as the *New England Quarterly Journal of Medicine.*

One of the country's leading obstetricians, Dr. Hugh L. Hodge, took immediate offense, and shot back with an article of his own, oppositionally titled "The Non-Contagious Character of Puerperal Fever." The very idea was preposterous, he countered, that physicians could "ever convey, in any possible manner, [anything as] destructive as puerperal fever." It was "cruel, very cruel," he went on, to suggest to a woman that her trusted doctor could possibly bring the deadly contagion. "It is far more humane," he explained in a burst of chivalry, "to keep her happy in ignorance of danger."[1]

At this point, another prominent obstetrician, Dr. Charles D. Meigs, leapt into the fray, accusing Holmes of "propagating a vile, demoralizing superstition."[2] It was impossible for doctors' hands to spread disease, he declared, because doctors were gentlemen.

Due to the refusal of the medical establishment to openly consider the evidence advanced by Semmelweis and Holmes, hundreds of thousands of women continued to die needlessly.

We can shake our heads in wonder at the blindness of the past. Of course, nothing like that could happen today. Our medical profession is devoted to the scientific method. Surely we can count on the practices of modern obstetrics to reflect our most advanced knowledge, and to produce the safest and best birth outcomes humanly possible.

Or can we?

The United States, with the highest per capita expenditure on health care of any nation in the world, now ranks 25th among Western industrial nations in infant mortality.[3] Almost every other industrialized nation in the world has better infant survival rates than we do.[4]

In the United States, physicians oversee 95 percent of all births.[5] In Europe, where infant mortality rates are superior to ours, midwives (nonphysicians, almost always women, skilled in the art and science of birthing) attend 75 percent of births.[6] In every single one of the nations where infant mortality rates are lower than ours, midwives are the principal birth attendants.

Nearly all birthing women in the Netherlands are cared for by midwives, and 35 percent of babies are born at home. As outdated and dangerous as this appears to our medical establishment, the results are hard to dismiss. Far more Dutch babies survive per capita than babies born in the United States.[7]

Doris Haire, past president of the International Childbirth Education Association (ICEA), has traveled worldwide investigating birthing practices, and she is not overly fond of what she finds in America: "Of all the 36 countries I have visited to observe maternity facilities, I am absolutely convinced that the United States has to be the most bizarre on earth in its management of obstetrics."[8]

BIRTH IN AMERICA

I have often thought that the way a society gives birth to its children speaks volumes about that society. If we were able to recognize the importance of birth, if we were able to honor its transforming power, spiritual nature, and long-term effects on both mother and child, I suspect that we'd be on our way to building a future with less war and violence.

A movement to humanize American childbirth care started in the early 1960s, partially triggered by a source that is not usually known for advocating radical social change—the *Ladies Home Journal*. Somehow in the midst of articles about knitting sweaters and redecorating the living room there appeared a bombshell aptly titled "Cruelty in the Maternity Ward." One nurse wrote, "I have seen doctors who have charming examination-room manners show traces of sadism in the delivery room. One I know does cutting and suturing without anesthetic. He has nurses use a mask to stifle the patient's outcry. Some doctors still say, 'Tie them down so they won't give us any trouble.'"[9]

The normally noncontroversial *Ladies Home Journal* hardly knew what it had unleashed. A torrent of letters came in that the magazine called "so shocking they deserve national attention." The May 1958 issue contained page after page of letters. One woman wrote, "Women are herded like sheep through an obstetrical assembly line, are drugged and strapped on tables while their babies are forceps-delivered. Obstetricians today are businessmen who run baby factories." Another woman complained, "I was immediately rushed into the labor room. A nurse prepared me. Then, with leather cuffs strapped around my wrists and legs, I was left alone for nearly eight hours."

A raw nerve had been struck. Month after month, the avalanche of letters continued. In December 1958, a woman wrote: "Far too many doctors and hospitals seem to assume that just because a woman is about to give birth she becomes a nitwit, an incompetent, reduced to the status of a cow. I was strapped to the delivery table on Saturday morning and lay there until I was delivered on Sunday afternoon. When I slipped my hand from the strap to wipe sweat from my face I was severely reprimanded by the nurse."

The effort to improve birth experiences in the United States has progressed considerably since those days, but I'm sorry to report that things have not become nearly as enlightened as most people believe. In fact, it has been during the last 30 years that the rate for cesarean sections (the surgical removal of infants from their mothers' womb by cutting through the abdominal wall) has become a national shame. During the early 1960s, the overall cesarean section rate in the United States was only 3 percent. Today it has risen to more than 22 percent.[10]

BIRTH CENTERS

To my eyes, one of the most positive changes that *has* taken place in the last 20 years has been the tremendous surge of growth in freestanding birthing centers (not to be confused with hospital-owned birth centers). In

1975, there were only 5 in the U.S., but by 1994, there were 140, with 60 more on the way.[11]

At nonhospital birth centers, birth is seen as a normal and healthy process that is respected rather than feared. Midwives provide constant support, and women are not made to fit into hospital routines and schedules. They can move around all they want, and labor in any position they desire. Interventions and drug use are minimal, although emergency equipment is available to handle common complications, such as maternal hemorrhage and babies who need resuscitation. Women's partners can hold them and comfort them, get into bed with them to cuddle if they desire, and any other family members or friends whom the mother would like present are also welcome. Babies remain with their mothers after birth, and breastfeeding is encouraged and supported. Nearly all women who give birth in out-of-hospital birth centers report great satisfaction with their experience.

When women are respected, and their rhythms are honored, they emerge with a sense of trust in their bodies. With fewer interventions, mothers feel a greater sense of personal responsibility and accomplishment. They know that they have achieved something momentous, and have a profoundly renewed belief in their own capacities. They undertake the responsibilities of parenthood from a position of enhanced self-respect and self-esteem.

As one new mother put it: "After I birthed my daughter, I knew there wasn't anything in this world I couldn't do."

How safe are birth centers?

The largest study ever done of freestanding birthing centers in the United States was published in the *New England Journal of Medicine* in 1989.[12] The results were telling. The infant death rate for all births begun at birth centers (including breech births, twins, and those which got into trouble and had to be transferred to hospitals) was much lower than that for births occurring in hospitals.

The study also found other advantages for birth centers. The cesarean rate was 4.4 percent—less than one-fifth the typical hospital average. Satisfaction with the birth centers was so high among the women in the study that 99 percent said they would recommend the birth center to friends. Costs averaged 30 percent less than hospital maternity care.

Impressed, the authors of the *New England Journal of Medicine* study concluded that "safety, satisfaction, and savings characterize freestanding birth centers."[13]

Grasping the significance of this and similar studies, the American Public Health Association endorsed freestanding birth centers, noting that births could be safe outside of hospitals.

That is not quite, however, how the obstetrical establishment saw the situation. Harkening back to the days of Ignaz Semmelweis, the American College of Obstetricians and Gynecologists issued a statement opposing all out-of-hospital births.

How did this organization justify its opposition? Its officials argued that the kinds of women who choose birthing centers are more motivated to take responsibility for their births, and so can't be reliably compared to the women delivering in hospitals. Women who choose birthing centers, the argument went, have better results simply because they are healthier and take better care of themselves.

The obstetricians' position was put to a test in 1986, when due to hospital overcrowding in Miami, a large group of women was assigned to a nearby freestanding birth center. These women were different from the self-selected women who are the usual clientele of birthing centers. They were poorer, less educated, and many were women of color—all factors that are typically associated with higher risk. If the obstetricians' contention that birthing centers get better results only because they handle self-selected women was correct, surely the women who were assigned to the birthing center would not show the same outstanding results as the center's typical patrons.

But that's not what happened. The assigned group's outcomes were found to be virtually identical with the results for the usual birth center clients. Interventions were few, complications were low, the cesarean rate was only 5 percent, no deaths occurred, and the satisfaction of the mothers was so high that many returned to the birth center for subsequent babies, and referred friends and family.[14]

The American College of Obstetricians and Gynecologists, however, kept its eyes conveniently closed to the evidence. Beginning to sound like a broken record, the obstetrical establishment continued to claim that only hospital births are safe.

THE BABY BUSINESS

Childbirth in America is a $20-billion-a-year business. Many American hospitals, eager to expand their share of the market, present potential customers with public relations campaigns advertising that they provide all the benefits of a home birth in a safe hospital setting. An ad from Eden Hospital in Castro Valley, California, shows a loving young couple with a smiling baby underneath the headline "Having my baby at Eden was so comfortable, almost like delivering at home." The HCA West Paces Ferry Hospital in Atlanta announces cheerily that their "birthing suites feature early American furniture complete with a four-poster bed and a charming cradle." The Alexandria Hospital in Alexandria, Virginia, tells expectant parents of its pink dining room, with fresh flowers on each table for two, where the new parents can choose between filet mignon, catch of the day, and chicken Kiev.[15]

Unfortunately, this is just advertising. Underneath the public relations, the reality of most hospital births remains distressingly high-tech and impersonal. Women are still far too often treated as objects from which babies are to be removed. The cesarean section rate is actually highest in the fanciest hospitals, where more affluent women can presumably pay (or have insurance that pays) for additional interventions. In some hospitals today, a white woman with insurance has a 50 percent chance of having a cesarean.[16]

Although many American hospitals today present a birth-friendly facade, they still view birth as a dangerous process that must be managed and controlled. It is true that husbands and other significant others are usually now allowed to be present, but the fear of something going wrong remains the dominant emotional chord. The furniture might be homey and the wallpaper cheerful, but the needs of the mother are still far too often subjugated to the routines of the hospital, the convenience of the obstetrician, the fear of malpractice suits, the vagaries of insurance coverage, and the personality conflicts of the staff.

There have been positive changes since the flurry of letters to the *Ladies Home Journal* revealed how America's mothers were feeling about their hospital birth experiences. But unfortunately these last few decades have seen an increasing reliance on technology and interventions. The result is that women giving birth in modern hospitals often still feel like passive victims of events that are occurring completely outside of their control.

MIDWIVES

For most women, it is difficult to feel safe in the typical obstetrician-managed, high-intervention birth climate of American hospital births. This is not merely a matter of emotional comfort, because a woman needs to feel safe for her labor to progress. Many mammals will actually stop their labor if they sense danger, waiting until the threat has passed before continuing.[17] Instinctively, they know that to bring forth new life in the midst of danger could place their newborns and themselves at great risk. It is remarkable how many women laboring in hospitals "fail to progress" because they sense that the situation is not safe for themselves or their offspring. Unfortunately, instead of responding in a way that would genuinely provide a climate of safety and support, obstetricians have been trained to react with aggressive interventions that make most women feel even more unsafe.

The contrast between the way of the obstetrician and that of the midwife is dramatic. Obstetricians are trained in surgery. They have seldom been taught to understand a woman's emotional needs. Midwives, on the other hand, are far more often versed in the art of helping a woman to feel safe. Appreciating a woman's birth experience as a natural expression of who she is, they care for her emotionally and spiritually as well as physically. Relying on their empathy and intuitive harmony with the woman's experience to help her open to the profound forces at work in her body and soul, they turn to obstetric technology only when necessary. Understanding that birth can be a beautiful, strengthening, and healing experience, they cherish the entire process as a sacred interaction between mother and child.

While few obstetricians are sensitive to the social aspects of childbirth, midwives are usually able to help the process become an event that unites a family. Many fathers-to-be approach birth with anxiety, seeing it as an emergency, and feeling uncomfortable when they can't "fix it." Obstetricians are often stuck in the same rut, and only reinforce the fathers' anxiety. Midwives, on the other hand, can often help a man to understand that though he can't have the baby for his partner, nor take away her pain, he can do something of enormous value—he can love his partner, be fully present with her, and touch her with his care. By providing constant respectful affection and support, he not only helps his partner to relax and express her birthing power, he also grows in respect for who she is and what she is accomplishing.

Midwives also often know how to involve siblings so they can feel part of things, and learn about birth as a natural and marvelous process. This is important, because children who are allowed to witness their mothers giving birth are far more likely to respect their mothers for what they have done, and develop positive relationships with the newcomer. "What we're seeing," says David Stewart, founder of the National Association of Parents and Professionals for Safe Alternatives in Childbirth, "is that [birth] is a biological prime time for attachment for all those who are present, regardless of age."[18]

Midwives often know how to help a woman to learn the subtle art of communicating with her baby before he or she is born. When fetal distress arises, obstetricians commonly assume the woman's body has failed and the time has come to call upon technology. Midwives are more apt to soothe the mother and ask her to send her baby messages of reassurance and love. Positive inner communication between mother and baby often translates into a deeper rapport that produces an easier birth, and a better relationship after birth.

SAFETY FIRST

Obstetricians typically say that all this talk about bonding and attachment and the woman's emotional experience is well and good, but *their* focus is on the safety of the baby. Sure, they say, nine out of ten women don't need the technology and the interventions, and might have a nicer time without them. But one in ten does, and they aren't about to let a baby die just because some wheat-germ-and-granola-eating young lady thinks birth is a way to attain cosmic consciousness. Birth can be dangerous, they say, and their job is to prevent catastrophes. They are there to save babies who would have died without their interventions. They are experts in technological birth, and they will not let themselves be bothered by the sight of normal, healthy women laboring on their backs with blood pressure cuffs wrapped around their arms, IVs stuck in their veins, belts wrapped around their bellies, catheters and electrodes hanging out of their vaginas, and looks of misery on their faces. "Look, this isn't a birthday party or a time for lovemaking," one obstetrician snapped. "Do you want your baby to die?"

If it were indeed true that modern obstetrical practices saved lives and delivered healthier babies, I would understand why they are routinely employed and would support them. But I have been astonished to discover that the medical literature is full of studies which reveal that the practices that lie at the heart of modern obstetrics, when used as a matter of course, do not save lives. In fact, study after study shows that they actually lead to higher death rates for both mothers and babies.[19]

This information is not a secret. It is found in the most credible peer-reviewed medical journals. The *British Journal of Obstetrics and Gynaecology*, for example, published a study which concluded that the historical decline in maternal and infant mortality (death) and morbidity (injury and illness) has not been due to obstetrical medical interventions.[20] Rather, these gains have been due to the development of antibiotics, the addition of vitamin D to milk (thus preventing rickets), advances in public health, sanitation, and nutrition, improvement in women's working conditions, and other measures that improved maternal health prior to birth. Remarkably, the study concluded that *maternal and infant mortality and morbidity would actually have declined even further without obstetrical interventions.*

When I first began to ponder these and many similar studies, I did not want to believe their implications. Could it really be that modern obstetrical practices, rather than saving lives, are in fact causing unnecessary deaths, injuries, and expense? Could it be the case that midwives are actually *safer* than obstetricians?

The sober truth is that the data does not speak well for contemporary obstetrics. A three-year experiment was undertaken at Madera County Hospital in California, during which time midwives managed the vast majority of births. The neonatal death rate during these three years was reduced to less than half of what it had been when obstetricians were managing births.[21]

What happened next was chilling, and is once again reminiscent of the days of Semmelweis. In their well-documented review of today's childbirth options, *A Good Birth, A Safe Birth*, Diana Korte and Roberta Scaer write: "The program was terminated, despite good results, because of opposition from the California Medical Association."[22]

Obstetricians again assumed control of births. During the next two and a half years, the hospital's neonatal death rate tripled.[23]

Studies in Kentucky, North Carolina, Missouri, Arizona, and other states likewise have shown superior outcomes for midwives.[24] A study by the Centers for Disease Control (CDC) found the death rate for home births attended by midwives in North Carolina to be only 57 percent of that for low-risk hospital births attended by obstetricians.[25]

The same pattern holds true throughout the fully industrialized world. In the Netherlands, in 1986, obstetricians delivering babies in hospitals had a mortality rate nine times greater than midwives delivering babies in the same hospitals. And midwives who delivered babies at home did better yet, with only 1 death for every 19 for obstetricians in hospitals.[26]

Staunch defenders of the obstetrical faith protest that these numbers could be misleading, because the Dutch babies born in hospitals with obstetricians in attendance might well include a greater percentage of high-risk situations. But the *British Journal of Obstetrics and Gynaecology* published a careful analysis of this data, finding that "[t]he average risk status [of women attended by obstetricians] at delivery was not much higher than that of midwives' deliveries. It could not possibly account for a perinatal death rate [nearly] ten times as high for obstetricians as for midwives."[27]

A comprehensive review of the medical literature by researcher David Stewart concluded that midwife-attended deliveries have neonatal death rates well below those for obstetrician-attended deliveries—even when "the midwives were attending the poor and high-risk clients, where one could expect higher neonatal death rates."[28]

The evidence testifying that maternity systems based on midwifery have better baby and mother outcomes is overwhelming. "The data base for these figures is in the millions, is global in scope, and spans almost a century, up to and including the present," says Stewart.[29] He estimates that if all American women had birth attendants with a midwife approach, mother and baby mortality would be halved, and the rates of brain-damaged children and other birth injuries and complications in newborns would be cut by three-quarters. Other authorities agree, adding that we'd save $8.5 billion a year.[30]

An outstanding demonstration of what can happen when midwives care for high-risk and economically disadvantaged women is taking place today in North Central Bronx Hospital in New York City. Here, 70 percent of the mothers are considered to be at medical or socioeconomic risk. Most are poor and women of color. One in ten arrive for labor with no previous care, and one in eight are addicted to drugs. Nevertheless, the prevailing philosophy is one of minimal interventions, respect for the mothers, and midwife-assisted birth. Complications are few, and the cesarean rate is only 11 percent, less than half what obstetricians as a whole average in the United States even when attending affluent and well-nourished women. The neonatal death rate for babies weighing 2.2 pounds or more at North Central Bronx Hospital is only 3.7 per 1,000 births—less than obstetricians as a group achieve even when dealing with lower levels of risk.[31]

It is troubling to acknowledge that obstetricians delivering babies in American hospitals consistently have higher infant death rates than midwives in out-of-hospital birthing centers. It is even more troubling that their infant death rates are higher than for births taking place in taxicabs. But the evidence is consistent. Study after study has found that births that take place in out-of-hospital birth centers yield better results for both mother and baby.[32]

A report in the prestigious British medical journal *Lancet* is typical.[33] It compared 500 women who used a birth center to 500 matched women who used a hospital. In the birth center, the women were allowed to move about, eat, and drink as they wished during labor. They used no intravenous drips (I.V.s) or electronic fetal monitors. Only a very few needed any pain-relief medication, and the women spoke glowingly of their experience of giving birth. The women in the hospital? All of them had I.V.s, and most were attached to electronic fetal monitors. Almost all needed high doses of pain medication. Some considered their birth experiences to be travesties.

The differences for the babies were equally dramatic. The *Lancet* study found that the hospital babies suffered 17 times more fetal distress. They were 3 times more likely to have neurological abnormalities, and 6 times more likely to have jaundice.[34]

Mothers have been telling obstetricians for years that when birth is violated, they lose hope and belief in themselves, and do not begin their parenting journey on the right foot. The *Lancet* study gave weight to their complaints, finding that 12 of the infants born in the hospital were victims of child abuse in the next year, while none of the infants born in the birth center were abused.[35]

There are times when the judicious use of medical interventions can be life-saving. Sometimes, if a woman's cervix is stuck at eight or nine centimeters dilation, it can be helpful to break the bag of waters. Once in a while, a catheter or a fetal monitor is useful. Prudent use of pain-relieving medication can be a great blessing. Cesareans have saved lives. But these interventions exist for the rare times when they are needed. To use them routinely, the data consistently say, is counterproductive.

Michelle Winkler, editor of *The Doula*, a journal dealing with birth and mothering issues, asks: **Why is it that when American midwives are interviewed by pregnant mothers, they are always asked, "Have you ever lost a baby that might have been saved by a real doctor? Have you** ever lost a baby at a home birth that would have lived in a hospital?" Why aren't obstetricians asked, "Have you ever lost a baby because of misuse of technology that might have lived if it had been born naturally at home? How many cesareans have you done that would not have been necessary if the birthing woman was supported in laboring naturally, following her own rhythm and timing?"[36]

HOME BIRTH

An obstetrical nurse who chose a home birth remarked: "People were very surprised I was paying out-of-pocket for a home birth with a midwife, when I was fully insured for a hospital birth with a doctor. I would tell them, 'It's worth it!' I knew the difference it would make in the kind of experience I had. I was talking to another nurse at the hospital where I worked, who wanted to know how much my home birth cost. I told her, and she said, 'That's all! It would be worth a lot more than that not to have it here.'"[37]

Women who choose to give birth at home often do so because they want an environment of peace and dignity where the process can unfold naturally. They make this choice despite knowing that they may be subjected to increased expense, suspicion, harassment, and ridicule. Most people believe that home births are dangerous.

Are they?

In rural Tennessee there is a community known simply as The Farm. In the 1970s and 1980s, more than 1,700 babies were born at home there, all attended by midwives. Statistics for these births were nothing short of spectacular. Interventions were almost nonexistent. Forceps were used in less than one in every 200 births (compared to one in every two births in some hospitals). Some 98 percent of the women gave birth without any drugs (while in many U.S. hospitals most women *are* drugged). Even twins and breech presentations were usually successfully delivered at home. The cesarean rate was less than 2 percent. Despite taking on high-risk situations, the neonatal mortality rate was far lower than the average American hospital.[38]

What are home births like? They are each unique, but here is noted author Joyce Vissell's story of one of hers:

"I graduated as a registered nurse from one of the top university nursing programs in the United States. I received an excellent education, including obstetrics. I left school with the firm conviction that I would never give birth in a hospital unless there was a medical complication (i.e., toxemia, multiple birth, or complicated fetal position). I never wanted to choose to place myself in such a humiliating and powerless position as I observed repeatedly in hospital births.

"All three of our children were born in our home. Each experience was totally fulfilling and beautiful. The third birth was perhaps the most memorable as our two daughters were present much of the time. My husband, Barry, and I chose a nurse-midwife who has an excellent reputation and who also honored the sacredness of husband and wife birthing their baby.

"In the months before birth I prepared our bedroom to greet our baby. I kept it spotlessly clean, with fresh flowers, and brought in pictures that inspired me. Every day I sat in this room and prayed for our baby. I visualized him coming into a sea of family love and acceptance. I placed his basket next to the bed with his first newborn clothes. Toward the end of my pregnancy the midwife came to my home and we sat in this room and talked about my highest hopes for the birth. She listened to what I wanted.

"I also worked on a 'birth-garden.' This was a place where I planned to spend the beginning of my labor. I planted flowers and herbs that I loved. I knew from experience how much energy nature can give a laboring mother.

"When I went into labor I immediately went to my garden for peace and inspiration. I spent several hours alone there enjoying the sun and the fragrance of nature. Barry and our daughters, ages 13 and 7, completed the final preparations for the house. They were excited and happy. I then spent time alone with each of our girls, telling them how much I loved and needed them during the birth. Then the girls played happily in the house while Barry and I spent time alone.

"This time with him was profound and loving. We renewed our love with each other and our commitment to parenthood. We felt held in an atmosphere of love, trusting fully that nature would bring through the baby in perfect timing. There was no worry about getting to the hospital on time. We were secure in our own home where everything felt safe and peaceful. To speed the labor along I took a walk in our woods. Barry supported me and the girls came along chattering joyfully about the new baby. The walk jumped me into strong labor, and the girls called the midwife to come.

"The midwife and her assistant arrived. Both women had given birth themselves. They honored my birth process. I loved and trusted these women. When I wanted to be alone with Barry and the girls, they stayed close and present in another room. I reflected on how in the hospital you never know who will walk into your room. You might establish a relationship with the nurse on duty in the beginning of your labor, and then when you really need the support, you've gone through a change of shift and have an entirely new staff.

"Barry knew I was depending on him and came through beautifully. All too often in the hospital I have seen husbands degraded to a secondary role. Their presence is tolerated as long as they keep quiet and stay out of the way of the doctors and nurses. They are not empowered in the hospital setting. At home, Barry was totally empowered and knew I really needed him to birth our baby. This greatly enhanced our relationship.

"I cannot describe the love, respect, and honoring that was shown to me during the labor and birth. I felt the eternal presence of my husband and daughters reaching out to support me in my time of need. It felt as if the door to heaven was opened for me, and I experienced the highest presence of our baby.

"Pushing our son out was a challenge since he weighed almost ten pounds. I took longer to push him than they usually allow in the hospital. In the hospital I would have been cut open. The extra time of pushing at home allowed the perineum to gently stretch. I didn't tear, and healed from the stretching very quickly afterwards.

"I wanted our baby to be born into a space of quiet and peace, for the first sounds he heard to be of love and tenderness. I have seen too many babies born in bright lights while the doctor shouts orders to his assistants. The midwives respected my desire for silence. In peace and gentleness our baby was born into the ocean of love of our family. The sounds he heard were whispers of love and adoration from his parents and sisters. The light was the full moon and several candles. He was tenderly held by his family.

"The midwives cleaned up and helped us all get settled for the night. The girls brought mattresses into our bedroom. We had all bonded so deeply that no one wanted to be apart from the family. Barry and I lay together with our newborn between us. The love and beauty of those 16 hours remain forever etched upon my heart.

"The three birth experiences at home have been among the highest and most fulfilling experiences of my life. Each left me feeling strong and inspired to care for the baby.

"Our insurance did not cover the midwife fee of $1,000. This money was well worth every sacrifice we had to make to get it. That fee allowed me to birth in total dignity and grace in a place of power and inspiration and allowed our baby to come into the world in peace, gentleness, and unconditional love."[39]

THE DATA SPEAK LOUD AND CLEAR

I have been privileged to be present at a number of home births, and I can vouch for the fact that they can be magnificent experiences. When my son, Ocean, was born at home into my waiting hands, I felt as though I was in the presence of all that is holy and good. I was filled with awe at the mystery, beauty, and power of life, and with unfathomable respect for my wife, Deo. I will always be grateful to have participated in that life-transforming event.

This experience was so profound that I find myself wondering how different our society would be if more fathers were fortunate enough to have the kind of experience I did. Would we see closer father-son and father-daughter relationships, fewer deadbeat dads, and less child abuse? Would we see more fathers involved in parenting, fewer mothers feeling unsupported, and less divorce? Would we see more children growing up feeling they have roots, and fewer aimless and alienated young people?

Although home births can be spiritually luminous, they are anything but popular with the obstetrical establishment. One obstetrician expressed the prevailing attitude rather colorfully. He said that home-birthers are "kooks, the lunatic fringe, people who have emotional problems they're acting out."[40]

I wish I could dismiss this remark as an extreme case, unrepresentative of the profession, but the man who made this statement was speaking as a past president of the American College of Obstetricians and Gynecologists.

What does the data say about the safety of home births? Lewis Mehl, M.D., director of the Institute for Childbirth and Family Research in Berkeley, California, compared matched populations of 1,046 women planning hospital births with 1,046 women planning home births.[41] The study was impeccably designed. The two groups of women were matched in terms of age, socioeconomic status, social parity, and risk factors.

The study found that women birthing in hospitals were five times more likely to have high blood pressure during labor; nine times more likely to tear; three times more likely to hemorrhage; and three times more likely to undergo cesarean sections.

Okay, say the hospitals, we can be pretty rough on women sometimes, but we do what we have to do in order to protect the babies.

Not quite. The hospital-born babies were six times more likely to suffer fetal distress before birth; four times more likely to need assistance to start breathing; and four times more likely to develop infections.

In every single category of comparison, home birth mothers and infants did vastly better. While 30 of the infants born in hospitals suffered birth injuries, not a single one of the infants born at home suffered this fate.

Nevertheless, the American College of Obstetricians and Gynecologists to this day continues to oppose home births. In 1992, its former president, Keith Russell, M.D., announced, "Home birth is child abuse."[42] To support this position, the organization frequently refers to a single study from the 1970s that appeared to find greater risk for home births.[43] But this study gave an inaccurate picture of the risk of home births because it included miscarriages and extremely premature births that took place unplanned at home!

It has not been easy for me to accept the implications of contemporary birthing statistics. The idea that all our expensive birth technology might only be creating worse outcomes has at times seemed almost unbelievable. Surely, I've thought, these must be isolated cases, or a few improbable studies.

An international team of researchers, led by Drs. Iain Chalmers, Murray Enkin, and Marc Keirse, took ten years to undertake the most thorough review in medical history of research assessing the safety of maternity practices. They evaluated more than 3,000 clinical research studies, and examined every report in 60 key journals published in the last 40 years. They also wrote to 40,000 obstetricians and pediatricians in 18 countries to find unpublished research. Their work culminated in the foremost encyclopedia of birthing practices in the world today, *Effective Care in Pregnancy and Childbirth*.[44] The data was found to justify this conclusion: "You may be shocked to find what little evidence exists in support of most obstetrical practices. . . . The evidence favors noninterventive management."[45]

I still feel troubled by the possibility that much of modern obstetrical practice could be so off-base. It's painful to consider that the medical profession could be botching things so badly. Surely, if the evidence was there, they would see the error of their ways and make the needed corrections. But then I remember Ignaz Semmelweis, and the reaction he received from the medical establishment of his time. Could it be that today's obstetricians are being just as closed-minded in their refusal to recognize the advantages of midwifery and the benefits of out-of-hospital locations for most births, as the obstetricians who refused to see that their own hands were spreading childbed fever?

THE WILL TO CHANGE

Raven Lang has been one of the most influential advocates of natural childbirth in the United States. It was her own childbirth experience that first gave her grave doubts about American birthing practices.

"I was at Stanford. I had to fight to keep my mate with me. I was in labor for five hours, and I was examined every 15 minutes, if not more. There was a whole host of interns that would come in. Sometimes I'd have intern A examine me, a vaginal exam, and then he would quit and intern B would put on his glove and examine me. They'd talk about it, and then intern C would come. I would beg them to leave me alone.

"Later they said, 'push your baby out,' but I didn't have the urge to push yet. I told the doctor I wasn't ready to deliver the baby. All of the staff were acting like I had to push the baby out instantly. I remember looking into my husband's eyes with tears, saying, 'Please, you must believe me. I am not ready.' I needed someone to know that what I learned about my body was the truth and what these bozos were doing was not the truth. The doctor gave me an episioproctotomy and cut through my anal sphincter. I was basically opened up from the top of my vagina through the posterior aspect of the anal sphincter. There was no reason to do it. Zilch. They were in such a hurry, the intern was inexperienced, nervous, and he simply did it. I was left in extraordinary pain.

"Some of the deepest pain that I have was in the fact that I was so bewildered by what they did to me, so bewildered and insulted. For the next two weeks I wept daily. I thought, if this is childbirth, how is a woman supposed to get up and care for her infant when she can hardly put one leg in front of the other from pain? It took me about six months before I could make love after this surgical insult."

Raven Lang eventually healed, and soon began to teach childbirth education classes, whereupon she had another experience of the obstetrical profession that was not particularly gratifying.

"A young woman asked me to be her midwife, but I wouldn't do it. (I'll call her Karen.) She sought the help of a doctor, and I was to go to the hospital with her. We met at the bottom of the road about four in the morning. She was in what looked like very early labor and I suggested we go back and do early labor at home. I knew she was going to have her baby in just a few hours. She was so relaxed and so in tune with the energy that she didn't act like a woman in strong advanced labor. She went to the hospital and was doing very well for about two hours. She was beautiful, completely in control of herself, and very happy. Then, the doctor called and said he wasn't going to come in for a few more hours and to give her a shot of demerol. Karen wasn't asking for it, she didn't need it. But it was given to her nonetheless. I remember being her advocate and saying, 'No, No, No, Don't do it!' But she got it and with that her labor changed. It slowed down and she got sleepy. The doctor called again, maybe two hours later, and said he wasn't going to be in until late afternoon and to give her another shot of demerol. I pleaded with the nurse not to follow his orders, that whoever was on call could deliver the baby. She got the second shot. Her labor stopped and she went to sleep. I watched her sleep for three hours.

"The doctor called around three or four P.M. to say he was coming in, and with this information the nurses came back to the labor room, woke Karen up, and put an I.V. drip in her arm. I didn't know it, but they were inducing her. They gave her a couple of shots in her vagina and kicked me out of the room because I had too many questions. They didn't want to be bothered. I remember saying, 'I won't leave you.' I had hold of her hand and she was weeping. As she got whisked away to the delivery room, she had big giant tears coming off her face. I went to the delivery room, which had a large window, and I watched the entire birth. It was very heavy. The baby was traumatized and delivered by high forceps. When the baby was born, the doctor hit the baby repeatedly because his breathing was depressed. The mother's arms were strapped down and you could see her neck reaching for the child. It took everything in my power and only my respect for this woman not to break the window in front of my face. I wanted to pick up a chair and throw it through, I was so enraged. Karen was weeping. I could hear her crying, 'Can I please just hold my baby. Please can I just take him.' The doctor was saying, 'No, No, No.' As he came out of delivery, I was right there. He walked out and I came right up to him and stood in front of him and said, 'Would you please just give her the baby?' He looked at me and asked, 'Do you think that giving the baby to its mother would be the best thing in the world?' I said, 'Yes, Yes.' And he said, 'Let me tell you that motherly love kills more babies than bullets.'

"I came home and had the biggest cry and told myself that the next lady who asked me to deliver her baby, I will help."[46]

And help she did. Raven Lang went on to become a midwife, teacher of midwifery, and one of the great leaders in the natural childbirth movement of our times.

The doctor, who is still practicing obstetrics today, went on to seek her arrest.

3
Birth, Hospitals, and the Human Spirit

In 1982, the state of California completed the largest study ever undertaken on the root causes of crime and violence. The number one cause was found to be medical interference with childbirth in our hospitals.

— Joseph Chilton Pearce

THE PROCESS BY WHICH BABIES ARE BORN has worked for untold generations, and is one of the great wonders of the human body. Every human being who has ever taken a breath has arrived on this earth through the womb of a woman. Though the many human cultures and races that have existed in the various parts of the world have spoken a wide array of languages and differed in a vast number of ways, every member of every tribe, society, and nation has this in common. The fact of our birth is one of the most fundamental connections we share with all humanity. Through this universal bond we are united in the miracle of life.

Every man and every woman since the dawn of the human experience has had a woman for a mother, and each of these women has given herself over to the creative process in order that we might be. In giving birth, women have known the agony, the ecstasy, and the mystery of creation. They have opened to the infinite and brought a piece of it here to earth.

What must it do to an aspiring physician to be repeatedly taught not that women are bringers of life, but that they are unpredictable containers from which babies are to be extracted? I can only imagine what happens to someone who, while preparing to spend years helping women give birth, is continually surrounded by the assumption that birth is dangerous, and women ill equipped for the task. If I were a practicing obstetrician, and had been trained as they have been, it is possible that I, too, would think that women should turn the experience over to me and the hospital staff. I, too, might come to view myself as the expert and expect to be in charge. Having been taught that it was upon my actions that the success and safety of the birth depended, I, too, might consider myself, not the laboring woman or the newborn, as the central figure in the drama of birth.

Almost everything in the training of obstetricians supports this kind of inflated self-importance, and almost everything in the hospital environment reinforces it. The kind of bed or delivery table that is used is designed for the doctor's comfort, not for the ease of the birthing woman. The position in which a woman's body is placed is chosen to give the obstetrician maximum access, not to facilitate her birthing process. Even the temperature of the room is set to accommodate the doctor's preferences, not the mother's, or the baby's.[1]

Obstetricians have been taught that a "safe" birth is one in which they, and they alone, are in control. As a result, many doctors believe they are providing optimum care by denying women a part in making medical decisions. If a woman asks too many questions, they may reply: "Just leave everything to me." Such doctors are behaving according to their training. They may think they are being reassuring. They do not realize they are being patronizing.

Even those obstetricians who would prefer to treat women as responsible and competent have been subjected to a form of medical education that points in a very different direction. Obstetrical textbooks consistently bespeak a lack of regard for birthing as a normal, safe, and natural process. One well-known medical textbook widely used in the 1970s, *Obstetrics and Gynecology*, did not exactly speak of women with reverence. "The traits that compose the core of the female personality," proclaimed this authority, "are feminine narcissism, masochism, and passivity."[2]

Surely, you might think, that sort of attitude belongs to a bygone day. Not quite. An obstetrical textbook widely used in medical schools during the 1980s, and still in use today, *Medical, Surgical and Gynecological Complications of Pregnancy*, could hold its own in any competition for the most chauvinistic textbook of all time. This textbook warns doctors not to be fooled by women who assert themselves. Particularly "dangerous," the text says, are "those patients who consider themselves 'socially aware.' They are not necessarily more mature but are trying, by their active interest in everything 'avant garde,' socially as well as medically, to persuade themselves and others that they are. . . . This is the patient who is interested in such methods as 'natural childbirth,' hypnosis, or using childbirth as an 'experience.'"[3]

Not content to stop with this glorious burst of insight, the textbook goes on to warn about the "occasional woman who is fanatic in her zeal for 'natural childbirth.'" Obstetricians-to-be are cautioned: "The intensity of her demands and her uncompromising attitude on the subject are danger signals, frequently indicating severe psychopathology." The textbook then concludes that the more a woman wants a natural childbirth, the less she should have it: "A patient of this sort is not a candidate for natural childbirth, and requires close and constant psychiatric support."[4]

Lest you believe that this way of thinking about women is no longer thriving in learned medical circles, an Ohio doctor in 1991 wrote in the *Journal of the American Medical Association* a short piece that displayed something less than passionate support for women as liberated beings. Choosing his words carefully, he said that women who tend to ask questions and otherwise show an "over anxiousness" about their health are suffering from "temperamental differences in gender-mediated clinical features . . . which are manifested by women's less active, more ruminative responses that are linked to dysfunction of the right frontal cortex in which the metabolic rate is higher in females."[5] As best I can tell, he's saying that women who seek to take charge of their health are inherently brain-damaged.

The standard obstetrical textbook in use today is *Williams Obstetrics*. The 15th edition of this classic is 923 pages long. In the index there appears an entry that was apparently slipped in unnoticed by some brave soul who, faced with the tedious task of preparing the index, wanted to voice his or her opinion about the book. The line reads: "Chauvinism, male, pages 1–923." The 18th edition of this illustrious text was a bit longer than previous editions, and the heading in the index was adjusted accordingly: "Chauvinism, male, pages 1–1102."[6]

I am not making this up.

AN AMERICAN SPECIALTY: CESAREAN SECTIONS

As a result of their training, obstetricians in the United States today often believe that vaginal births are unpredictable and risky. A few of them actually believe that all babies should be born by cesarean sections. In a 1991 issue of *Ob-Gyn News*, a doctor wrote, "Maybe the obstetrician should be charged not to justify a cesarean section, but rather to justify a vaginal delivery."[7]

If a woman is older than 35, in most obstetricians' minds she is a high risk, and they will be that much quicker to bolt to surgery rather than allow her labor to develop. Actually, whether or not a woman is more at risk due to her age is an individual matter. An older woman who smokes, never exercises, is overweight, and diabetic, would certainly be at higher risk. But a healthy woman is quite capable of a safe and natural birth, regardless of her age.

And then there is the matter of women who have had previous cesareans. Beginning in 1916, and continuing for the next 72 years, the obstetrical establishment held fervently to the belief that "once a cesarean, always a cesarean." Even as an avalanche of international research was proving that women who have had previous cesareans can usually succeed in giving birth vaginally,[8] the American College of Obstetricians and Gynecologists remained unfazed. The organization did not change its policy in 1980, when the National Institute of Child Health and Human Development called for vaginal births after cesareans (VBACs). Nor when research showed that cesarean-born infants are at increased risk for respiratory problems and distress caused by the anesthesia that must be employed in surgical deliveries. Nor when articles in leading medical journals showed the risk of maternal death from cesarean section to be 3 to 26 times greater than with vaginal delivery,[9] and that 50 percent of all new mothers who have undergone cesareans have some serious illness such as infection or hemorrhage.[10]

The American College of Obstetricians and Gynecologists was simply not about to budge from its stance of "once a cesarean, always a cesarean," even when the *New England Journal of Medicine* reported: "Morbidity and mortality are greater among infants delivered by cesarean section."[11] It did not stir when even its own *American Journal of Obstetrics and Gynecology* concluded: "Our data support the view that the policy of 'once a cesarean, always a cesarean' should be abandoned."[12]

Meanwhile, some practicing obstetricians were getting fed up with the results of such unrelenting stubbornness. In 1986, Chicago's inner-city Mount Sinai Hospital instituted programs to encourage VBACs. Within two years, its cesarean rate dropped to less than half the national average, with no rise in complications or neonatal mortality.

Finally, on October 16, 1988, the American College of Obstetricians and Gynecologists lumbered into action, officially recommending that women who have had previous cesareans should be encouraged to birth their subsequent babies vaginally, belatedly noting that 35 percent of current cesareans are "performed not because of . . . medical need, but merely because the mother had previously delivered by cesarean."

Obstetricians, however, like all of us, can be creatures of habit, and despite the change of policy many of them continue to believe "once a cesarean, always a cesarean." Even when they don't insist on a repeat cesarean, they speak of "allowing" a woman a "trial labor," a choice of words that doesn't exactly ooze confidence. Should they bestow their permission for a woman to "attempt" a vaginal birth, they still stand poised and ready to perform a cesarean at any moment.

Today, the United States has one of the highest cesarean rates in the developed world—and one of the worst infant mortality rates. It wasn't always this way. In 1962, when cesareans were still rare in this country, our standing in the world community for infant mortality was much better than it is today. As our cesarean rate has soared, our ranking in infant mortality among other nations has plummeted.[13]

Why is the rate of cesarean sections in the United States so high?

For one thing, U.S. judges usually hold physicians liable when they don't use technology. More than three-quarters of obstetricians in the U.S. have been sued, disproportionately more than any other medical specialists. In 1994, Jeffrey Phelan, M.D., editor-in-chief of *OBG Management,* wrote of how scared he was by the many lawsuits involving claims that a cesarean was not done or was done too late. The current legal climate, he warned, might well push the cesarean rate above 50 percent.[14]

Another reason is that there is far more money to be made from cesareans. No one wants to think of babies as a business, but it's naive to deny the role that financial motives play in the decisions made by doctors. In the state of Washington, the cesarean rate in nonprofit hospitals is 20.3 percent; the rate in for-profit hospitals is 36 percent.[15] When a Kansas health maintenance organization, Total Health Care, changed its policies and began to reimburse doctors equally for cesareans and for normal deliveries so that there was no longer a financial incentive to do cesareans, the cesarean rate dropped from 28.7 percent to 13.5 percent in one year.[16]

And there is yet another reason that obstetricians may choose to do unnecessary cesareans. Natural births can take place at any time, day or night. There is no telling how long the labor will last, nor predicting when the baby will emerge. Cesareans, on the other hand, can be arranged to take place at the convenience of the obstetrician and the hospital.

In short, if an obstetrician schedules a pregnant woman for a cesarean, he (and in the vast majority of cases it is a "he") makes more money, does so at his convenience, and is covered in case he's sued.

The U.S. Has One of the Highest Cesarean Rates in the Developed World, and One of the Worst Infant Mortality Rates.

*Cesarean Section Rates**		*Infant Mortality Rates***	
Japan	7%	Sweden	4
Czechoslovakia	7%	Finland	4
Netherlands	10%	Japan	4
England and Wales	10%	Singapore	5
Hungary	10%	Hong Kong	5
New Zealand	10%	Denmark	6
Switzerland	11%	Germany	6
Sweden	12%	Ireland	6
Norway	12%	Switzerland	6
Spain	12%	England and Wales	6
Denmark	13%	Austria	6
Greece	13%	Canada	6
Italy	13%	Norway	6
Portugal	13%	Netherlands	6
Scotland	14%	Italy	7
Bavaria	15%	Australia	7
Australia	16%	Slovenia	7
Canada	19%	New Zealand	7
UNITED STATES	23%	Israel	7
Brazil	26%	France	7
		Korea (Rep. of)	8
		Spain	8
		Greece	8
		Belgium	8
		UNITED STATES	8

*Source: Francis C. Notzon, "International Differences in the Use of Obstetric Interventions," Journal of the American Medical Association, June 27, 1990, vol. 263, no. 25, pp. 3286–91.

**Source: The State of the World's Children, 1996, UNICEF. (Countries are listed in ascending order of their infant mortality rates.) All of the nations with better infant mortality rates than the U.S. spend less on health care, and use midwives as their principal birth attendants.

Infant Mortality Rates are measured in infant deaths per 1000 births.

The results are not pretty. According to the World Health Organization's Marsden Wagner, "At least half of all cesareans performed in the U.S. are unnecessary. And a good number of them are life threatening, or at the very least, significantly debilitating. . . . The fact that cesareans pose serious risks to both mother and baby is one of America's best-kept secrets. . . . Most importantly, women are not told, as part of their informed consent, that the

As the U.S. Cesarean Rate Soared, the U.S. Rank in Infant Mortality Among Other Nations Plummeted.

U.S. Cesarean Rates*	U.S. Infant Mortality Rank Among the World's Nations**
1962 5%	1962 12th
1978 14.7%	1970 15th
1992 22.6%	1975 17th
*Source: Esther Zorn, *Profile of the Cesarean Epidemic.*	1980 18th
**Source: Myron E. Wegman, "Annual Summary of Vital	1985 19th
Statistics," *Pediatrics,* 1994, 94(6):792803, and other	1990 21st
annual summaries.	1996 25th

procedure increases the likelihood of mothers dying and babies experiencing life-threatening problems."[17]

Mortimer Rosen, M.D., head of obstetrics at Presbyterian Medical Center and the College of Physicians and Surgeons, is uncomfortable with the fact that mothers are rarely told that "the [cesarean] patient will inevitably face certain complications."[18] He lists some of them as follows:

"She won't be able to eat for a day or more. She will be in considerable pain and will continue to have some pain for about six weeks; she will often find it painful to urinate, defecate, or move freely. She will have a urinary bladder catheter for a day or so. She will probably need painkillers. She will have up to four or seven days hospital stay. She will have a good chance of developing some sort of infection, which will need antibiotic treatment."[19]

Such birth experiences can also affect a mother's feelings for her newborn. In their powerful book on cesarean sections, *Silent Knife*, Nancy Wainer Cohen and Lois Estner point out: "The cesarean mother and child are at a decided disadvantage as they begin life together. Often the mother is medicated, sluggish, depressed, angry, disappointed. . . . The baby is groggy and fussy because of the effects of the anesthesia and other complications. And these two are supposed to be gazing into each other's eyes with everlasting love? Add to this the hospital procedures that routinely separate cesarean mothers from their newborns, and this couple is off to a very difficult start."[20]

Although many women who give birth via cesarean section are able to overcome these obstacles and become wonderful mothers, it is not uncommon for women who undergo the procedure to lose a sense of trust in themselves and their bodies, and to feel disconnected from their babies. Often, the experience depletes their self-confidence, and leaves them unprepared for the challenges involved in caring for a newborn. **Perhaps this helps to explain the sad fact that women who give birth via cesarean are three to nine times more likely to abuse their children than mothers who give birth vaginally.**[21]

BONDING AND BECOMING

Authors of books on the subject of postpartum depression have been struck by how often the phenomenon follows disappointing birth experiences.[22] Mothering instincts do not simply arise suddenly after a baby is born; they develop over time, becoming stronger through the pregnancy and rising to a climax through the birth process itself. If a woman's experience of giving birth provides her with feelings of fulfillment and self-worth, these will be among the first feelings she associates with her newborn. On the other hand, if her maternal instincts are thwarted in the birth process and her bonding with her newborn is disrupted, feelings of frustration and depression may seep into the relationship.

The obstetrical establishment does not believe, however, that there is any connection between the quality of women's birth experiences and postpartum depression. A recent account in the *New York Times* reads: "While nearly two-thirds of new mothers experience the blues for a brief period in the days or weeks after childbirth, for about ten percent of women, depressive symptoms are far more severe and prolonged. . . . Postpartum depression often comes out of the blue, literally and figuratively. Most women who experience it have nothing in their past or present to account for it."[23]

Is that so? At The Farm in Tennessee, where nearly 2,000 home births have taken place, postpartum depression is virtually nonexistent. The rate is 0.03 percent.[24] This incidence is 300 times less frequent than similar sized populations experience after typical hospital births.

Some women are able to weather unfulfilling birth experiences and still emerge as loving, connected, and joyous mothers. The experience of birth is certainly not the only factor involved in a woman's relationship with her baby. The kind of support she receives from others is one of many factors that play a part. Some women have disappointing births, and end up bonding beautifully with their infants. But how can any mother be assisted by a birth process that leaves her feeling disappointed and degraded?

It is painful for me to see how often the type of birth that obstetricians have been taught to perform causes new mothers to feel disempowered and humiliated. What could be for them an opening to the monumental powers of motherhood very often becomes, in the hands of modern obstetrics and today's hospitals, a violation of their natural trust in who they are.

There are today in America tens of millions of women who have given birth by cesarean section, and I want to make it clear that there is no reason for them to blame themselves or feel guilty. Many of these women are courageous souls who loved their babies so much that they were willing to be cut open because they believed this was best for their infants. But when they discover how unnecessary most cesareans are, they may wonder what they might have been capable of if they had been supported and helped to give birth naturally. Even those women who look back on their cesareans with a sense of pride and accomplishment may question how their experience might have been different, and how what happened has affected their relationship with their offspring.

One such woman handled this concern by speaking to her grown son of his birth and of her experience. She told him of her hopes, fears, dreams, and pain, and said that it had always been her heart's desire to be the very best mother she could possibly be. She added that she hoped that her sharing could be a step toward healing any wounds or separation that had originated at his birth.

Her grown son, a professional comedian, listened to her with appreciation and thanked her for her love. He then proceeded to write a new joke which, with her permission, he now uses in his nightclub routine. "I was born by cesarean," he tells audiences. "But it didn't affect me at all. Just that when I leave home, I always go out the upstairs window."

AMERICAN HOSPITALS

Today, 97 percent of American births take place in hospitals. Let's say you're a woman in labor. Here's what you're likely to find at a typical American hospital:

When you arrive at the hospital, you may be offered a wheelchair.

Pregnant women are sometimes put in wheelchairs even if they are not in labor and have come to the hospital for something else. You might be told that it's hospital policy for laboring women to be wheeled to the labor and delivery floor. Do you feel taken care of and supported? Or do you have an uneasy feeling that you are now in the hospital's territory, and must follow its rules? Do you sense that you have just lost your status as an independent person? Have you begun to internalize the message that you are to be passive and obedient? Does anyone here realize that walking and an upright posture are among the best ways to help labor progress?

Next there are admission procedures, in which you must sign papers prepared by the hospital for its own purposes. You probably don't understand all the implications of what you're signing. Things don't get a whole lot better when you read the hospital form that states, "We expect total cooperation from the husband and from the patient at all times."

Next, you are given a hospital ID bracelet to put around your arm. Oh well, you might think, I've got to trust the system here, or I'll never get through this.

When you get to the labor room, they may take your clothes and make you wear a flimsy gown affording the world a full rear view. So much for dignity. One woman I know who is inclined to take charge of her own health was handed a hospital gown and told to put it on. "Why?" she asked. "Hospital policy," came the answer. "I'm quite comfortable dressed as I am," she replied, "and fully intend to remain so."

Of course, some hospitals have taken steps to be more appealing. They have changed the wallpaper, added a few cushions, and may offer you a form to fill out, asking: "Do you want to wear your own nightie or a hospital gown? Do you want to hold your baby immediately after birth? Please check the appropriate box."

This is very considerate of them, but it may take more than checking the right boxes to insure that you remain in control here. In 1996, Marshall Klaus, M.D., a pediatrician and neonatologist at the University of California, San Francisco, said that many hospitals still routinely separate mothers from their newborns, and send the infants to the nursery soon after birth, where nurses sometimes give them bottles. This can cause feeding difficulties in the newborn and feelings of distance and lowered confidence in the new mother. Even more troubling, this early separation creates touch-starved infants, and sets the stage for a higher risk of child abuse and parental abandonment.[25]

During labor, some hospitals still sometimes want women lying down on their backs, even though researchers are unanimous that this is the worst possible position (short of hanging upside down like a possum) for labor to progress. The reason is gravity. Lying on your back lessens the flow of blood and oxygen to your uterus and your baby, reducing the effectiveness of the contractions, increasing pain, and contributing significantly to fetal distress. Lying in bed on your back directly contradicts the basic principles of anatomy and physiology. Have you ever tried to have a bowel movement lying on your back, with your legs in the air?

One reason they've got you lying on your back is for the convenience of the hospital staff, who will come in from time to time and insert their hands into your vagina. This is called "doing an exam," and is a reliable way to introduce infections into your uterus. Some women have eight or ten exams during the course of a labor. The reason doctors do it is so they can tell you how you're doing.

I picture a woman grabbing her physician's arm and demanding his full attention. "Excuse me, but I'm sure that from now on you will ask my permission before examining me, and will only do so when absolutely necessary." I see her getting up and starting to move around. He objects, but she is unfazed. "I'm sure you realize," she continues, "that an upright posture dilates the cervix faster, and leads to less pain, less drug use, and babies in better condition at birth."

THE PRESSURE TO PERFORM

Most women, however, are not sufficiently informed or confident to stand up to "hospital policy." So if yours is a typical hospital birth, you are now about to undertake what may be the most demanding physical exertion of your life (one woman runner said the Boston Marathon was nothing by comparison to her child's birth), and yet your only sustenance may be a solution of sugar, water, and various electrolytes. Many U.S. hospitals still forbid women from eating during their labor. "Nothing by mouth," they say. They don't tell you that without food, you may feel weaker and more exhausted as the labor continues, and lose confidence, as your strength wanes, in your ability to successfully give birth.

The reason you may not be permitted to eat during labor is that the hospital is already planning what to do if you need to suddenly be put under general anesthesia. The irony is that treating all laboring women as candidates for surgery, and not letting them eat, makes surgery far more likely. When women become famished and tired, their uterine contractions are often weakened. This process is called by a variety of names— failure to progress, uterine inertia, failure to dilate, dystocia—and is seen as justification to perform cesarean sections.

Hospital "nothing by mouth" policies are a classic example of how fear can create a self-fulfilling prophecy. In the course of labor, unfed women can become uncomfortable and exhausted, which increases the rate of obstetric interventions, which increases the use of anesthesia, which leads to more problems.

A study at Jubilee Maternity Hospital in Belfast, North Ireland, found that women who eat and drink during labor request less pain-relieving medication and other drugs, have much shorter labors, and give birth to babies with higher Apgar scores (indicating healthier outcomes).[26]

Without food, you are deprived of a sense of comfort, your uterus is deprived of nutritional support, and the chance of complications increases. Meanwhile, your doctor will probably tell you that you have to produce the baby in a certain length of time, or a cesarean will be necessary. Hospitals usually have clocks on the walls that are large enough to be read by the legally blind, helping you to remember that time is passing. Pressuring a woman to have her baby in a certain length of time is a great way to make her feel anxious, slowing down her labor.

I picture a woman telling her obstetrician, "Okay, to help you to understand what you're putting me through, I'm going to give you exactly five minutes to get an erection and ejaculate. We're going to put you under these bright fluorescent lights, and I'm going to stand here watching. We're going to put an I.V. in your arm, a blood pressure cuff on your other arm, and we're going to have interns coming in regularly to examine your penis and measure your progress. We're also going to place electronic straps on your penis so that we can continuously monitor the angle of erection. And if you don't make it in the next few minutes, we'll cut you open and remove your sperm surgically."

Doctors consult the "Friedman Curves" to decide whether a labor is progressing normally. When a woman's labor is not progressing as rapidly as the curve says is normal, they may call an end to the labor and perform a cesarean. But the man who developed the Friedman Curve, Emanuel A.

Friedman himself, is strongly opposed to this use of his work. "There is no magic number of hours beyond which labor should not continue," he says. "The Friedman curve is being abused. . . . To intervene with a cesarean for prolonged labor is unthinkable."[27]

Unthinkable, maybe, but it's standard operating procedure in most American hospitals today. By the way, in the early 1990s, staff members at Burnaby General Hospital near Vancouver, Canada, decided to experiment and dispose of all the clocks in the hospital's birthing rooms. Was it a coincidence that the cesarean rate dropped immediately?[28]

INTERVENTIONS UNLIMITED

Now with all this going on you might possibly feel a tad inhibited, and your labor might not be speeding right along to hospital standards. Never fear, though, for your obstetrician has up his sleeve a drug called pitocin. This is a synthetic hormone that mimics oxytocin, the body's natural labor stimulant. Doctors use it to induce or to augment labor. An alternative would simply be to leave things be, and let nature take its trusty course, but that's not what obstetricians are trained to do. They have been taught to administer pitocin, which speeds up uterine contractions. It does have a slight drawback, however. It produces contractions, sometimes violently, that are difficult for women and babies to tolerate. They are sudden, abrupt, and offer no time for adjustment or preparation. The contractions frequently become overwhelming, and even if you had fully committed to an undrugged birth, you may find yourself begging for pain relief. Many women who are given pitocin become frightened and unable to cope, and require drugs to endure the process.

Giving pitocin carries other serious consequences, including increased rates of neonatal shock and fetal distress. Infants born after pitocin-augmented or induced labors are more often in need of help to breathe, and more likely to end up in intensive care.

The risks of pitocin are well known. The *American Journal of Obstetrics and Gynecology* reports that pitocin and similar drugs invariably lead to greatly increased rates of cesareans and forceps deliveries.[29] A *Lancet* article stresses that these drugs cause excessive uterine activity and uterine rupture.[30] The *International Journal of Gynecology and Obstetrics* finds that pitocin puts dangerous pressure on the fetal head that can cause cranial hemorrhage.[31]

Obstetricians know that these drugs are powerful and risky. Does this mean they hesitate to use them? Not quite. It means they have felt obliged to come up with still more interventions to try to control things—such as electronic fetal monitors.

The internal fetal monitor requires rupture of the bag of waters, which opens the door for infections and deprives your baby's head of its cushion of water during contractions. This is necessary so that two electronic catheters can be inserted through the vagina. One is inserted into the fetal scalp. The other is inserted between the fetus and the wall of the uterus.

Dozens of studies have been published in medical journals on internal fetal monitoring.[32] Most agree that the monitors cause greatly increased rates of fetal and maternal distress, and triple the number of cesarean sections, with no improvement in infant outcome.[33] On the brighter side, if the obstetrician is sued, being able to say he used the latest technology will serve him well in court. You can feel good knowing that, although the monitor is restrictive, uncomfortable, and greatly increases your odds of undergoing a cesarean section and giving birth to a brain damaged baby, you are doing your part in the greater cause of protecting your obstetrician's relationship with his insurance company.

The external fetal monitor is a little different, in that no one has to reach into your vagina and screw electronic wires into the scalp of your fetus. Instead, straps are placed around your belly, which use ultrasound to obtain information that is sent to a noisy machine that sits next to your bed. The situation may be a little disconcerting at first, but everything will be fine as long as you get used to the noise and don't move. One woman wrote: "When the monitor was attached to me, I was made to be flat and told that the monitor wouldn't work if I didn't keep still. I was yelled at several times because I tried to change positions. I felt like a caged animal."[34]

She was not being a good sport. Perhaps she was not able to appreciate the wisdom of hospital policy. Fetal monitors are obligatory in almost all hospital births in the U.S. today, even though they give 30 to 50 percent false positive results.[35]

What happens in case of a false positive? All kinds of things, none of them fun. In Massachusetts recently, a fetal heart monitor signaled distress and was unable to locate any fetal heartbeat. The obstetrician panicked, and declared that a cesarean had to be done immediately, even though there was no time to administer an anesthetic. He cut the poor woman open, and pulled out a perfectly healthy baby while the mother screamed at the top of her lungs. A nurse who was present said that if the physician had taken the time to listen for the heartbeat with his ears, he would have known the baby was fine. "It wasn't fetal distress," she said, "it was physician distress. And now I'm distressed from working at this hospital!"[36]

Many doctors have become so dependent on the monitors that they no longer know how to listen to a baby with their own ears, or how to use a simple hand-held stethoscope, or fetoscope. This, despite the fact that in 1989 the American College of Obstetricians and Gynecologists evaluated data from eight studies covering 50,000 births, and declared that use of these simple procedures is at least as effective as the monitors. All eight studies, by the way, reported a significant increase in cesareans when monitors were used.

It is extremely common for a cesarean to be performed because the monitor indicates that something might be wrong, only for the surgeon to find out afterwards that the baby had been doing just fine. And when a baby is found to have been in distress, much of the time it is only because the woman was lying flat on her back, which cut off the oxygen to the uterus and the baby. In one study, 96 percent of babies born by cesarean due to monitor-perceived fetal distress had Apgar scores of eight to ten, suggesting that the only significant stress these infants were experiencing was caused by the monitors themselves.[37]

The man who invented electronic fetal monitors is an obstetrician named Edward H. Hon. You would think that at least he would have a kind word for the way the technology is used. But no. "Most women in labor are better off at home than in the hospital with the electronic fetal monitor," he protests. "They're assaulting the mother."[38]

If there were a contest held to determine which modern medical technology was the most frequently misused, I wouldn't want to bet against fetal monitors. Many studies emphatically state that monitoring causes the very distress it is supposed to detect. One researcher, writing in the *American Journal of Epidemiology*, says that the information obtained from monitors is about as accurate as "tossing a coin."[39]

THERE'S MORE

At this point, with your doctor, nurses, and even your husband staring fixedly at the monitors, waiting for something to go wrong, you may not be feeling entirely loved, supported, and connected to those around you.

But are you ever grateful to the hospital when pain medication is offered! Later, you might say, "Thank God I was in the hospital. I couldn't believe the pain. I couldn't have made it without the drugs." It is not likely that either the obstetrician nor any of the hospital staff will tell you how much of your pain was caused by hospital procedures. They won't tell you that emotional stress triggers the release of catecholamines, stress hormones that constrict the blood vessels, particularly those in the uterus, depriving your uterus of oxygen, and causing you excruciating pain.

If you express qualms about the drugs, the hospital staff will probably just smile sweetly, wondering what planet you're from. "You haven't seen anything, yet," they'll warn, implying that you're being foolish to even think about trying to undergo the ordeal without painkillers. They aren't familiar with the many proven alternative approaches that midwives know are helpful in reducing labor pain—things like maternal movement and position change, touch and massage, the use of heat or cold, baths and showers, acupressure, visualization, self-hypnosis, and music.

And so soon you will probably receive what has delicately been called a "barrage of analgesics and anesthetics" that will be fed to you, dripped into your veins, and jabbed into half a dozen locations, including your cervix and your spine. These drugs relieve pain, all right, but they also relieve you of the capacity to make conscious, rational decisions, or to protest what is being done to you. Not that you're likely to be told that the drugs you're taking will cross the placenta and reach your baby. Or that your baby's brain is still growing, and these drugs can adversely affect its development. Your baby's liver, needed to metabolize toxic materials, is not mature enough to do so yet. Your baby's kidneys, needed for the elimination of toxins, are not yet ready for the task.

Do these drugs really affect babies? When researchers with the National Institutes of Health and the University of Florida analyzed 53,000 births, they found that children as old as seven still suffered from noticeable negative effects due to obstetrical drugs used at their birth. They discovered that older children whose mothers had received drugs during labor and delivery scored lower in reading and spelling, and showed other signs of neurological impairment. **One researcher testified before the U.S. Senate, "There is no doubt in my mind and in the minds of many other individuals working with brain-injured children, that a large proportion of brain-injured and learning disabled children are the result of ob-**

stetric drugs administered to women to relieve discomfort or pain, or to induce or stimulate their labor. Most women are unaware that obstetric drugs diminish the supply of oxygen to the unborn baby's brain and can result in brain damage."[40]

THE RUSH TO CUT

I wish I could speak more positively about modern hospital birth, but the reality is not particularly inspiring. Doctors frequently do not ask women's consent before performing episiotomies (surgical incisions to enlarge the vaginal opening), because they take the procedure so for granted. Episiotomies are performed in most U.S. hospital vaginal births. The rate is particularly high for first-time mothers. In many hospitals, the rate approaches 100 percent.[41] And yet, in Scandinavian countries the episiotomy rate is only 6 percent.[42]

Are U.S. perineums different from Scandinavian ones? They are all made up of elastic tissue, able to stretch and open. Obstetricians are trained to believe that cutting a woman will prevent her from tearing, but many women will not tear at all if allowed to ease the baby out, particularly if the vaginal opening is massaged or soaked in warm water. At The Farm in Tennessee, more than 70 percent of the thousands of home births have involved no tearing at all, and when tearing has occurred, it has usually been minimal. The midwives there, like midwives in general, are well versed in helping the mother to relax and stretch around the emerging baby's head, thus greatly reducing the need for episiotomies and the incidence of tears.

Obstetricians, however, are not typically masters of the art of patience. In fact, the atmosphere in a typical American labor around the moment of birth frequently borders on pandemonium. Everyone is shouting, "Push! Push! Go for it! Push!"—which is probably not the best way to help a woman giving birth to relax and surrender to the inner workings of her body and soul. As a culture, we seem to have some difficulty differentiating between a birth and a football game.

What are the advantages of routine episiotomies? There actually aren't any. Studies published in *Lancet* and other major medical journals have consistently found that the procedure has no noticeable medical benefits, and often causes harm.[43]

In performing an episiotomy, the doctor cuts through muscles and nerves. When no episiotomy is performed, if tears do occur, they tend to take place where the perineum has stretched to its fullest, along the lines of least resistance and easiest mending. A 1990 study in the *American Journal of Obstetrics and Gynecology* found that women who undergo episiotomies are 50 times more likely to suffer from severe lacerations.[44] Another major study concluded that women with episiotomies undergo far more pain than those with tears, and that the pain lasts longer.[45]

Botched episiotomies are frequent. Sometimes perineums remain numb for years, and there can result a permanent loss of sexual pleasure. Nurses I have spoken with refer to a particular obstetrician as "the butcher" because he routinely cuts women open from vagina to anus. This procedure (called an episioproctotomy) can lead to permanent loss of sphincter control and anal incontinence. Unfortunately, this man is not an isolated case. In fact, he is the head of obstetrics at a major hospital.

Today's obstetricians have been taught to routinely perform episiotomies, just as they have been taught to routinely perform all the other interventions that can mutilate a woman's experience of giving birth. They do what they were taught to do, and most believe that what they do is necessary and helpful.

Episiotomies might make sense if nature had designed perineums defectively. Current obstetrical practice might make sense if women were not equipped for birth, if the process was, as many doctors still believe, inherently pathological and in need of constant medical management.

But women are beautifully designed to give birth, and need loving support and wise guidance far more often than they need pitocin, electronic fetal monitors, cesareans, and episiotomies. The medicalization of childbirth has turned something that can be glorious and magnificent into something comparatively obscene. It's like the difference, says Michelle Harrison, M.D., between "the beauty of those moments when sexuality takes on a spiritual quality and pornography."[46]

When birth technology is truly needed, it can save lives. In extreme situations, medical and surgical interventions have an important place. If a mother is experiencing a serious outbreak of primary genital herpes when she goes into labor, it makes sense to do a cesarean. If a baby is presenting in a breech position and cannot be turned, it may be useful to do an episiotomy. The trouble is that most births are normal, and obstetricians are not trained to do normal births.

JUST HAND ME THE BABY WHEN IT'S ALL OVER

It is not only obstetricians who often believe that birth is a dangerous and foreign process from which women need to be rescued. Many women believe this as well, and pass this crippling mythology on to other women. Some mothers tell their pregnant daughters, "Now you'll see how I suffered with you." Others seem to think it is their duty to tell pregnant friends the most frightening stories they can about pain and tragic outcomes. The belief that childbirth is virtually unbearable has gained credibility every time it has been passed on to the next emotionally porous pregnant woman. Television and movies frequently add to this terror by depicting birth as a nightmarish experience where mothers and babies often die.

This conditioning does not help women to feel confident, or to focus on birth as a miraculous process of creation and transformation. Some women are so scared of labor that they have a hard time imagining themselves going through it.

One such woman pleaded, "Knock me out. I'm not an Indian."

"I don't want to feel a thing," moaned another. "Just hand me the baby when it's all over."

Women who are frightened of labor often believe that they would never be able to give birth without chemicals, drugs, tools, monitors, and machines. They assume that they would be lost without experts to do it for them. They have lost trust in themselves, and in their bodies' abilities to actively and successfully birth their babies. They believe that someone else must get their babies out for them.

Although the *Ladies Home Journal* did much in the late 1950s to expose what the medical model of childbearing was doing to women and to babies, the popular women's magazines have more often counseled women to obey their doctors and put their faith in medical technology. In 1982, an article in *Family Circle* explained, "The single factor most responsible for recent advances in helping mothers and infants . . . is sophisticated technology. It allows physicians to closely monitor fetal development through pregnancy and labor. If the . . . delivery is totally uncomplicated, the full weight of this technology need not be brought to bear, although it sometimes is."[47]

Fortunately, more and more women today are shifting from helplessness to power, and converting their anger into passion for change. They know they are capable of going through the process with consciousness, love, and courage. They are proud of themselves. They are reminding one another, and telling the world, that their bodies have evolved over millions of years and are exquisitely capable of giving birth.

ANOTHER POSSIBILITY, ANOTHER WAY

What would happen, I wonder, if we had a medical system that helped people to understand and befriend their bodies? What if women were told by their doctors that birth is essentially safe for both mother and baby, and that both are perfectly designed for the task? What would happen if doctors communicated a set of beliefs that helped women to respect and appreciate the natural design? What if women were treated with trust in their ability to make informed and responsible choices? What if they were helped to understand that every birth is unique and precious? What if their needs for emotional support were validated and met?

Not every woman would choose a natural childbirth. Not all women would see labor as a dance with the great forces of life, as a journey of personal and spiritual power. Some would still want all the technology a hospital could offer. But all could make informed choices that expressed their values and affirmed their lives. They'd be in charge of their births. And a great majority would choose not to miss what could be one of the most meaningful experiences of their lives.

Increasing numbers of women would step off the obstetric table and reclaim the power of their bodies. There'd be a lot fewer operations, and a lot more celebrations.

Mothers would be learning about the depths of their resilience and power. They would be learning that they are stronger and more passionate than they ever knew. And in subsequent years, at times when being a mother was difficult, they could remember their labors and how they gave birth to this child, how they had been tested in the fire and found the strength to fulfill this sacred trust, and they would in the remembering feel an upwelling of renewed confidence.

There'd still be a need for hospitals, to take care of those births where high-tech support was needed. But hospitals would be more like the National Maternity Hospital in Dublin, Ireland, where nurses are trained to touch the mother, to have eye and hand contact, and to use positions in which nurse and mother are eye-to-eye on the same horizontal plane. In this hospital, interventions are minimal, the cesarean rate has never risen above six percent, and labors typically last half as long as they do in the United States. A woman in labor is always given continuous loving support, and every effort is made to help her "feel that she will be able to handle her labor, that she will be safe, that her dignity and experience matter, and that her body's responses are natural and normal."[48]

If hospitals recognized that birth is not an illness, maybe they could actually start to become the humane places their advertisements make them out to be. They would be eager to have midwives attend births, and would be supportive of women who chose out-of-hospital birth centers, or home births. Their policies would reflect the study published in the *Journal of the American Medical Association* in 1991, which found that when women in labor are continuously attended by a caring person the result is 68 percent fewer cesareans, and 85 percent less pain medication.[49] No woman would ever again labor in a hospital without being surrounded by an atmosphere of loving support.

There'd still be a place for obstetricians, but they would be taught to be more like Michel Odent, M.D., who for many years directed the obstetrical unit at Centre Hospital in Pithiviers, France. Thousands of women from every social class and economic background have given birth at this public hospital, including many high-risk women. Here, labors are never artificially induced, and there is no use of pitocin to speed labor, medication, or anesthesia (except for cesareans). The results put most hospitals to shame. The episiotomy rate is less than 6 percent. The cesarean rate is less than 7 percent.[50]

How do they do it? Everything possible is done to enhance a woman's capacity to have pleasure and a sense of well-being. Supported and cared for in a safe, quiet place, she can turn inward and listen to what her feelings tell her to do in labor and birth. As Michel Odent says, "What we try to do at Pithiviers is to rehabilitate the instinctive brain, the emotional brain, the brain which is close to the body, in a world that generally only knows and takes into account the other brain, the rational brain."[51]

Michel Odent has found that helping laboring women to reach a deep, feeling level of consciousness results in safer, smoother, faster, and less painful labors and births. The average first-time mother labors less than half the average time for American first-time mothers. Yet a short labor is a byproduct of helping a woman to feel supported, nurtured and safe, not a goal in itself. When asked how long he is willing to wait for a birth, Michel Odent replied, "As long as it takes. We have no clocks anywhere in the birth rooms."[52]

Michel Odent is world famous for his groundbreaking work in the use of warm water in labor. "We observe many times," he says, "that a good bath in warm water with semidarkness is the best way to reach a high level of relaxation." Some women shower, others immerse themselves in the pools. If a woman's labor stalls, she will often enter the pool, and find that within an hour she is fully dilated. Sometimes women feel so comfortable in the pool that they give birth there. Writing in *Lancet,* Odent reported no complications or infections in more than 100 underwater births at Pithiviers.[53]

Visitors to Michel Odent's hospital are often struck by the feelings of joy and friendliness they observe. Pregnant women and their partners can attend weekly groups which validate the happiness that naturally surrounds birth. Many women who have given birth here have called it one of the most meaningful and beautiful experiences of their lives.

RECLAIMING BIRTH

A woman does not need to give birth in order to be a fulfilled and complete human being, nor to express her love and nurturance into the world. But if a woman does give birth, she deserves an opportunity to do so in a way that is emotionally and spirtually meaningful to her. In every woman who gives birth there is a meeting of the intimate and the infinite.

Maybe someday we will all know a world of birth in which women are respected, and given the opportunity to deliver their babies in an atmosphere of total love and support. Maybe we will yet know a world where every birthing woman receives comfort and guidance from her attendants, be they midwives, family members, or wonderful obstetricians like Michel Odent.

I like to believe that someday our medical profession will understand what Kazantzakis's immortal character Zorba the Greek learned so poignantly:

"I remember one morning when I discovered a cocoon in the bark of a tree, just as the butterfly was making a hole in its case and preparing to come out. I waited a while, but it was too long appearing and I was impatient. I bent over it and breathed on it to warm it. I warmed it as quickly as I could, and the miracle began to happen before my eyes, faster than life. The case opened, the butterfly started slowly crawling out, and I shall never forget my horror when I saw how its wings were folded back and crumpled; the wretched butterfly tried with its whole trembling body to unfold them. Bending over it, I tried to help it with my breath. In vain.

"It needed to be hatched out patiently, and the unfolding of the wings should be a gradual process in the sun. Now it was too late. My breath had forced the butterfly to appear, all crumpled, before its time. It struggled desperately and, a few seconds later, died in the palm of my hand.

"The little body is, I do believe, the greatest weight I have on my conscience. For I realize today that it is a mortal sin to violate the great laws of nature. We should not hurry, we should not be impatient, but we should confidently obey the eternal rhythm."[54]

I like to believe it possible that someday our medical profession will help women labor and give birth according to the rhythms and timings of their inner being; that the conflict between the medical mind and human nature will be over. When that day dawns, more women will be able to forever remember their children's births as events that brought them closer to themselves and to what they hold dear.

Fewer babies will be born to mothers who are bewildered and humiliated, too groggy and weak to hold their babies, and too drugged to care. More babies will be born to mothers who feel that their choices matter, and who have been helped to take active responsibility for their lives and their health. Born into an atmosphere of love and respect, these babies will arrive fully alert and able to breathe, to nurse, and to undertake life. They will be greeted by mothers who have been prepared, by the enormous forces of birth itself, to parent them with love, understanding, and joy.

4
A Modern-Day Witch-Hunt

Every president of the United States except Jimmy Carter and Bill Clinton was born at home.

W HEN AN ELEPHANT went into labor in an American zoo, the zoo-keepers put her in her own enclosure, isolating her from the other elephants. As her labor progressed, however, the elephant became distressed and began thrashing about violently. Recognizing that something was going terribly wrong, the zoo officials quickly telephoned a European zoo where an elephant had recently given birth successfully. When the Americans described what was happening, the Europeans were shocked. "Where are the midwives," they demanded. "Where are the other female elephants to help with the delivery?"

The Americans immediately complied with the Europeans' instructions. As soon as they were allowed into the area with the birthing mother, the other female elephants rushed to her and began to assist her, stroking her with their trunks, calming her with their presence, and helping her to complete her labor. After the newborn elephant emerged, the midwives cleaned the baby and took care of her while the mother rested.[1]

Birth educator and author Nancy Wainer Cohen comments, "It is no wonder to me that so many women in hospitals 'thrash about' and are disoriented, upset and traumatized at birth when we are deprived of women—midwives and friends—whom we know and trust."[2]

We can perhaps chalk up a female elephant's frightening isolation from her caring sisters to the well-intended ignorance of zoo keepers. But to what can we attribute the attitude of the American medical establishment toward midwifery?

A HEROINE IN HANDCUFFS

"I've been placed in handcuffs three times in my life. The first two times were in the 1960s; when I was giving birth I was handcuffed to the delivery table—like other women in labor in those days—to keep me from touching my baby. And then in August 1991, I was arrested at my home—my youngest daughter had to watch it happen—and taken to jail for assisting women who give birth at home."[3]

These are the words of Bonnie Faye "Faith" Gibson. A practicing obstetrical nurse in Florida for 15 years, she left the profession after being part of too many births in which invasive procedures were employed too often and with too much harm to the mother and baby. Having tried to change the system from within, she came to a point where she simply could no longer in good conscience continue to be part of it. At the time of her arrest, she had been a practicing midwife in Palo Alto, California, for more than ten years.

Not that long ago, when I heard about the arrest of a midwife, I assumed she must have done something seriously wrong that caused significant harm to a mother or a baby. But I have learned that this is rarely the case.

Faith Gibson is a good example. In the 20 years prior to her arrest, she had attended over 4,000 births. Her record as a midwife had been flawless. She had presided over 350 home births without a mishap. There had never been a single complaint registered against her by a client, and no mother or baby had ever suffered a birth injury associated with her care.

Yet on August 9, 1991, armed medical board agents burst into her home, catching her smack in the dastardly act of teaching a breastfeeding class.[4] After arresting and handcuffing her, they completed this noble performance of their civic duty by dragging her off to the county jail. The charges? Practicing without a license. The penalty if she were found guilty? A year in prison, and a sizable fine.

The arrest had been in the works for months. A series of covert operators had visited Faith Gibson. One had pretended to be a woman interested in home birth; another had posed as a salesman who said his wife was eight and a half months pregnant. There had been at least five entrapment calls. The medical board spared no expense in plotting the capture of this dangerous criminal.

Unfortunately for the medical board, the case drew the attention of Paul Halvonik, a nationally renowned constitutional lawyer. His statement was telling:

"Faith Gibson is not charged with doing something that is, in itself, illegal. Midwifery is not illegal in California. Faith Gibson is not charged with performing poorly as a midwife. Faith Gibson is charged with not having a license. At the same time, it is forbidden that she have a license [to practice traditional midwifery]. California's midwife license is available only as a renewal to one who possessed one in 1949. Faith was born in 1947, and, unforehandedly, made no application when she was two. . . .

"Faith Gibson is challenging a law, flatly, that the only people competent to function as [traditional] midwives are those who were honing their skills during the Truman administration. And yet, one does no dishonor to tradition by entertaining the possibility that, since 1949, someone has come along who can handle the task."[5]

The case dragged on for almost two years, with Faith Gibson and her attorneys having to attend no fewer than 16 different court hearings. Between the activities of the medical board and the court costs, more than a million dollars were spent prosecuting this woman, much of it at taxpayers' expense. Finally, on April 9, 1993, Paul Seidel, the deputy district attorney of Santa Clara County, decided enough was enough. He dismissed the last of the charges against Faith Gibson in a three-minute hearing.[6]

The ordeal, however, had left the midwife badly bruised. The publicity had severely stained her reputation. And despite the many contributions she had received from grateful former clients to help pay her court costs, she was left with a heavy personal debt. She had done nothing wrong, but the California Medical Board had ruined her career.

THE WITCH-HUNTS

As I've learned about the plight of modern midwives, and sought to understand the roots of this strange persecution, I've often been reminded of one of the greatest shames of European history—the murder of women as witches. We don't really know how many women were burned to death as witches in Europe during the 16th, 17th, and 18th centuries. Estimates range into the millions.[7] But two things are certain. Of the people burned at the stake as witches, most were women. And the women who had it the roughest were the midwives.

It all began in 1484, when the not-so-aptly-named Pope Innocent VIII made an official declaration against the crime of witchcraft. Two years later, a pair of Dominican monks, Heinrich Kramer and Jakob Sprenger, published an extremely influential book titled *Malleus Maleficarum*. This treatise became the official doctrine of the witch-hunt. With the pope's blessing, it was required reading for all Roman Catholic judges and magistrates, and functioned as the indispensable authority for 300 years of mass terror and persecution throughout Europe.

The authors of the *Malleus* were not overly fond of women. "What else is a woman," they wrote, "but a foe to friendship, an inescapable punishment, a necessary evil, a natural temptation, a desirable calamity, a domestic danger, a delectable detriment, an evil of nature painted with fair colors!"[8]

It wasn't only women who were burned. Those men who dared to stand up for the women who were being persecuted were called "witch lovers," and frequently executed along with them. In addition, homosexual men were burned to death. In fact, the cruel use of the word *faggot* to mean a male homosexual stems from this time. Homosexual men were bound and placed at the foot of witch pyres, their bodies used as "faggots" to kindle the flames.[9]

But it was women, according to the authors of the *Malleus*, who were the cause of most if not all of the world's problems. And among women, they repeatedly emphasized, midwives were "the worst offenders."[10] Lest there be any confusion in the matter, these esteemed authorities declared: "Midwives cause the greatest damage, either killing children or sacrilegiously offering them to devils. . . . The greatest injury to the Faith are done by midwives, and this is made clearer than daylight itself by the confessions of some who were afterwards burned."[11]

The "confessions" in which midwives acknowledged the horrible things they had done were obtained, however, in a manner that was not the greatest example we have ever beheld of the Christian ethic of compassion. Although judicial torture was not allowed under native European law, the *Malleus* made an exception in the case of witch-hunts.[12] "Let her be often and frequently exposed to torture," its authors wrote, speaking of the woman accused of being a midwife/witch, "and while this is being done, let the notary write it all down, how she is tortured and what questions are asked and how she answers. If, after being fittingly tortured, she refuses to confess the truth, he should have other engines of torture brought before her, and tell her she will have to endure these if she does not confess."[13]

It has been terribly difficult for me to comprehend the sadism that dominated Europe, and I admit that I have at times wanted to look away when confronted with the facts. Some of the simpler torture instruments, according to Monica Sjoo and Barbara Mor writing in *The Great Cosmic Mother*, were "eye-gougers, branding irons, metal forehead tourniquets, and spine-rollers with sharp metal protrusions. There were also the usual thumbscrews and leg vises, stocks with iron spikes, and boards with nails on which people were forced to kneel for hours. One of the more exotic instruments was called the 'pear.' It was roughly the size and shape of a pear, constructed in two metallic halves, each attached to a handle and hinged to open—like scissors or forceps. The pear was heated to red hot, then inserted in the prisoner's mouth, anus and/or vagina, and spread as far as it would go."[14] Of course, the torture instruments were always to be blessed by the priests before they were used.

If an accused woman succumbed to torture and confessed to being a witch, then her confession stood as proof of her guilt, and she was put to death. If, on the other hand, she did not confess despite the relentless torture, then the only possible explanation for her fortitude was that she had powers derived from the devil. This then constituted proof of her guilt, and so she was burned to death.

In the relentless endeavor to discover which women were witches and kill them, some men made their living as "prickers."[15] It was their job to go from town to town, sticking needles in women who were stripped naked and exposed in public for this purpose. If a woman did not bleed, then this proved she was a witch and she was burned to death. The "prick" these professional gentlemen used was a tool with a hollow shaft and a retractable needle, which allowed them to appear to prick a woman and yet guarantee, if they wished, that she would not bleed. "Prickers" were paid by the local churches and town governments for each woman thus confirmed as a witch and put to death. It is from the activities of these chivalrous gentlemen that we have inherited the word *prick* to denote a man who treats women with something less than generosity and kindness.

The flames spread from Germany to Italy and to France, and finally to England. Whole villages blazed with the fires of women being burned to death. Executions averaged 600 a year for many German cities.[16] In some villages, virtually every female was murdered, even little girls and elderly women. In 1585, two villages in the Bishopric of Trier were left with exactly one female inhabitant each.[17]

As Monica Sjoo and Barbara Mor write: "While Michelangelo was sculpting and Shakespeare writing, witches were burning. . . . Renaissance men were celebrating naked female beauty in their art, while women's bodies were being tortured and burned by the hundreds of thousands all around them."[18]

I had always believed that, although the witch-hunts were surely one of the most hideous periods of our history, the church only meant to execute the bad witches, women who they believed had seriously injured or poisoned their fellow beings. But I was wrong. In fact, the reason midwives were the women who were most heavily persecuted was precisely because it was not merely murdering or poisoning that was considered a crime, but also helping and healing.[19] As a leading English witch-hunter put it, "For this must always be remembered . . . that by Witches we understand not only those which kill and torment, but all . . . wise women. In the same number we reckon all good Witches, which do no hurt but do good, which do not spoil and destroy, but save and deliver. . . . It were a thousand times better for the land if all Witches, but especially the blessing Witch, might suffer death."[20]

One medieval scholar estimates that more than one million midwives and healers were executed for the crime of helping other women.[21]

When a midwife/healer named Jacoba Felicie was brought to trial by the Faculty of Medicine at the University of Paris, the chief accusations against her were that, "she would cure her patient of internal illness and wounds or of external abscesses. She would visit the sick assiduously."[22] No fewer than six witnesses testified that this woman had cured them, even after numerous doctors had given up all hope. One patient declared that Jacoba Felicie was greater in the art of medicine and healing than any master physician or surgeon in Paris. But these testimonials were of no use to her; in fact, they were used against her, as proof of her guilt, for she was charged, as California midwife Faith Gibson was in 1991, not with incompetence or harming anyone, but simply for daring to practice her healing art, when the authorities wished her not to do so. Unlike Faith Gibson, however, Jacoba Felicie's "crime" was punished with torture and murder. After all, according to the holy men who wrote the *Malleus*: "If a woman dare to cure . . . she is a witch and must die."[23]

One witch-hunt authority proclaimed that the good witch was "a more horrible and detestable monster" than the wicked one. And the worst of the good witches were the midwives, he said, because by helping a woman to be self-reliant they were reducing her dependence on God.[24]

"No one," bellowed the *Malleus*, "does more harm than midwives."[25] It was the midwife who went about her community, using herbs that could reduce a fever or stop a hemorrhage. The *Malleus* called, accordingly, for the destruction of "the ancient and secret knowledge" of herbs, "both healing and hurtful."[26]

How on earth, I have wondered again and again, could such cruelty ever have happened? I recognize that individual human beings can become psychopathic and sadistic, and I know that for fleeting periods such a mentality can tragically overtake an entire society, but to see such traits embodied for hundreds of years in the church and in the legal structure of the culture from which our own has developed can be almost too much to bear.

Today, many people are learning about the witch-hunts from an outstanding historical documentary produced and directed by Montreal filmmaker Donna Read, called *The Burning Times*. **When asked if she sees any sort of historic parallel between the medieval witch-hunts and the medical establishment's efforts to drive midwives from their profession, she replied that it is not exactly a parallel. "It's more of a continuum."**[27]

It is painful for me to even imagine what living in constant terror did to 300 years of European women. I have wanted to push the horror of it away, to say the witch-hunts are ancient history, products of a terrible and insane time that we have fortunately left behind us. Most history books hardly mention it, as if also wanting to deny that such a thing could have occurred. But what residue from this holocaust lives on in the depths of the human psyche today?

I doubt that it's possible to overestimate how much damage the witch-hunts did to the possibility of sexual peace. How could a man have felt safe loving a woman, when she might at any time be accused of being a witch and burned at the stake? And how could a woman trust any man, when he might, should he become displeased with her, accuse her of being a witch and cause her to be tortured and killed?

The terror lasted for centuries. What did women learn to pass on to their daughters in order for them to survive? Could it be that from these times today's women have inherited a fear of speaking out, asserting themselves, and expressing their healing powers? Did women learn that, in order to survive, they must never speak their mind, but must be compliant, submissive, and deferential?

What vestiges remain deep in the collective unconscious of our culture? Does some vague sense of awful foreboding still cling to the midwife, the herbalist, and the female healer? The average schoolgirl today has no idea what a midwife is, but she "knows" what a witch is—an old, ugly, and evil woman. She may even have innocently played a part in perpetuating the myth, dressing in black on Halloween with a broomstick and pointed hat.

I've often wondered why so few famous historical figures are women. Given that women are half of our species, how is that their actions and ideas are hardly discussed in our history books? No doubt historians have selectively recorded the activities of men. But could it also be that many of the most gifted, inspired, and powerful women were killed? When women did arise as prominent historical figures, what happened to them? How many of them, like Joan of Arc, were burned at the stake?

And in case anyone thinks that witch-hunting is a thing only of the medieval past, we have televangelist and former presidential candidate Pat Robertson to remind us otherwise. When an Equal Rights Amendment was proposed in Iowa in 1993, he declared: "The feminist agenda is not about equal rights for women. It is about a socialist, antifamily political movement that encourages women to leave their husbands, kill their children, practice witchcraft, destroy capitalism, and become lesbians."[28]

CONTINUING A TRADITION

In the United States, witch burning never caught on to the extent that it had in Europe, but this continent certainly did not escape its horrors. A woman named Anne Hutchinson was one of the most socially prominent women in colonial America. She was known as a "woman very helpful in the times of childbirth, and other occasions of bodily infirmities, and well-furnished with means for these purposes." That may have been all right, but she crossed a line when she "believed that God's grace could be found in every person, rather than being reserved for the favored few."[29] After it was discovered that she had been present at the birth of a deformed child, she was accused of witchcraft, and forced to flee for her life from her hometown of Boston. When she died, the church fathers decreed that the church bells in the city were to ring for 24 hours to celebrate her death.[30]

For the most part, however, midwives were practicing their arts and attending virtually all births in the United States until the late 19th century, when organized medicine took up the cause of prohibiting their activities. Doctors wanted pregnant women, or at least those with money, to depend on them for childbirth assistance. One physician actually went to the trouble of calculating all the fees "lost" to doctors on account of midwives.[31]

The public campaign against midwifery was, of course, never presented as a grab for market share. Instead, it was couched in a language of benevolent concern for women giving birth. Midwives, the public was told, were the enemies of progress. Never mind that their rates of both infant and maternal mortality were superior to doctors. Nor that, unlike the male obstetricians, they understood what the laboring mother was experiencing.

The voices of organized medicine proclaimed that midwives were "hopelessly dirty, ignorant and incompetent, relics of a barbaric past." One physician railed that midwives "may wash their hands, but oh, what myriads of dirt lurk under their fingernails." The elimination of the midwife was presented by doctors as a necessary part of the effort to sanitize society. The midwife, explained one distinguished physician, "is the most virulent bacteria of them all."[32]

Name-calling was a key part of the campaign. Midwives were called *mammies, old wives, hags,* and *crones.*

The campaign worked. Women came to fear the dangers of childbirth to the point that no amount of precautions could be considered excessive. Upper- and middle-class American women who had money to spend became the territory of the new obstetrical profession. In 1847, when the AMA was founded, midwives were attending nearly 100 percent of the nation's births. But by 1915, the number dropped to below 40 percent.[33]

Not that this improved results for women or babies. In 1916, Julius Levey, M.D., of the New Jersey Department of Public Health did a major study in Newark. Midwives, he found, actually had far better birth outcomes than physicians. As well, he found that midwives were sometimes charged unfairly with a death, "even where it appeared that the result was due to unnecessary interference or negligence on the part of the doctor."[34]

But the attack on midwives was not deterred. In 1921, shortly after women had received the right to vote, a group of midwives and citizen reformers proposed legislation providing funds for childbirth education, prenatal classes, and better training for midwives. The AMA responded by pledging its full might in the effort to stop the bill. The editor of the *Illinois Medical Journal* explained that the bill was the work of "endocrine perverts, derailed menopausics, and a lot of other men and women working overtime to destroy the country."[35]

Organized medicine's attack on midwifery was extraordinarily successful. By 1960, midwives were attending less than one percent of American births. By then, the medical profession's efforts appeared near to achieving total success in the United States, with midwifery seemingly on its way to being forever banished from the land. But just as the nation's pitifully few remaining midwives were about to be eliminated, there began to arise in the late 1960s a counterculture movement that revived the time-honored tradition. People were interested in learning how to live off the land, build houses by hand, grow food without chemicals, keep themselves healthy, and care for one another's ailments in natural ways. With this emphasis on self-reliance and community spirit, midwifery fit right in. Naturally it was in California, where the counterculture movement was strongest, that the resurgence of midwifery began.

And it was in California that the medical profession struck back.

THE FIGHT

In the small California town of Santa Cruz, about 70 miles south of San Francisco, midwives, led by Raven Lang, were becoming increasingly popular in the late 1960s and early 1970s. When physicians realized that increasing numbers of women were going to midwives to give birth, they declared the whole thing a public health menace. In a maneuver not unlike pouting children saying "If you don't play my way, I'll take my ball and go home," the local medical society decided by unanimous vote that henceforth obstetricians would refuse to provide prenatal care to any woman intending to have a home birth. They would no longer perform blood tests or offer any other form of care during pregnancy.

The doctors did not seem troubled that their strategy might deprive patients of needed care and could endanger their lives. Perhaps they thought that their decision would crush the midwifery movement. But Raven Lang and the other midwives were a far hardier and more responsible sort than the medical society had anticipated. They learned how to provide many of the services the doctors were no longer willing to offer.

In response, the doctors grew more obstinate. Raven Lang and the other midwives had always sought medical help in those few situations where it was needed. They had always taken birthing women to the hospital when the situation called for medical technology or obstetrical expertise. But now local physicians refused to help her or any other midwives, and would not provide any follow-up after home births.

There were, of course, some physicians who wanted to help, but they were made virtually impotent to do so by the professional organizations that dominated medicine. In 1975, Yale University Hospital issued a written policy that any doctor who attended a home birth would lose the right to practice in that hospital. Other hospitals and institutions throughout the country followed in short order. Bowing to organized medicine's lobbying efforts, insurance companies refused to cover doctors or nurse-midwives who attended home births, or even those who worked in licensed birth centers.

Meanwhile, in California, things were heating up. In early 1974, a pregnant investigator for the California Department of Consumer Affairs, acting on behalf of the California Board of Medical Quality Assurance, dressed herself up as a hippie and went a number of times to the midwife-run Santa Cruz Birth Center. Then, on March 6, she called the center saying she was in premature labor, and pleaded with the midwives to come to her aid.

Although the midwives, Jeanine Walker and Linda Bennet, had been uncomfortable with this woman and did not trust her, they responded to her call for help. When they arrived, however, they were arrested. At the same time, police descended on the Birth Center, and were not only ransacking the place but also tearing apart the home of another midwife, Kate Bowland. In their zeal to find hidden evidence of misdeeds, they left no drawer or cupboard unsearched.

Envisioning the police rampaging through every nook and cranny of Kate Bowland's home at the behest of the medical profession, it's hard not to be reminded of the witch-hunts. In fact, the police's behavior almost uncannily reflects instructions found in the witch-hunt rule book, the *Malleus:* "Her house should be searched as thoroughly as possible, in all holes and corners and chests, top and bottom; and if she is a noted witch, then without doubt, unless she has previously hidden them, there will be found various instruments of witchcraft."[36]

When Raven Lang learned what was happening, she called the press, and went to Kate Bowland's house to meet them. She was standing in the front yard, watching police carrying out diapers, blood pressure cuffs, bandages, stethoscopes, and virtually anything else they could find as "evidence," when a police officer came up to her. He was evidently not entirely alert, for he showed her a picture of herself and asked if she knew where he could find the ringleader. Amazed, Raven shook her head, and then watched him flounce off in hot pursuit of the woman to whom he had just spoken.

Seemingly unconcerned with expense, the authorities in Santa Cruz culminated a year and a half investigation by employing 13 persons and eight cars to arrest three women on a misdemeanor.[37] The police report acknowledged the excellent prenatal care the pregnant female "special operative" had received while paid to represent herself as a client of the Birth Center for several months. Not mentioned was the fact that in the previous three years, the Birth Center had been involved with over 300 births, with a zero percent mortality rate, while during the same time period more than 3 out of every 300 babies delivered by doctors in Santa Cruz County hospitals had died.[38]

When the cases came to court, supporters of the midwives filled the courtrooms, and in one instance the overflow crowd spilled out onto the lawn all the way down to the banks of the nearby San Lorenzo River. Finally, more than three years after the arrests, the district attorney announced that he would drop the charges.

But the Medical Board did not need a conviction to succeed. The goal had been to make life miserable for midwives, and to send fear into the heart of any woman even contemplating such a career.

The midwives were finally free from prosecution, but the court battles had taken a terrible toll on them, both emotionally and financially.

CHARGED WITH MURDER

Meanwhile, the proponents of organized medicine's assault on midwifery knew that sooner or later a baby would die at a midwife-attended home birth. They waited, hoping that when the inevitable occurred they could convict the midwife, settling the midwifery question once and for all.[39] What midwife would attend home births if by so doing she risked being tried for murder if the baby died?

The unlucky midwife who happened to be in the wrong place at the wrong time was Marianne Doshi of San Luis Obispo, California. Marianne had always been a pioneer. In college, she was the first woman to ever run for any kind of office at Cal Poly, where she was student body vice president. In July 1978, however, she could not resuscitate a newly born child. Despite being whisked by ambulance to Mt. Zion Hospital, the child died. On July 6, Marianne Doshi was arrested and charged with murder.[40]

In a situation eerily reminiscent of the witch-hunts, where midwives were accused of killing babies and burying them where they would never be discovered, some local authorities claimed she was "a member of a criminal midwifery ring responsible for an unknown number of backyard burials."[41]

No evidence of anything of the sort was ever found. And as far as the child that died, the grieving parents stood steadfastly by the beleaguered midwife, saying she had done all she could to help them and their baby.[42] Nevertheless, the midwife was in a battle for her life.

The parents of the dead infant, a young, devoutly Christian couple who were well-respected citizens of Los Osos, a tiny coastal community ten miles north of San Luis Obispo, pleaded with the sheriff's department and the Board of Medical Quality Assurance to drop the case. But to no avail. According to the father, Robert M. Gannage: "The investigators had an axe to grind. It was obvious. Their attitude was, 'Ah ha! We've been waiting for a case like this!'"[43]

The trial was intense and hard-fought. Although the midwife had done everything correctly, it was nevertheless true that a baby had been born dead, and the district attorney sought to create the suspicion that the infant might have lived if the birth had taken place in a hospital. In the end, though, Judge Richard C. Kirkpatrick declared Marianne Doshi innocent of all charges. The evidence, he said, was that the baby had died of natural causes.

In a stinging rebuke to the war on midwifery, the judge ripped into the San Luis Obispo doctors who refused to support traditional midwives. "The only reason the D.A. is going on this sort of case," he told the press, "is that he's getting the screws put to him by the medical profession. Doctors don't want to see those midwives out there. They don't want someone stealing all their business."[44] He also said, "The medical profession wants to run the show, period. They don't want the patient or parents having any part of it."[45]

The chief of obstetrics at San Luis Obispo County Hospital was not pleased. He had been a key figure for the prosecution. After the verdict, he announced that although he might possibly be able to tolerate working with a nurse-midwife, his colleagues would certainly not be so generous. They would allow a nurse-midwife in one of their hospitals, he said, only "over their dead bodies."[46]

Although they did not get the desired conviction, the doctors delivered another punishing blow to midwifery. Being jailed and tried for murder can take a lot out of any person, and even brave Marianne Doshi felt the impact. In time, she closed her practice. Asked why, she said, "I always felt like I was sitting on a time bomb. Having been through the murder charge, I was scared. Every month in the *California Association of Midwives Newsletter,* I read about someone else getting arrested, and about defense funds being started to help them. Endless defense funds. Such a drain. I think the California Board of Medical Quality Assurance and the obstetricians were very effective. They drained our energy. They discouraged us. And that was their intention."[47]

IF AT FIRST YOU DON'T SUCCEED . . .

Though failing to get a conviction in the Marianne Doshi case, the advocates of the war on midwifery remained poised, ready to pounce on the next home birth death. Sure enough, one came along in November 1979, when midwife Rosalie Tarpening of Madera, California, delivered an infant that had trouble breathing. A deeply religious woman who believed in the sanctity of birth as a family event, she had built up a large following of grateful women during her years of practice. At the time, poor women were in a bind, because few California obstetricians would accept Medi-Cal patients, and many of them came to her. Her record was outstanding, even though she frequently took high-risk mothers who could not afford hospital care. When Gracellia Villa, an undocumented alien, had come seeking her aid, saying that she could not pay very much but she had no where else to turn, the midwife did not turn her away.

When Rosalie Tarpening was unable to resuscitate Gracellia Villa's newborn, she did the correct thing and sent the baby immediately to Madera Community Hospital. In the emergency room, the infant was pronounced dead after resuscitation efforts failed.

Several days later, an agent of the California Board of Medical Quality Assurance led an armed posse to the midwife's home, where they arrested her on charges of murder.[48] She was jailed, and the bail set at $100,000. The bail was finally reduced to $25,000, but she and her husband were able to post bond only by mortgaging their home.

The pretrial hearings were the longest in Madera County's history. Tarpening's supporters rallied around her, and sought to raise money for her defense. "Do not let the District Attorney, at taxpayers' expense, make Madera the medical witch-hunt capital of the nation," read one of their mailings.[49]

The prosecution brought forth physicians to testify that home births are dangerous, and midwives incompetent. They implied that the infant would have lived had the birth taken place "properly, in a hospital." Things were not looking good for the defense. Finally, Rosalie Tarpening's attorneys presented their lone witness, a white-haired woman named Edith Potter, M.D. Then 79 years old, she was considered one of the seven top pathologists in the world. Her major work, *Pathology of the Fetus and Infant*, had been cited repeatedly by the prosecution. She was not an advocate of home births or even of midwifery, and she made that clear.

But she made something else clear, too. A former professor at the University of Chicago Medical School, Edith Potter said the autopsy that had been performed on the infant would have earned an F if one of her students had done it. It was clearly an attempt to cover something up. After a thorough analysis of the electrocardiograms and other evidence, she stated firmly that the resuscitation efforts of the midwife had been correct and helpful, that the baby had been alive when it reached the hospital, but the resuscitation efforts at the hospital emergency room had been vastly too forceful. The cause of death was not anything Rosalie Tarpening had done or failed to do. It was the clumsy efforts at resuscitation performed by the hospital staff. The infant's liver and diaphragm had been displaced, and his abdomen distended when air was pumped into his lungs at far too great a pressure. "No baby can survive under these conditions," Edith Potter said. As a result of this stunning and indisputable testimony, the entire atmosphere of the trial was reversed, and the murder charge promptly dismissed.[50]

The district attorney was embarrassed, but was not about to give up the fight. In the months that followed he proceeded to once again arrest Rosalie Tarpening, this time putting her on trial for two felony counts of practicing medicine without a license.

Almost two years after the event, he managed to get a conviction on one of the counts, though it was reduced to a misdemeanor. Judge Clifford Plumley, noting that the midwife had never before in her 55 years had any difficulties with the law, gave her a suspended one-year jail term, and forbade her to attend any births for two years.[51]

The midwife now had a criminal record. She was deprived of her livelihood, after having been subjected to more than two years of accusation, fear, and substantial financial loss.

Remarkably, no action was taken against the emergency room staff that had mangled the resuscitation efforts, caused the death of the infant, and then sought to hide the facts behind the death. The California Board of Medical Quality Assurance, relentlessly intent on prosecuting midwives, simply looked the other way. The people who were responsible for the infant's death were not even subjected to a disciplinary inquiry.

THE CALIFORNIA MEDICAL BOARD — ALWAYS AT YOUR SERVICE

What, you may wonder, is the California Board of Medical Quality Assurance? This organization, which changed its name in 1991 to the Medical Board of California, supervises the licensing of physicians in the state, and is charged with policing the profession for the protection of the public. Most of the members of the board are practicing physicians.

Over the years that this agency was devoting itself to the harassment of home-birth midwives, California's doctor-discipline system was becoming the object of national ridicule.[52] Dissatisfied patients could not find the Medical Board's phone number, and those complaints that were registered often lay idle for years. When citizens took pains to track down the board, and then to fill out reports protesting unethical, incompetent, and illegal behavior on the part of physicians, the reports were generally filed away, without investigation. Every so often, the department brought itself up to date—by dumping the files into the trash. Even convicted murderers escaped professional sanctions.

In April 1989, the Center for Public Interest Law in San Diego issued a devastating report, stating that the agency was doing virtually nothing to protect the public from even the most blatantly criminal of physicians.[53] One physician, who admitted to multiple acts of oral copulation on an 11-year-old girl, was left free to practice.[54] The report concluded that the board "provides less of an effective remedy for public protection than does the current rate of death from natural causes for those [physicians] who should be disciplined."[55]

One obstetrician who continued to practice while the agency devoted itself to the great task of persecuting midwives was Milos Klvana, M.D., from Valencia, California, who found himself standing trial in Los Angeles Superior Court in 1989 for the murder of nine babies. The Medical Board had allowed him to continue to practice for ten years after his initial conviction on 26 criminal counts, and for eight years after the first infant death due to his incompetence had been reported to the agency.[56] The agency had performed a stunningly inept inquiry into four of the deaths—according to the *L.A. Times*, the agency had simply "relied upon Klvana's version of events to close the investigation"—allowing Klvana to continue practicing.[57] In the meantime, six babies had died as a result of Klvana's misuse of pitocin, putting deadly pressure on babies' heads as they were forced through the birth canal.[58]

Richard A. Leonard, Klvana's attorney, said his client was "tough" to defend. "There were no facts for the defense. Everywhere we checked we came up dry. I didn't have one doctor to put up on the stand."[59]

On December 18, 1989, a Los Angeles jury found Dr. Klvana guilty on nine counts of second-degree murder, as well as 38 other felony counts including insurance fraud, perjury, and conspiracy. On February 5, 1990, Superior Court Judge Judith Chirlin sentenced the doctor to 53 years to life.[60] Author Jessica Mitford noted, "In a rare display of courtroom unanimity among the frequently warring elements in a criminal trial, defense, prosecutor, judge, and jury all tore into the Board of Medical Quality Assurance for its negligence."[61]

The jury foreman sent a scorching six-page "open letter" to the agency and to California legislators, saying that the agency was criminally negligent. "We find the Medical Board's performance so irresponsible that we wish there were a way for them to share in the verdicts."[62]

Judge Chirlin also had a few things to say about the Medical Board. "The case is a testament to the abject failure" of the agency, she said. "How many more dead babies or dead patients of other incompetent doctors will it take before the Board of Medical Quality Assurance is forced to take a serious look at its procedures?"[63]

You or I might have hoped that the Medical Board's woeful performance in the Klvana situation would have forced the agency to recognize the need to pay more attention to truly incompetent physicians with serious complaints lodged against them, and to spend less of its resources and money harassing midwives with impeccable records. But this was not to be the case.

On April 5, 1990, Sally Wright, a midwife in Roseville, California, was at home with two of her three children. Suddenly, she heard loud banging on the front door, with angry shouts of "Open up! Police!" Before she could get to the door, six armed men burst in. Waving guns and wearing bullet-proof vests, these Board of Medical Quality Assurance "investigators" proceeded to ransack the house.[64]

Sally's three children became hysterical when they were all ordered to remain in the living room, and Sally was told she was under "room arrest" and could not go into her bedroom.

The resemblance to the witch-hunting instructions of the *Malleus* is eerie: "If she be taken in her own house, let her not be given time to go into her room; for they are wont to secure in this way some object or power of witchcraft."[65]

After three hours of searching, the Board of Medical Quality Assurance team departed, carrying with them no less than 38 boxes of Sally Wright's possessions, including her books and magazines, toilet articles, and even a hair-curling iron. These were all, presumably, evidence that she had been practicing medicine without a license.

Five days later, 100 of Sally Wright's friends and supporters staged a rally in her defense at the state capitol. The case dragged on for some time. Eventually, the Medical Board had to admit it had no case, and went off in search of other midwives to prosecute.

It didn't take them long to find one. In 1994, Medical Board personnel kept the 13-year-old daughter of a southern California midwife on the floor at gunpoint while they searched the house for evidence of a midwifery practice.[66]

As I've learned of case after case in which agents of the Medical Board have broken into midwives' homes, guns drawn and pointed, I've had to wonder about their degree of connection to reality. Who do they think they are dealing with? Mafia drug lords? Do they think that these women and their children are armed and dangerous? Personally, I haven't heard of a great many shoot-outs between medical authorities and midwives.

Meanwhile, the Medical Board hasn't been making a great deal of progress in actually performing the task for which it purportedly exists—

following up on serious complaints lodged against physicians. In 1992, a front page story in the *San Francisco Examiner* reported: "A San Diego doctor is charged with raping five patients based in part on complaints, some going back to 1983, filed with the state Board in charge of policing physician conduct, but never acted on."[67] Evidently, the Medical Board considered a physician repeatedly raping his patients less worthy of investigation than a midwife safely helping mothers give birth to their babies in their own homes.

I wouldn't try to tell the relatives of Magdalena Ortega-Rodriguez that the California Medical Board was doing its job properly. On December 8, 1994, the 23-year-old woman paid $1,000 to Suresh Gandotra, M.D., to perform an abortion in his San Ysidro, California, clinic. Gandotra botched the procedure badly, and perforated the woman's uterus. The doctor then waited three hours to summon an ambulance. By the time she reached the hospital, Magdalena Ortega-Rodriguez was dead.[68]

She had no way of knowing that the physician she hired was a convicted felon, accused of nearly killing a 1991 patient who, like her, had sought an abortion. Nor did she know that the Medical Board had taken more than three years to file disciplinary charges against him based on his 1990 conviction for 17 different crimes. When she placed her life in his hands, more than four years had gone by since the conviction, and still a hearing had not been held.[69] The agency responsible for policing the medical profession had been too busy to deal with the situation.

THE TWO KINDS OF MIDWIVES

There are two types of midwives. Most of the midwives who have been prosecuted are traditional (also called "direct-entry") midwives, as opposed to "nurse-midwives" (who are now licensed in all 50 states). Traditional midwives are not schooled as nurses. They learn their skills through apprenticeship and rigorous training, and typically have a profound respect for birth as a natural process.

Nurse-midwives, on the other hand, are products of medical training. They are used to relying heavily on diagnostics, lab work, monitoring, and other technology. They are trained to defer to physician authority.

One midwife who went to nursing school so she could become "credible," was sure that she could survive her nurse's training without absorbing the fear of birth and the need to control it that tends to characterize the medical model. She had attended many beautiful home births, and had a strong sense of birth as beautiful and normal. But she found it impossible not to be affected. "I found myself thinking that something was bound to go wrong, whereas before, I just knew that things generally went right."[70]

Another nurse-midwife explains that the arts of nursing and midwifery are really quite different, and that what she learned in nurse's training is quite irrelevant to attending births. Nurses help sick people get well, and also to some extent help to prevent them from getting sick. Midwives, on the other hand, help healthy women have babies. "Nurse-midwife has the same ring to me as ballerina-carpenter."[71]

Nurse-midwives are often in a position to do a great deal of good. They are versed in prenatal, postpartum, and normal newborn care, and in routine gynecological care. Compared to obstetricians, they are far more able to teach women to trust that their bodies can deliver healthy babies naturally. And, being more "credible" than traditional midwives, they are often allowed to practice where traditional midwives are not.

Yet even nurse-midwives are frequently harassed and impeded by the medical profession. Many rural counties in the United States have no obstetricians practicing in the area, and yet, amazingly, obstetricians have frequently joined together to block nurse-midwives from practicing even in these areas.[72]

Most of today's licensed nurse-midwives work for hospitals, HMOs, and other types of managed health-care plans. Trained in hospitals and accustomed to the technology, many of them rarely leave the hospital environment. If they do, if they dare to attend home births or work in non-hospital birth centers, they are often denied hospital privileges and physician backup for their patients. This, in spite of the fact that the statistics for nurse-midwives in birth centers are superior to those for nurse-midwives working with obstetricians in hospitals.[73]

In fact, nurse-midwives are still today sometimes subjected to the same witch-hunt tactics as are traditional midwives. In 1994, for example, armed police forced their way into the home of certified nurse-midwife Lynn Amin, the licensed owner of Natural Birthing Services, the only out-of-hospital birth center in Riverside, California. They arrested her on charges of practicing medicine without a license, put her in handcuffs, took her to jail, and chained her to a wall with her hands cuffed behind her back for many hours. Lynn had very recently had disc removal surgery in her neck, and had not yet recovered. She spent the night in enormous pain, frightened, and handcuffed. Shivering cold, she asked for a blanket. The jailer replied, "That's how it is."[74]

Eventually, they locked her in a shower room. When she told them she had a valid license, they snickered, "Yeah, that's what everybody says." When she repeatedly told them about the recent surgery on her neck, they sent in a male nurse, to whom she spoke of the excruciating pain she was enduring. His response was not entirely helpful. "I know guys who have discs removed, and they go out to the rodeo the next day."[75]

Lynn Amin was not only terrified and in enormous pain; she was completely bewildered as to why this was happening. She had always done everything by the book, and always worked well within the legal limits imposed on her profession by California law. She and the other midwives at Natural Birthing Services all had impeccable records.

Meanwhile, one of Lynn's associates at the birth center, another registered nurse practitioner by the name of Lorri Walker, was receiving similar treatment. Undercover officers, at California taxpayers' expense, made two visits to Lorri Walker's home pretending to be expectant parents, where they sought to entrap her by persistently asking leading questions.[76] Lorri had a very strange feeling about the couple, because they said a number of things that made no sense, and also because the woman kept having to go to the bathroom over and over again.

Lorri learned later that the reason the woman made so many visits to the bathroom was that she and the male officer were carrying concealed weapons, and every time the woman thought Lorri was going to examine her, she'd go to the bathroom to hide her gun so Lorri would not discover it during the exam; then, each time she thought it might be a few minutes yet before an exam took place, she would go back to retrieve it.

When Lorri Walker, a registered and licensed nurse practitioner, took the "pregnant" woman's blood pressure, she was ordered to put her hands behind her back, handcuffed, arrested, shoved out the door and into the police car, and subsequently charged with a felony offense of practicing medicine without a license.

Neither of these women had done anything harmful or illegal, yet they were now faced with many thousands of dollars in attorneys' fees. According to Lorri Walker, "Every birthing option but hospital birth has been eliminated in Orange County, except for our birth center. Several birth centers have lost their licenses or been closed down. My phone was tapped and my three children were scared to death I was going to jail. I've worked very hard to get through nursing, ob/gyn practitioner, and nurse-midwifery school. I believed that if you played by the rules and got your license, followed your protocols, you didn't risk going to jail. Now I realize that it is not true, particularly for midwives who work outside of institutions. It's so scary. It's like the Middle Ages. It's a witch-hunt."[77]

I'm not a great fan of intentional conspiracy theories. I prefer not to attribute to malice what can be adequately explained by ignorance. But what is happening to midwives in the United States seems to go beyond the random actions of confused people. It appears to be something more than a series of unfortunate mistakes.

THE TIDE BEGINS TO TURN

Some midwives think the motivation behind the effort of many physicians to wipe them out is economic, an instance of trying to destroy the competition. Others think it is sexist, yet another case of males wanting to dominate women. Still others think it is simply a toned-down replay of the witch trials.

But whatever the intent behind the targeting of midwives, it is beginning to create results very different from what the doctors have had in mind. The publicity is serving to bring attention to the fact that the statistics for midwives doing home births and working in birth centers are consistently superior to those obtained by obstetricians doing hospital births.

Nurse-midwives are now legal in all 50 states, although in many states there is still no way for traditional midwives to legally obtain training and certification. When hearings were held in California on the status of health care for mothers and their newborns, with a view toward the licensing of traditional midwives, the state's medical societies were not pleased. The chief deputy director of the California Department of Consumer Affairs recalls: "In four hours of testimony, the only opposition was from the California Medical Association and the local chapter of the American College of Obstetricians and Gynecologists. Both groups took the position that women should not have the option of a midwife-attended birth."[78]

In the matter of supporting women's right to self-determination, the American College of Obstetricians and Gynecologists came up a little short. An editorial in the organization's newsletter fumed, "We must reassert our control over the patient and insist that we exclusively make the decisions."[79]

But despite such opposition, a bill passed and was signed in October 1993, granting California traditional midwives the right to obtain licensing. Although the legislation, as a compromise to the state's medical establishment, required that those who pass the licensing exam work under the supervision of a physician, and placed their licensing in the hands of the very Medical Board that had long been persecuting them, it nevertheless represented a giant step forward for the birthing community.

EXTRAORDINARY COURAGE

The resolve of the medical profession to squash midwifery has only been matched by the determination of the midwives to persevere, to carry on the ancient art of midwifery, and to help women give birth with joy, self-confidence, and love. The tenacity of these women has moved me, at times, to tears.

Kate Bowland, whose Santa Cruz, California, home had been torn apart when she was arrested back in 1974 (while pregnant herself), explained what has given these women the strength to carry on. Midwifery, she says, is "one of the few places we can use all of our aspects as a working woman—our intelligence, our logic, our intuition, our endurance, our love, our caring, our compassion."[80] She added, "I have the privilege of being with women as they labor, open up, and give birth. I am a greeter. I greet new beings at the edge of the ancient ocean and first air. And I see women at their best. I know their strength and endurance. I know what women will do to sustain life."[81]

Ironically, 17 years after her arrest, Kate Bowland won the Charley Parkhurst Award from the Santa Cruz County Women's Commission for the very work that had once made her an outlaw. In 1996, having spent more than two decades attending more than 1,000 home births in Santa Cruz, she had reason to be proud. The county was filled with Bowland babies, some of them now old enough to be mothers themselves. The sign on the office she shared with midwife Roxanne Potter said simply: "Since 1972—Midwives of Santa Cruz."

What kind of women has it taken to persevere in midwifery despite the oppression? These women do not make much money, and so when they are taken to court they typically have few financial resources with which to fight. Author Margaret Atwood once said, "We all have this little fantasy of ourselves that we'd be brave and daring, but when the witch-hunt is on the rampage, it takes extraordinary courage."[82] These women are more than brave, more than self-sacrificing. Some of them, I believe, are truly heroic. They make me proud to be human, and give me hope for our world.

In the late 1960s, there were only a few hundred practicing midwives in the United States. By 1996, the profession was 15,000 strong, and growing rapidly.[83]

RECLAIMING BIRTH—STATE BY STATE

In 1996, each of the 50 states had its own unique set of licensing and practice requirements for midwives. Although the war against midwifery continued in most states, in some—most notably Alaska, Arizona, Tennessee, Florida, New Mexico, Pennsylvania, Washington, Oregon, and much of New England—it was at least beginning to subside.

Pennsylvania stood as one of the more midwife-friendly states, but it did not achieve this status without challenge. In 1989, the parents of a baby delivered by midwife Lucille Sykes were arrested by police, and charged with child abuse by the Mercer County Children and Youth Services. The agency director, Eugene Montone, explained that the charges were brought against the parents in order to force them to speak against the midwife. The charges against the couple would be dropped, he said, as soon as they "were honest and said what happened."[84]

The parents were frightened and outraged. Their baby had been born perfectly healthy, and they were delighted with the midwife's care. Lucille Sykes had successfully delivered over 600 babies during the previous 13 years, and her reputation was outstanding. Montone, however, contended that he had to put a stop to her practice "because we are going to do everything under the sun to protect the children."[85]

In April 1989, Lucille Sykes was arrested. But after 700 of the midwife's supporters attended the hearing, the charges were dismissed. Not wanting to let midwifery off the hook, the State Board of Medicine proceeded to file an injunction against her, but this, too, was dismissed by a judge.

The rulings gave a tremendous boost to the Pennsylvania home-birth movement. Far from being defeated by the ordeal, Lucille Sykes told me in 1995 that she was then delivering 130 babies a year at her clinic, the

Cradle Time Birth Center, near Stoneboro, Pennsylvania. Many of her mothers were Amish women. Lucille's 24-year-old-daughter, Cyndee Sorrell, having attended births since she was nine, had herself delivered more than 150 babies.

And Montone? He came under severe public fire, and was removed from office.

In Florida, family-based maternity is beginning to flourish, and the state now leads the nation in the number of birth centers. Health officials want to see half the state's babies delivered by midwives.[86] To accomplish this task, Florida has begun steps to produce more midwives.

In 1991, the Florida legislature considered a bill that would legalize three-year training schools for traditional midwives. The Florida Medical Association and the Florida Obstetric and Gynecologic Society, as you might imagine by now, were not overly enthusiastic. They wrote a joint letter to Florida senators strongly opposing the bill, and calling the practice of traditional midwifery the "deliberate endangerment of the lives of mothers and infants."[87]

"Oh grow up already!" said one prominent senator who read the letter.

In the state of New York, a midwife named Julia Lange Kessler is fighting back against the persecution. She was arrested in 1994, despite having no bad outcomes with a mother or child in more than 1,000 home births. In 1995, she and her attorneys sued the state for restraint of trade and to protect the right of privacy regarding birth choices. If her class-action suit against New York State proves successful, it could be used as a case law in any other state where a similar challenge might be mounted.[88] Ultimately it could be used to change the law on a federal level, creating protection for women's right to choose, and home birth as a civil right. As of early 1996, this landmark case was still pending.

The state of Oregon is already providing a supportive legal climate for midwifery. Many traditional midwives already get reimbursement from the state health-care plan for birth center births.

Legislators in Florida and New Mexico have recently required insurance companies to reimburse licensed midwives for home births. But the champion of the 50 states is probably Washington, the first to grant true professional autonomy to traditional midwives. In this state, 4 percent of all births now take place at home. While this may not seem like a lot compared to the Netherlands, where 35 percent of births are at home, it is 16 times the national U.S. average, and it is growing.

LIVES ON THE LINE

Throughout the country, the battle continues for freedom of choice in birthing options. In many states, a midwife has to attend a certain number of births with a physician in order to become certified. I can't help but wonder what would happen if things were reversed, and instead doctors were required, in order to become licensed, to attend a certain number of home births under the supervision of midwives.

One physician who would like to see that happen is Patte Coombes, M.D. In 1987, this remarkable 62-year-old woman had been practicing medicine for 23 years in Twain Harte, a small town in the foothills of the California Sierras. An exemplary physician, she never asked about insurance before lending a helping hand. She made innumerable house calls, often getting up in the middle of the night in the dead of winter when she was needed. She spent decades caring for her people, bandaging heads, setting broken bones, tending to flus—and helping women to give birth.[89]

However, in 1988 the executive committee at Sonora Community Hospital called her kind of doctoring "substandard," and "in flagrant violation of good standards of care." Although unable to find a single patient or nurse who would testify against her, the hospital authorities, led by the local obstetricians, met in secret, proclaimed Dr. Coombes "incompetent," and forced her out of practice.[90]

As J. L. English wrote in *Midwifery Today*: "If there had been good cause, if she had been responsible for the deaths of newborns, for unnecessary injury due to inept emergency responses, we could commend the committee for its integrity in identifying an incompetent member and excising her from their ranks."[91]

Yet nothing could be further from the truth.

In her 23 years of practice, Dr. Patte Coombes had not once been sued for malpractice. At a hospital where the cesarean rate ranged month to month from 25 to 33 percent, hers had remained close to 2 percent. She never lost a single baby or mother in the more than 4,000 she attended.

When the hospital attacked Dr. Patte Coombes, the reaction from the community was sudden and overwhelming. The local newspaper, hospital, and doctors' offices were besieged with letters of disbelief, all of them brimming with love and support for this woman who had given so much to so many for so long. The local newspaper, the *Sonora Union Democrat*, ran pictures of hundreds of picketers, mostly couples with their Coombes-delivered children, carrying banners surrounding the hospital. More than 400 people immediately signed a petition addressed to the hospital, demanding that she be reinstated, citing her for exceptional kindness and skill, and describing her as a friend who was always there "any time of the day or night." Day after day, both the *Union Democrat* and the *Modesto Bee* published dozens of eloquent letters from her patients, supporters, and friends.

When newspaper reporters questioned hospital authorities about Dr. Patte Coombes's zero infant mortality rate in more than 4,000 births, a record so outstanding it may not be matched by any practicing physician in the United States today, the response was not totally convincing: "She was just lucky."[92]

What could possibly have caused such a beloved and outstanding physician to be attacked? A local midwife, Gennette Ohlatt, explained, "There was a crackdown on midwives here, and Dr. Coombes was the only doctor who stood up for us. They thought that by getting rid of her, they could get rid of us."[93]

The formal complaints against Dr. Patte Coombes were revealing. One was that she rarely performed episiotomies. "I don't like them, not at all," she said. "How ridiculous to cut a woman all the way through and down to her anus. Doctors try to make women believe that if they don't have one, they will rip to bits. The truth is that most women only tear a little bit, and it heals right up. Many women don't tear at all. There is a technique to it. You massage the perineum, you let the woman open gradually, and you ease the baby out."[94]

Another complaint was that Dr. Coombes did not routinely administer vitamin K injections to newborns. "Some mothers don't want their babies stabbed at birth. I don't insist. If we were in Ethiopia, it would be another matter—babies born to severely malnourished mothers need it. But with a baby born to a healthy mother, there's no reason."[95]

Dr. Coombes was also faulted for not routinely using sonograms. "We don't know enough about them. They should only be used when medically indicated," she replied.

She was called "stubborn" and "rigid," because in her birthing practice she did not routinely employ drugs, fetal heart monitors, IVs, and cesarean sections. "The only reason most of these are done," she said, "is because of impatience. Birth is a celebration; it's not something to be got over with as quickly as possible. It's hard to get that through to many doctors. To them it may just be one more birth, but to the mother, this is an experience she will carry with her for the rest of her life. When we hurry, when we control and manipulate, we make that experience much less than it can be."

Behind all the criticisms was a simple fact. Dr. Patte Coombes had rubbed some of her colleagues the wrong way. She delivered babies at home when the mothers wanted her to do so, billed her patients less than any other doctor, and accepted poor patients on MediCal insurance when the other doctors chose to reject them.

She also dared to speak out when she saw her fellow physicians treating patients with a lack of respect. "I had a case," she recalls, "where I had called in an obstetrician for a second opinion. These two had never met before, but he marches in, throws off her covering, and makes to plunge [his hand into her vagina]. I caught his hand in midair. I said, 'Dr. So-and-So, this is Mrs. So-and-So.'"

In another case, she explains: "I had a young woman at the hospital who was nearing the end of her labor and everything was going lovely. She was rocking back and forth and chanting. There were several other women in the room and they were chanting with her. There was such a sense of peace. Then a knock came at the door. I stepped into the hall, and there was the head obstetrician. He said he had something he must read to my patient. It was a form stating that by refusing to consult with [an obstetrician], she freely and willfully jeopardized her own life and the life of her unborn baby."

The obstetrician marched into the room, interrupted what was going on, read the statement to the laboring mother, and demanded that she sign it. He subsequently ordered Dr. Coombes to obtain signatures on similar forms for every woman planning a home birth, or a vaginal birth after a previous cesarean. She never did.

Dr. Patte Coombes had an attitude about birth that just didn't fit into the system. "When I go to a birth I go as a servant. I'm there to provide love and nurturance and to make her birth as comfortable as possible. There is a sisterly kinship, the mother, myself, the midwives—I love the midwives! We make up hot ginger compresses and shepherd's purse tea, we brush the mother's hair, talk to her baby, and we have a lovely time."

But her love for home births and midwifery was not consistent with the mentality of the other doctors in town. In fact, her attendance at home births and her willingness to provide backup for midwives was presented as damning evidence that she was "anachronistic" and "dangerous." Her low cesarean rate was labeled "a reluctance to employ medical technologies." To this charge, she defended herself, saying she was not shy to use them *when* they were necessary. "The instruments developed through technology," she said, "are a marvelous adjunct to the physician's artistic abilities. However, they should never be used as a substitute for close observation, for the capabilities of the physician's hands, eyes, ears, and nose. . . . The most important factor in an uncomplicated birth isn't the presence of high-tech, isn't the size of the baby or the age of the mother, it's the soul of the mother, and the soul of the mother must be comfortable with the environment."

When the hospital kicked her out, they gave her a form to sign, saying that if she left quietly, the "matter would never be mentioned again," and "it would never be used against her." They were trying to buy her silence, but Dr. Patte Coombes did not sign. "I never said I wasn't going to talk. I want the public to know what has happened here."

She knew what her crime had been. "I plowed in and upset the establishment. There are certain rules; I didn't obey them. I have fought . . . to protect the right of every woman to have a non-interventionist birth experience. . . . I served all patients regardless of financial status."

When the prestigious World Health Organization learned of Dr. Patte Coombes's ordeal, they immediately sent from Copenhagen an impressive letter of unqualified support. "You have been providing the best type of primary health care that can be provided to women during pregnancy and birth. . . . Indeed, the best epidemiological data suggest that your type of care is in general safer than the hospital-based care typically available in the United States."[96]

Dr. Patte Coombes is one of untold numbers of women who have sacrificed greatly in order to help the birth experience be as beautiful and life affirming as possible. They believe that our mothers deserve the best possible birth experiences, and our newcomers deserve the safest and most loving possible welcome into the world.

For this cause, they have put their lives on the line. I honor them for their courage. And I join them in the struggle.

Part Two

5
Awakening From Patriarchal Medicine

This is a time of a monumental shift, from the male dominance of human consciousness back to a balanced relationship between masculine and feminine. The resistance to this is stronger than most people know. The invalidation, the crucifixion, of feminine power is one of the most emotionally violent and subversive forces at work today. The fate of every woman alive today, whether she likes it or not, is that the story of her life shall be played out against this panorama.

—Marianne Williamson

AS A MAN, it is not always easy for me to understand how deeply most women in our culture are challenged by the centuries of oppression to which women have been subjected. I am coming to learn, though, that in these times it is every woman's unique struggle to keep from internalizing this oppression, so that she does not fall prey to seeing herself as less worthy or capable. As I realize what women are up against, I am heartened to see so many women rising up strong, powerful, and loving. It is thrilling to see the women who are reclaiming their innocence and beauty, even in a world that so often sees them as inferior and treats them as objects.

Despite sometimes still being treated as second-rate people, increasing numbers of women are now finding their voices, proclaiming their worth, and rejoicing in their love. Courageous and compassionate, they are healing the hurts that have come their way, and turning their experiences into opportunities for growth. Just 80 years ago, American women couldn't vote. Today, women are not only voting but winning elections, and one day soon, I am sure, a woman will be president.

Most important, women are increasingly realizing that they deserve to be respected and appreciated, and are learning to honor themselves.

Every day, more women are finding their integrity and value, and showing the world how magnificent women can be. They know who they are, and they live in their bodies in order to heal the world. Their joy in discovering their magic moves us all to a higher plane of possibility. In their glory they nurture all humanity.

MEDICAL CHAUVINISM

Though American medicine today is not about to win many awards for honoring women, it has come quite a way in the last century. Only 100 years ago, U.S. physicians treated "female masturbation" and other evidence of "undue female sexual desire" by removing women's clitorises.[1] Female masturbation greatly alarmed doctors, who formally pronounced that the activity led to menstrual dysfunction, uterine disease, lesions of the genitals, tuberculosis, dementia, syphilis, and other calamities. Warning that in women the slightest amorous thoughts "could upset the entire physiology," doctors proclaimed that the reading of romantic novels was "one of the greatest causes of uterine disease in young women."[2]

Women were evidently not supposed to have any kind of autonomous sexuality. They were also not supposed to think very much—and the medical profession was there to see to it that they didn't. At the beginning of the 20th century, women were being told by their doctors that too much reading or intellectual stimulation would result in permanent damage to their reproductive organs. If they sought to develop their minds, doctors cautioned gravely, it would certainly be at the expense of their reproductive health. Women were commonly told that if they persisted in the foolish struggle to express their intellect, they would end up sterile, or if they did manage to give birth, it would be to unhealthy babies.

Nevertheless, some women wanted to enroll in institutions of higher learning. As the movement to allow women access to higher education gained strength, a prominent professor of medicine at Harvard University named Edward Clarke, M.D., responded with a book entitled *Sex in Education*. His volume was widely read, racing through 17 editions, all the while providing medical authority to the belief that women are innately frail and ill equipped for mental work. Higher education was not for women, declared the learned doctor, because it would cause the uterus to atrophy.[3]

He was not an isolated case. At that time, it was a basic tenet of the medical profession in the United States that women's bodies made them unfit for thinking. As if that wasn't enough, American medicine also held that the female body was to blame in those cases where women were unable to recognize that their proper and appropriate role was a subservient one.

Early in the 20th century, it was medically fashionable to remove women's ovaries to "cure" various "disorders of the personality." Countless women had their ovaries removed because they displayed a desire to eat more than was judged seemly, because they experienced a sexual appetite that was viewed as socially incorrect, or because they had the audacity to argue with their doctors and husbands.[4]

Almost anything—backaches, irritability, indigestion, and so forth—could be used to justify a medical assault on the female sexual organs. In 1906, a leading gynecologist estimated that 150,000 women had lost their ovaries to surgery. Doctors boasted of how many they had removed, some notching claims for as many as 2,000 ovaries. Patients were often brought in by their husbands, who complained of their unruly behavior. "The operation was judged successful," say historians, "if the woman was restored to a placid contentment with her domestic functions."[5] One leading advocate of the removal of women's ovaries explained why he was so happy with the procedure. "The moral sense of the patient is elevated," he said, "and she becomes tractable, orderly, industrious and cleanly."[6]

THE GREATLY ESTEEMED DR. MITCHELL

The paternalistic side to American medicine did not develop merely by historical accident. The American Medical Association Code of Ethics, officially adopted at the organization's inception, specifically called upon doctors to embody in their persons the twin traits of "condescenscion" and "authority."[7]

These highly-esteemed qualities of "condescenscion" and "authority" were perhaps most fully embodied in the person of S. Weir Mitchell, M.D., a man who early in the 20th century was considered the leading (and was apparently the highest paid) gynecologist in the United States. When female patients came to him and tried to tell him of their symptoms, he scoffed at the very idea that they could possibly understand their own bodies, and dismissed their attempt to communicate with him as "self-conceit." According to Mitchell's biographer, the doctor did not want information from his patients; he wanted "complete obedience."[8] Typically, he forbade his female patients from reading or from asking any questions. Their role, he explained, was simply and without question to follow his commandments.

His advice was not on the cutting edge of women's liberation. "Live as domestic a life as possible," he told one woman. "Have but two hours intellectual life a day. And never touch a pen, brush, or pencil as long as you live."[9]

This particular patient, Charlotte Perkins Gilman, believed that she was fortunate to have the famous doctor's counsel, and tried dutifully to follow his directives. But the result was not a happy one. "I came perilously close to losing my mind," she wrote later. "The mental agony grew so unbearable that I would sit blankly moving my head from side to side. . . . I would crawl into remote closets and under beds, to hide from the grinding pressure of that distress."[10]

Finally, in what she later described as a "moment of clear vision," Charlotte Gilman understood intuitively why she was sick, and what she must do to become well. Her perception of the situation, however, could hardly have differed more dramatically from that of the illustrious Dr. Mitchell. Feeling that her deepest desire was to be a writer, she did indeed pick up her pen, and babe in tow moved to California, where she regained her health as she began to express herself. In 1915, she wrote a successful utopian novel, *Herland*, about a peaceful and highly creative society in which women held power.[11] For the rest of her life, she spoke out for the rights of women to take responsibility for their own bodies and lives.

To many in the medical profession at the time, however, the sight of a woman acting independently was not only socially unacceptable; it was an indication that she was ill and should be treated. Some doctors actually advised suffocating or beating such women until they became compliant.[12]

Obviously, many things have changed for the better since then, and the mistreatment of women in medicine today is far less extreme than it was in times past. Yet a study of how women were portrayed in gynecology textbooks as recently as the 1970s, when many of today's practicing physicians were being trained, found that paternalism had not exactly disappeared. An analysis of the textbooks found that the volumes "were more concerned with the well-being of a woman's husband than with the woman herself. . . . Women were consistently described as . . . designed to reproduce, nurture, and keep their husbands happy."[13]

PATERNALISM TODAY

While the number of women doctors is steadily increasing, even the branches of medicine that deal exclusively with female issues are still dominated by males. **Some 80 percent of today's gynecologists and obstetricians are men.** And these are for the most part men who think and act in their relationships with women patients the way men typically think and act toward women in this culture. There is nothing about being physicians that makes them immune to the typical prejudices and patterns that characterize men's relationships with women.

As a man, I recognize that many men in our society believe that they are more important than women, that their time is worth more, that their judgment is superior, and that women are in need of and should be grateful for their advice. Male gynecologists are not exempt from such assumptions. Like other men, they have rarely been exposed to respect either for female consciousness, or for the female body. The difference is that they stand in a socially sanctioned position of power and authority over women.

Even those special gynecologists and obstetricians who go out of their way to treat the women in their care with respect must work within a system that views women as inherently prone to malfunction. There have always been a few brave professors who dared to buck the tide, but for the most part, as today's male gynecologists were preparing to spend their lives serving women as their physicians, they were given no classes in the ethics of sexual issues, no sensitivity training, nor any other help in overcoming the chauvinism that is pervasive among men in our society. Very few learned how to recognize and help women who have been victims of physical, emotional, and/or sexual abuse. Instead, there was continual reinforcement for the belief that it is acceptable for men to be dominant and controlling in their relationships with women.

There are, of course, many gynecologists and obstetricians who rebel against this kind of thinking, and do not want to be under its influence. But there are few places in their profession to which they can look for support, where they might learn to encourage women to trust in their bodies and rejoice in their wisdom.

Male gynecologists are men and part of our society. Though some of them would like nothing more than to renounce chauvinistic attitudes, others still today commonly expect women to ignore their dreams in deference to men and the needs of their families.

THE FATE OF THE FEMALE HEALING COMMUNITY

That such a large percentage of our medical profession are males is an historic aberration. For centuries, it was to women that people turned for help when they were ill. Women were the primary repositories of the healing traditions. They were the nurturers and the counselors, the ones who understood how to use native plants, who knew ancient methods of birth control and taught them to other women, who could, if necessary, perform abortions. The arts of healing primarily lay in the female domain, linked to the spirit of motherhood, combining wisdom and caring, tenderness and skill.[14]

It was not that long ago that the arts and practices of healing were neighborly and familial services, intimately interwoven with all of the rest of life. The skills and knowledge of healing were not held exclusively by a particular profession; they were shared freely and belonged to the community as a whole.

The United States and Canada are today the only nations in world history where male obstetricians have almost totally replaced female midwives as birth attendants. But Barbara Ehrenreich and Deirdre English have shown that the destruction of midwifery beginning in the late 19th century caused the loss of much more than female birthing attendants.[15]

Before then, the tradition of female healers existed through informal networks of information-sharing and mutual support. The war against midwifery, and the exclusion of female healers from practice, caused the destruction of these networks. As healing became detached from personal relationships and a sense of community, it became, almost exclusively, a commodity to be sold. It was the destruction of the web of community and healing that had been sustained by women for centuries that enabled the practice of healing to become a profession, its powers concentrated in the hands of the few.

While the grassroots traditions of female lay healers were no doubt prone to superstition, they nevertheless contained bodies of wisdom and practice that had stood the tests of time, that had been discussed and revised for generations. They did not have an in-depth anatomical understanding, modern technology or pharmaceutical wonder drugs to fight disease, but they knew how to harvest and prepare herbs, how to work with and encourage the natural healing forces in the human body, and how to soothe and nurture. Their healing work was part of an ongoing community of involvement. People in need were not dependent upon someone who made more money if they were sick than if they were healthy. Rather, they were ministered to by someone who was part of their community of support, who knew their families, understood their feelings, and came to them when they needed help.

The physicians of the time, on the other hand, were businessmen who were prone to some rather bizarre practices.

Some of the leading medical voices advocated that women wear tight-laced corsets. In being fashionable and looking her best, they explained, a woman kept her spirits up and attained the full flowering of her femininity. They were apparently not dismayed that a fashionable woman's corset exerted 21 pounds of pressure on her internal organs. Nor that the pressure from the corset on the body was compounded by the 37 pounds of clothing that the "well-dressed" woman wore in the winter months. Tight-laced corsets caused difficulty breathing, constipation, indigestion, and profound weakness. In the longer run, bent and fractured ribs, displaced livers, and uterine prolapse were common consequences. Sometimes, uteruses were actually forced, by the continual pressure of the corset, out through the vagina.[16]

The 19th century was not the most enlightened phase in Western medicine's history. Most physicians advised that exposure to fresh air and bathing were dangerous and unhealthy activities.[17] At their behest, houses were unventilated and closed, and hung with heavy draperies to keep out sunlight and air. Women were told to keep their skin covered at all times.

One woman wrote: "Under a popular allopathic [regular] doctor, I was fast sinking under a fever. On a feather bed, windows and door closed on a hot summer day, pulse and breath nearly gone, I lay roasting. Friends stood around, 'looking at me to die.' At this critical moment a woman was called in to see me. She ordered both doors and windows thrown open, and with a pail of cold water and towel, she began to wash me. As the cold water towel went over me, I could feel the fever roll off and in less than five minutes I lay comfortable, pulse and breath regular, but weak, and soon got well."[18]

THE AMA RISES TO PROMINENCE
BY OUTDOING THE POPE ON ABORTION

From its inception, the American medical profession dreamed of obtaining licensing laws that would exclude their competition, and allow only themselves to practice medicine. In seeking to gain economic proprietorship over the health of the American public, doctors banded together in 1847 to form their first national organization. Their choice of name—the American Medical Association—expressed their desire to be seen as the voice of American medicine, and disguised the fact that they were merely forming a trade lobby to look after their own economic interests. The AMA name falsely implied that the organization existed to further the public interest. It was as if the American Bar Association called itself the American Justice Association, and claimed to represent the ideal of justice itself rather than being a partisan advocate for the interests of its lawyer members.

One of the original goals of the AMA, according to the actual language of its charter, was "to eliminate the competition."[19]

How was this to be accomplished? In order to achieve market dominance, the AMA deliberately set about destroying the community of female healers.

Since the female healing network was the primary source for contraception information and abortions, AMA officials reasoned that they could undermine their competitors if they could manage to get abortion made illegal.

In the 1850s, a Boston obstetrician/gynecologist by the name of Horatio Robinson Storer, M.D., launched the AMA crusade to outlaw abortion. In 1857, the AMA House of Delegates appointed a committee to investigate abortion "with a view to its general suppression," and Storer was named committee chairman.[20]

The ensuing antiabortion crusade was the fledgling AMA's first national lobbying effort, and it became the campaign that put the organization on the political map. While the organization's public statements opposing abortion were typically presented in ethical terms regarding the sanctity of life, internal documents revealed that the AMA's actual motive was to rid itself of the female healers once and for all. The AMA's goal was to consolidate its power and launch itself as a political force. To accomplish this objective, it sought to outlaw abortions and the women who performed them.[21]

Before the AMA's campaign, abortions were legal in the United States up until the mother could feel the fetus move or kick, an event that typically takes place in the 16th to 18th week of pregnancy. Up until then, even the Catholic Church was relatively tolerant of early abortion. It was not until 1869 that Pope Pius IX declared the church opposed to abortion at any time.[22]

The AMA, however, beat the pope to the punch. In 1864, the AMA published and promoted a book by Storer designed to persuade the general public that abortion at any stage and for any reason was evil and should be outlawed.[23] Shortly thereafter, the AMA published similar books aimed at lawyers, legal scholars, and lawmakers.[24] As the years went by, the campaign built up steam—and began to achieve its intended results.

Abortion historian James Mohr of the University of Oregon explains: "The pressure of [the AMA] crusade pushed state legislators beyond expressions of cautious concern about abortion and its possible excesses to straightforward opposition to the practice."[25]

As the AMA campaign continued, state after state passed laws making abortion a felony, making abortions illegal at any stage of pregnancy, and turning women who underwent abortions into criminals. Between 1857 and 1900, every state except Kentucky passed laws restricting abortion. Kentucky finally followed suit in 1910.

In 1871, the AMA issued an official policy statement on abortion which referred to those who performed abortions as "executioners" and "paid assassins."[26] This proclamation would remain in place as the organization's statement on the issue for nearly the next 100 years.

During that time, hundreds of thousands of women in the United States died from abortions performed under unsanitary conditions. There is no calculating the number of abortions that continued to be performed, illegally and underground, sometimes with disastrous results. Emergency rooms saw a seemingly endless stream of mutilated women, victims of self-induced and back-street abortions.

And yet for most of that time, the AMA not only stridently opposed abortion, but actively thwarted doctors in the United States from providing contraceptives or even information about fertility and birth control to their patients.[27]

In 1973, the Supreme Court's Roe vs. Wade decision declared that the state laws against abortion that had been prompted by the AMA were unconstitutional. In the next 20 years, as a result of abortion being legalized by Roe vs. Wade, abortion-related maternal deaths in the U.S. dropped more than five-fold.[28] Countless women were spared disabling, long-term health consequences from unsafe abortions.

Many people today want to outlaw abortions in order to prevent them from occurring, but history has repeatedly shown that women get abortions even when they are illegal, and even when they have to risk their lives to do so. Making abortion illegal pushes the practice underground, making what can be one of the safest of all surgical procedures highly dangerous.

For 14 years ending in December of 1989, Romania under dictator Nicolae Ceausescu made abortions not only a criminal offense, but one punishable in some instances by death. No woman under 45 with fewer than five children could obtain a legal abortion under any circumstances. The effort to prohibit abortion was so massive that it involved a special arm of the secret police force, called the "Pregnancy Police," who administered monthly checkups to female workers and monitored pregnant women. Nevertheless, the country exceeded virtually all other European nations on rates of abortion and abortion-related maternal mortality.[29] Some 3,000 women a year came to Bucharest Municipal Hospital after botched abortions, even though doing so subjected them to terrifying legal consequences. There is no telling how many women died without seeking medical aid, but conservative estimates are that more than 1,000 women died each year in Bucharest alone from bungled abortions.[30]

In western Europe, by contrast, legalization of abortion coupled with public education efforts on planned parenthood has not only produced the world's lowest abortion-related maternal mortality rates, but also reduced the number of abortions performed.[31] On the Swedish island of Gotland, abortions were cut by 50 percent in three years by providing improved family planning services. One of the most dramatic examples of this trend is the Netherlands, where abortions are not only legal, but are paid for by the state. This nation, where contraceptives are widely available and comprehensive sex education is an accepted part of the school curriculum, enjoys one of the lowest rates of abortion in the world.

Worldwide, the most abortions occur in those nations where there is limited access to contraceptives. In 1990, the Soviet Union was home to 70 million women of childbearing age, yet did not have a single factory producing modern contraceptives. The result was that the average Soviet woman was terminating between five and seven pregnancies during her reproductive years.[32] Researchers in Soviet health at Georgetown University in Washington, D.C., estimated that there were three abortions for every live birth.[33]

Similarly, when access to contraception for couples in Hungary was poor, the country had one of the highest abortion rates in the world—even though abortions were illegal. But when Hungary undertook a campaign to reduce the abortion rate by distributing condoms, birth control pills, and IUDs, and educating people about their use, the results were stunning. Even when abortion was legalized, there was a substantial decline in the number performed. Henry David, director of the Transnational Family Research Institute, a group that studies trends in abortion and family planning worldwide, says that Hungary went from being "an abortion culture" to one relying on education and modern contraceptives.[34]

The lesson seems to be that the most effective way to reduce the number of abortions is to provide couples with the means to understand their fertility and to prevent unwanted pregnancies.

In the United States today, there are many political and religious factors involved in the abortion controversy, and the AMA is certainly no longer the leading voice opposing legal abortions. In fact, the organization now does what it can to side-step the issue. But the self-serving tactics of the AMA, as it sought over the years to eliminate competition from the female healers, helped to create our current highly polarized and volatile situation. Today, many of those desperately wanting to reduce the number of abortions seek to do so by outlawing the procedure, rather than by supporting birth control, family planning, education, and other means to improve the health and welfare of women and children. The fact that the most effective way to reduce the number of abortions is to reduce the number of unwanted pregnancies seems almost to have gotten lost in the shuffle.

Currently, a remarkably high percentage of all U.S. abortions—about a third of the total—are undergone by teenage girls. The lack of education regarding family planning methods is one of the primary reasons that we now have one of the highest rates of unintended pregnancy among teenagers in the industrial world.[35] And yet in 1994 the AMA issued a policy statement declaring that physicians "should be free to . . . withhold contraceptive advice" from "teenage girls whose sexual behavior exposes [them] to possible conception."[36]

WHAT ABOUT BIRTH CONTROL?

In every land and every time, it has been female healers and midwives who have taught women how to be aware of their cycles and how to tell when they were fertile. But as the AMA campaign to destroy the network of female healers gathered strength in the late 19th and early 20th centuries, these traditional activities were ridiculed as "old wives' tales" and criminalized.

When it was pointed out that the destruction of the community of female healers was leaving poor women with nowhere to turn for contraceptive information, the medical profession did not allow itself to become overly concerned. "The poor have only themselves to blame," announced one prominent physician. "They indulge their appetites too much."[37]

The American medical profession's support for family planning has never been entirely overwhelming. In 1905, Augustus Gardner, M.D., professor at the New York Medical College, called contraception a "detestable practice." He proclaimed that "all methods to prevent pregnancy . . . [cause] moral degradation, physical disability, premature exhaustion, and decrepitude."[38]

Things have changed since then, of course, but until 1937, the AMA opposed doctors giving any kind of contraceptive advice to patients.[39] And it wasn't until 1970 that the organization got around to mentioning birth control in its service guidelines.[40]

Americans are repeatedly told that they receive the finest medical care in the world. Yet, in western Europe today, contraceptive options are much greater than they are in the United States. Accurate information is far easier to come by; diaphragms and cervical caps are more available and of higher quality; research into "morning after" pills, reversible vasectomies, long lasting contraceptive vaccines, and male birth control pills is more advanced and better funded; and a greater variety of oral contraceptive formulations is available. In short, couples have many more options and women are more empowered.

Remarkably, even women in some Third World countries have more options than American women, according to the National Research Council's Committee on Population and the Institute of Medicine's Division of International Health.[41] Carl Djerassi, the Stanford University chemist who helped develop the first birth control pill, adds: "The United States is the only country other than Iran in which the birth-control clock has been set backward."[42]

Today, even as global population growth threatens to overwhelm the natural resource base of the earth, bringing with it disastrous consequences to human health, the AMA has still not become an effective voice for contraceptive research and development.

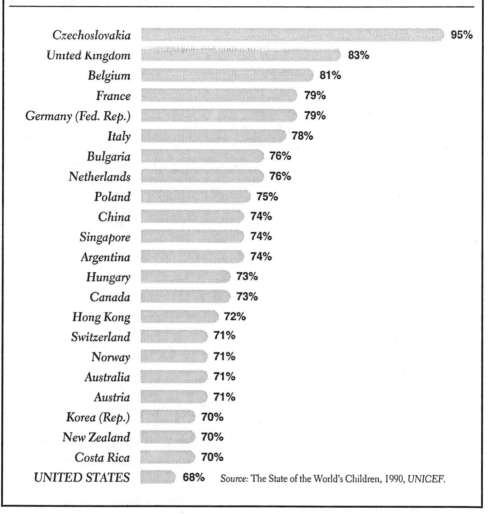

Percentage of the Population Using Contraception: U.S. Ranks Surprisingly Low

Czechoslovakia	95%
United Kingdom	83%
Belgium	81%
France	79%
Germany (Fed. Rep.)	79%
Italy	78%
Bulgaria	76%
Netherlands	76%
Poland	75%
China	74%
Singapore	74%
Argentina	74%
Hungary	73%
Canada	73%
Hong Kong	72%
Switzerland	71%
Norway	71%
Australia	71%
Austria	71%
Korea (Rep.)	70%
New Zealand	70%
Costa Rica	70%
UNITED STATES	68%

Source: The State of the World's Children, 1990, UNICEF.

BIAS? WHAT BIAS?

After the medical profession accomplished its initial task of excluding midwives and the other traditional female and folk healers, there continued to arise the possibility that some women might take it upon themselves to want to become physicians. In response, the gentlemen doctors became extremely solicitous of women's "delicate sensitivities." How, they asked, could a refined lady possibly expect to survive the realities of medical training, the vulgar revelations of anatomy class, the shocking truths about human reproduction?[43] How, in short, could she expect to face life? Didn't she realize that she needed male experts to handle the task for her?

In 1871, the president of the AMA, Alfred Stille, M.D., expressed the organization's opinion of women who sought to practice medicine: "Certain women seek to rival men. . . . In doing so, they may command a sort of admiration such as all monstrous productions inspire, especially when they tend toward a higher type than their own."[44]

In case words like that were not sufficient to deter women from trying to become physicians, the influential editor of the *Buffalo Medical Journal* explained that women, for their own good, simply must be protected from such desires: "If I were to plan with malicious hate the greatest curse I could conceive for women, if I would . . . make them as far as possible loathsome and disgusting to man, I would . . . propose to make doctors of them."[45]

From the male-dominated medical profession's point of view, there were tremendous commercial advantages to regarding the female body as flawed, and women as inferior. Defining women as inherently dysfunctional generated a perpetual supply of patients, and thus a steady source of revenue. At the same time, if menstruation, pregnancy, and menopause were physical and intellectual liabilities, then women were ill equipped to become doctors. The male medical establishment was only too pleased to have women depend on its members for help, while presenting neither competition nor challenge to their privileged status and self-importance.

It was not until 1915 that the AMA begrudgingly accepted its first female physician member. Not until 1989 did the AMA elect its first woman board member. In its 148-year history, the largest organization of physicians in the world has never had a woman president.

Only when World War II created a heightened demand for doctors, along with a decreased supply of available young men (with so many entering the military), did some medical schools begin admitting women. Harvard Medical School refused admittance to women until 1945.

And once women began to be admitted to medical schools, there were still a few remaining obstacles to be surmounted. The first females accepted into Johns Hopkins Medical School were allowed only to examine male patients from the neck up.

In 1970, less than 8 percent of all U.S. physicians were women, a figure lower than that of any other country in the world. Fed up with this injustice, the Women's Equity Action League filed a class-action suit in October 1970 against every medical school in the country. The action proved to be dramatically successful. In the next five years, the number of female medical students tripled. Today, 40 percent of all American medical students are women. Nevertheless, only 18 percent of practicing physicians today are women, and they still make only 63 cents to every dollar made by their male colleagues.[46]

Of the 126 medical school deans in the country today, only 4 are women. Even in pediatrics, where more than half of all residents are women, women are conspicuously absent from leadership positions. Of the 126 academic pediatrics departments, only 6 are chaired by women.[47]

Perhaps the most telling example of the bias against women in modern medicine is the American College of Obstetricians and Gynecologists, whose patients are exclusively women. In its 43-year history, the executive board of this organization has never been less than 75 percent male. Only once has a woman been president.[48]

MR. FIX-IT

It has not been comfortable for me to comprehend the degree of sexism that still remains in modern medicine. Dimly aware that many women are unhappy with how they are treated, the AMA's *American Medical News* sought in 1993 to advise doctors how to create "women-friendly" practices. This learned voice of organized medicine instructed physicians to pay particular attention to "seating, lighting, and wall decorations."[49] Somehow I think they might have missed the point. Most women don't list "ugly interior decorating" as their chief complaint against modern medicine.

The real problem is that most male gynecologists have been taught that female anatomy is inherently problematic, and are conditioned as men to act like experts and play Mr. Fix-It. Under the circumstances, it was probably inevitable that modern medicine would produce a doctor like James C. Burt, M.D., of Dayton, Ohio.

For 22 years, until he relinquished his medical license in 1989, this obstetrician/gynecologist performed an operation of his own design on more than 4,000 women. Although these women did not give their permission or consent, Dr. Burt was of the opinion that he knew better than they what was best for them, and so he took the liberty of performing what he called "love surgery." While women were heavily anestheticized and unconscious just after giving birth, he rearranged their sexual organs in a manner that he believed would improve their sex lives. Many of his patients were left mutilated, in pain, and sexually impaired.[50] Meanwhile, James Burt drove around town in a white Rolls-Royce with the license plate: "C-Section."

I have wanted to dismiss Dr. Burt as a grotesque aberration who somehow managed to slip by and get into medical practice. But he continued his assaults on women for 22 years, during which time other gynecologists knew about his activities and did nothing to stop him. "Doctors would put women in stirrups, take a look and say, 'Ha, ha, looks like Jim Burt got hold of you,'" says Harvey S. Wachsman, M.D., a practicing neurosurgeon and president of the American Board of Professional Liability. "If somebody was doing something to men's genitals, something would have been done about it in an hour. Or if Burt had cut someone's arm on the street, he would be in jail. But because the victims were women (and he was a doctor), he was able to mutilate them and still be free."[51]

Why is it that the many male gynecologists who saw Dr. Burt's thousands of mutilated patients over a period of 22 years did not try to stop him? How is it that the network of physicians protecting each other can become so tightly woven that even such a flagrant ethical violation can go so long unchecked?

Gynecologist John M. Smith, M.D., explains, "Many physicians feel that if a fellow physician, especially one in their own specialty, is threatened with a suit, it could just as well be them the next time, so they refuse to render an honest opinion. . . . Physicians are being pressured by malpractice insurance carriers to refrain from giving expert opinion against another physician who uses the same insurance. . . . The threat to physicians is twofold: one, that their malpractice coverage could be canceled, and two, that premiums will go up for all doctors if everyone doesn't cooperate in this obstruction of patients' rights. . . . Where is the patient in all this? Totally disregarded and kept largely in the dark because of the complete autonomy and authority that physicians in our country have managed to acquire."[52]

AWAKENING FROM PATRIARCHAL MEDICINE

James Burt is certainly an extreme case, but a great number of today's physicians still tend to look at women's bodies as accidents-about-to-happen or as problems-to-fix. That's what they learned in medical school. It is a tragedy that they have been taught to control and intervene, but have not been taught to appreciate the marvelous healing powers of the human body.

In the face of this imbalance, however, there are women today who are doing something spectacular. They are beginning to stand up to this exploitation and affirm the dignity of the human body. Everywhere women are taking charge of their own health, and insisting that their physicians serve them as supportive resources rather than as dominating authorities. They are saying no to unnecessary drugs and surgery, and using safe and natural methods for themselves and their families. They are getting in touch with their inner resources, and learning how to listen to what their bodies are telling them. They are expressing their health needs and celebrating their wholeness. Their lives are messages to us all, male and female, of hope and inspiration.

The medicine that women are calling for, and calling into being, will touch us all with hands of love, not hands of superiority. It will speak to us in a fashion that enhances our self-confidence and honors our inner light. It will not only serve the unfolding of our health, but the blossoming of our truth.

In their work to free and honor their essential selves, women today are doing more than liberating themselves. They are calling forth a new form of medicine, one that is less arrogant and more wise, one that will help us all to understand and trust our natural bodily processes. The medicine of the future will give us the information we need to reclaim and rejoice in our wellness. It will replace body fear with body awareness. It will honor the extraordinariness of every human being, and help every one of us to value our unique personhood and experience of life.

In reclaiming their health and their lives, women are taking back their power, but they are doing far more. They are being midwives to a new kind of healing profession, one that will help all of us, male or female, to experience our bodies as wellsprings of creative intelligence. They are helping our society to awaken from a patriarchal form of medicine, so that we all might become more appreciative of the wisdom of our bodies and more open to our inner joy.

The awakening may seem slow, but that's only because we've been asleep for so long. We may yet all know our bodies as allies on life's journey. We may yet all know our bodies as sources of light and love.

6
Cycles, Fertility, and Personal Power

A vibrant, healthy woman is an unstoppable force for positive change on the planet.
— Carolyn DeMarco, M.D.

THE GREAT CYCLES AND RHYTHMS OF NATURE are among the most fundamental realities of physical life. The ebb and flow of the tides, the waxing and waning of the moon, and the alternation of night and day, are but a few of the eternal patterns by which nature renews itself and life is sustained. As human beings, our in-breath and out-breath, our waking and sleeping, are among the many rhythmic alternations that connect us to the great cycles of the living universe, and are intimate to our being. Understanding and honoring the way our personal cycles interplay with the vast forces of the planet and the wider universe is part of our glory. And yet few normal bodily experiences have been treated quite so disdainfully as one of women's most basic and earthly cycles—menstruation.

"Nothing in our society, with the exception of violence and fear," says Christiane Northrup, M.D., "has been more effective in keeping women in their place than the degradation of the menstrual cycle."[1]

Many women find it hard to imagine that their menstruation could be anything but a source of discomfort. A young woman told me recently, "I learned to be ashamed of my bleeding, to not talk about it, to basically try to ignore it, plug it up, and get on with things. I would harshly judge women who complained and talked about how uncomfortable they were. So what, I thought, we all go through that. Just get on with your life."

As a man, I of course have no experience of menstruation in my own body, but I wonder what would happen if women were supported in finding ways to honor their menstruation, not as a time to function as usual, but as a source of connection to themselves, to their cyclic natures, and to the earth. What if more women came to see their periods as a process of renewal, vital to the maintenance of a healthy uterus and reproductive system?

There is a purpose behind the body regularly shedding the uterine lining and letting the blood flow away. By this means, the uterus is cleansed of any unhealthy microorganisms that might have gained entrance and taken up residence during the preceding cycle. By ridding the uterus of cells that might have become infected, the immunological integrity of the body is protected, the incidence of sexually transmitted diseases is reduced, and the uterus is kept clean in anticipation of a potential pregnancy.

If this cleansing function of menstruation were more fully appreciated, we would certainly see far fewer cases of Toxic Shock Syndrome, a serious and sometimes fatal disease that has afflicted tens of thousands of American women in recent years—almost all of whom used superabsorbent tampons.

In a typical period, a woman releases between two and four ounces of blood.[2] A single superabsorbent tampon is capable of soaking up an ounce or more of fluid, more than most women actually have in their vaginas at a given time.[3] As a result, these tampons tend also to absorb the normal secretions of the healthy vaginal walls, causing vaginal ulcerations, lesions, and lacerations. To make things worse, they are often left in place far longer than regular tampons, thus serving as a medium for the growth of pathogenic bacteria and becoming a source of infection. When left in the vagina for five or six hours, they swell to press against the vaginal walls, which they cause to dry out and to which they then may adhere. Removal can actually cause cells to be torn off the vaginal wall. The combination of injury to the vagina and buildup of bacteria that is characteristic of frequent use of superabsorbent tampons is the primary cause of Toxic Shock Syndrome.[4]

Most women who use these tampons do not develop full-fledged or identifiable cases of Toxic Shock Syndrome, but many of them feel awfully lousy every month. There is increasing evidence that superabsorbent tampons, effective as they are at blocking the blood flow, can cause a variety of immune system disruptions, including increased risk of autoimmune diseases.[5] These problems may be compounded by the chlorine bleaching of tampons, which exposes women to carcinogenic chemicals, including dioxin.

I can't help but feel that Western medicine contributes to the problem when it fails to help women learn to cooperate with the marvelous workings of their bodies. The medical system could, for example, support women in understanding that their bodies are essentially purposeful, that they are symphonies of energy and function orchestrated by a natural wisdom. Then women would more often pass on to their daughters and other women the understanding that menstrual cycles are rhythmic expressions of self-care and hygiene.

A young woman friend of mine recently told me that just before she had her first period, her mother took her to the doctor for a checkup, where she was told to take off her clothes and wait on a sterile table. The doctor, a man she had never before met, came in and examined her, then coldly asked whether she had noticed any discharge in her underwear. Mortified that this strange man was asking her questions about her vagina, she immediately answered no and tried to change the subject. Having no idea whether she was supposed to have a discharge or whether this meant she had some sort of disease, she left the physician's office feeling frightened and ashamed.

How different it would have been, I thought, if her mother, a nurse, or a doctor she knew and trusted had said to her: "At around your age, every young girl begins to have her periods. This is a beautiful process that your body undertakes to keep itself clean and healthy. Have you noticed how the moon goes through cycles, and how there is a full moon about once a month? Your body is as much part of the beautiful earth as the moon is part of the sky, and about once a month you too become full. By having periods, your body renews itself, and keeps your uterus clean and healthy. You'll probably notice that you'll have different feelings and thoughts at different times during your cycle. This is natural, and part of the beauty of becoming a woman."

What would happen if the medical profession provided support for women guiding, educating, and initiating other women into puberty? What if women were helped to initiate their daughters into the beauty and mystery of being women? Could it be that what has become for many women a reservoir of shame might be converted into a source of self-understanding? Might it be that a more life-positive relationship to the menstrual cycle would allow women to more fully grasp the connection between their bodies and their consciousness? What might women find within the ebb and flow of dreams, creativity, and hormones associated with different parts of the cycle? Might they find, instead of pain and confusion, opportunity and possibility?

In the first half of a woman's cycle, the time between bleeding and ovulation, her estrogen levels predominate, building to a peak at ovulation. In the second half of her cycle, from ovulation until bleeding, progesterone predominates, with estrogen still present (unless pregnancy occurs). Before bleeding begins, the levels of both estrogen and progesterone subside.

The timing of the menstrual cycle often corresponds to the phases of the moon, which rule the ocean tides and affect the flow of many bodily fluids, including the cycle of ovulation. More ovulations and conceptions occur around the full moon than at any other time, particularly when women live in natural settings. During the new moon, ovulation and conception rates decrease, and more women start their menstrual bleeding. A study of 2,000 women with irregular menstrual cycles found that more than half of the subjects attained regular menstrual cycles of 29 days length by sleeping with a soft light on near their beds (simulating the full moon) during the three days around ovulation.[6]

"Our creative biological and psychological cycle parallels the phases of the moon," explains Christiane Northrup, M.D., Assistant Clinical Professor of Obstetrics and Gynecology at the University of Vermont College of Medicine, and Past President of the American Holistic Medical Association. "Scientific evidence suggests that biological cycles as well as dreams and emotional rhythms are keyed into the moon and tides as well as the planets. The moon and its tides interact with the electromagnetic fields of our bodies, affecting our internal physiological processes. The moon itself has a period when it is covered with darkness, and then slowly, at the time of the new moon, it becomes visible to us, gradually waxing to fullness. Women, too, go through a period of darkness each month, when the life-force may seem to disappear for a while [the premenstrual and menstrual phase]. This is natural."[7]

Not only do the phases of women's menstrual cycles frequently correspond to the phases of the moon and the tides, they also correspond to different states of mind, different emotional states, and different ways of being. Women relate to the world differently at various times in their cycles.

Dr. Christiane Northrup continues: "From the onset of menstruation until ovulation [the follicular phase], we're ripening an egg and—symbolically, at least—preparing to give birth to someone else, a role that society honors. Many women find that they are at their 'best' from the onset of their menstrual cycle until ovulation. Their energy is outgoing and upbeat. They are filled with enthusiasm and new ideas. At mid-cycle, we are naturally more receptive to others and to new ideas—more 'fertile.' Sexual desire also peaks for many women at mid-cycle, and our bodies secrete hormones into the air that have been associated with sexual attractiveness to others. . . . Our male-dominated society values this very highly, and we internalize it as a 'good' stage of our cycle. One patient, a waitress who works in a diner where many truckers stop to eat, has reported to me that her tips are highest at mid-cycle, around ovulation. . . .

"If we do not become biologically pregnant at ovulation, we move into the second half of the cycle [the luteal phase], ovulation through the onset of menstruation. During this phase, we quite naturally retreat from outward activity to a more reflective mode. We turn more inward, preparing to develop or give birth to something that comes from deep within ourselves. Society is not nearly as keen on this as it is on the follicular phase. Thus we judge our premenstrual energy, emotions, and inward mood as 'bad and unproductive.' Our society generally appreciates only what we can understand rationally, so many women tend to block the flow of unconscious 'lunar' information that comes to them premenstrually or during their menstrual cycle. Lunar information is reflective and intuitive. It comes to us in our dreams, our emotions, and our hungers. It comes under cover of darkness."[8]

Many women today are learning to cooperate with their monthly cycles. If they can, they take time off as they would for any other important event in their lives, cutting back on obligations in order to allow more time to be with the process and receive the special feelings that come to them. They may take baths, quiet walks, rest, read, draw, use hot compresses, spend time in nature, or do whatever else relaxes and nurtures them. Many women continue working, but they might put a flower on their desk, take more breaks, or consciously use the hours they are not working to rest and replenish themselves. They may experience no need to restrict their normal activities. Being more sensitive does not make them less capable. Their sphere of action is not in any way decreased. For them, it is not a question of doing less, but of honoring themselves more.

When women listen to their bodies, many find that they need more sleep just before and during their periods. Studies have found that women's dreams are more frequent and vivid during the premenstrual and menstrual phases of their cycles.[9] Other studies have shown that women are more emotional during this time, and more apt to become angry and to cry.[10] Could it be that this upsurge of emotion is not a sickness to be pushed away in the haste to "be normal" and "get on with business," but an opportunity, a bearer of balance and wisdom if it be heeded?

There is little doubt that premenstrual women tend to be more in touch with their personal pain and the pain of the world. Healthy contact with this pain can generate healing by breaking up patterns of avoidance and psychic numbing, by giving rise to compassion, and by generating the courage to change anything in a woman's life that is out of alignment with her highest good.

In many traditional cultures, premenstrual and menstruating women would often take time to be alone, time to rest, time away from their daily duties. This was not an act of shame or inferiority, not a banishment because they were less than normal, but a way of honoring their cycle and their need to replenish themselves. They did not feel an obligation to be active, peppy, and cheerful every day. They knew that in their fragility they were vulnerable, and with the support of their community they found the gifts and renewal that come with respecting the ebb and flow of the inner tides.

In contrast, many women in our society have such a difficult time before and during their periods that they find it hard to even imagine that the process could be part of their system of inner guidance and healing. They may think, "Why would I want to be alone with myself at *that* time? I feel horrible then. Why would anyone want to hang out with cramps, irritability, bloating, and low energy?"

ANSWERS

The conventional medical response for premenstrual syndrome (PMS) and menstrual cramps is drugs—diuretics for the bloating, painkillers for the headaches, and Valium for the anxiety. In the long run, though, this approach creates more problems than it solves. Fortunately, there are many natural alternatives that do not lead to adverse side effects. A more enlightened medical community would educate women about these options:

- Women who eat a low-fat, whole-foods, vegetarian diet almost invariably have healthier menstrual cycles, with periods that are more regular, lighter, and easier. A study published in the *American Journal of Obstetrics and Gynecology* found that women suffering from PMS who switched to a low-protein, low-fat diet experienced substantially reduced levels of depression, tension, anger, confusion, sadness, and fatigue.[11] In another study, women ate a diet that derived 40 percent of its calories from fat for four menstrual cycles, then switched to a diet that derived 20 percent of its calories from fat for their next four menstrual cycles. On the lower-fat fare, they showed significant decreases in weight gain, bloating, and breast tenderness.[12]

Why is a low-fat vegetarian diet so beneficial? Animal fat and animal protein lead to increased levels of the hormone prostaglandin F2 alpha, the hormone associated with menstrual cramps. They also contribute to a syndrome called "estrogen dominance" in which the ratio of estrogen to progesterone is too high. Women who eat healthy vegetarian diets typically have much lower blood levels of estrogen compared to women who eat meat.[13] They have far less PMS, and much easier periods.

There is another reason, too. By eating lower on the food chain, vegetarian women consume fewer of the artificial hormones fed to modern livestock, and subject their bodies to fewer residues of the toxic pesticides that are sprayed heavily on land growing animal feed. Many of these pesticides mimic estrogen in the body, throwing off the body's hormonal balance.

* Women who eliminate dairy products from their diet often experience great improvement in their menstrual cycles. One study found that women with PMS consumed five times more dairy products than women without PMS.[14] One explanation for this dramatic difference is that the increased calcium from dairy products can upset the balance between calcium and magnesium in the body and interfere with magnesium absorption, leading to cramps and heavy periods. (Craving for chocolate is often a sign of magnesium deficiency.) Another explanation is that dairy proteins cause inflammatory allergenic reactions in many people.

* Avoiding sugar and white flour products, and eating plenty of whole grains, fresh vegetables, and fruits is fundamental to a healthy diet. Refined foods frequently do not carry the essential nutrients needed by the human body for optimum health. They leave the cells still hungry for nutrients, thus promoting overeating and excessive weight gain. The increased body fat in turn produces higher blood levels of estrogen, and more PMS.

- Since the liver requires the B vitamins (especially B6 and B12) to break down and inactivate estrogen, it is important that women obtain these in sufficient quantities. Vitamin B supplements, along with vitamins C and E (which are also required in the metabolism of estrogen) provide tangible benefit to many women. One British study found that women taking 100 IU of vitamin E experienced a 27 to 42 percent reduction in the severity of PMS symptoms, particularly depression and anxiety.[15]

- The body requires linoleic acid to metabolize hormones. Walnuts, pumpkin seeds, flax seed oil, and soy products are good dietary sources of this essential fatty acid. Supplementing a healthy diet with capsules of evening primrose oil, borage oil, or black currant seed oil can be of additional help.

- As well as the dietary approach to optimizing health and reducing menstrual problems, studies have consistently shown that regular aerobic exercise (such as brisk walking) decreases menstrual symptoms, and increases the body's natural endorphins (hormones that function as mood elevators and pain relievers).[16]

- Women who practice stress reduction, such as meditation, yoga, or other methods of deep relaxation, are often able to noticeably reduce premenstrual and menstrual difficulties. A 1989 study at Harvard University found that women who practiced relaxation techniques experienced a 60 percent reduction in PMS symptoms.[17]

- Contrary to the advice espoused by physicians of a century ago, exposure to natural or full spectrum light is also important. In one study, women with PMS were exposed to two hours of bright light a day. Their symptoms improved dramatically, including the reversal of weight gain, depression, food cravings, fatigue, and irritability.[18] Living under conditions of artificial light, without regular exposure to natural light, has been repeatedly shown to disturb the menstrual cycle and cause PMS.

- A very careful placebo-controlled 1993 study published in *Obstetrics and Gynecology* found that women suffering from PMS who received a 30-minute reflexology (a form of pressure-point therapy applied to the feet, ears, and hands) session once a week showed a 46 percent reduction in both physical symptoms (including headaches, backaches, nausea, insomnia, and menstrual cramps) and psychological symptoms (including mood swings, anxiety, depression, irritability, confusion, and difficulty concentrating). Unlike the drugs that are commonly prescribed for PMS, reflexology produces no unwanted side effects.[19]

• When coupled with lifestyle and dietary changes, natural progesterone often yields impressive benefits in cases of PMS.[20] Joel Hargrove, M.D., of Vanderbilt University Medical Center has achieved a 90 percent success rate in treating PMS with oral doses of natural progesterone.[21] John R. Lee, M.D., of Sebastopol, a clinical instructor at the University of California Medical School, Department of Family Medicine, has obtained similar results with smaller doses of natural progesterone skin creams.[22]

Most doctors are not aware of natural progesterone, thinking it to be the same as the synthetic progestins such as Provera. However, unlike the progestins, natural progesterone has no side effects at the usual doses, and is often more effective. Because it is a natural substance (usually derived from soybeans or a type of wild yam), it is not patentable, and is of no interest to the pharmaceutical companies. Many physicians and researchers only have experience with patented drugs, and thus know nothing about this remarkable substance.

The Women's International Pharmacy (1-800-279-5708) provides information about natural progesterone. The pharmacy compounds individualized dosages, and answers questions or concerns women might have. Doctors can call the pharmacy and gain assistance in determining dosages. Women can call for the names of physicians in their area who are knowledgeable about natural progesterone, and understand its usage.

LISTENING WHEN THE BODY SPEAKS

The evidence for the ability of diet, lifestyle, and other natural measures to help heal women's menstrual difficulties is powerful and well documented. But even following the best diet and jogging every single day won't bring complete healing to a woman who is living in a sexually exploitive relationship, is in a job or family that undermines her health, or has been the victim of incest or any other form of sexual trauma and has not yet been able to work through her feelings and come to emotional resolution.

When any of us, male or female, is living with substantial emotional or spiritual wounding, this pain will come eventually to be expressed in our bodies. The difference is that men are often more able to ignore their unresolved issues and deny the messages of their bodies, which may partially account for the fact that men typically die younger. Women, on the other hand, experience their emotional nature most vividly during certain phases of the menstrual cycle.

What dietary and lifestyle changes can do for women who are carrying unresolved emotional or spiritual trauma is make it easier for them to be in touch with themselves, to learn to cherish their bodies, and to move in a healthy direction. Eating thoughtfully and exercising consistently can break up self-defeating patterns, enhance self-esteem, and support a positive attitude toward life. In time, with discipline and tenderness, many women are able to make the changes in their personal lives and careers that are needed in order to heal emotionally, bringing them healthier functioning and a higher quality of life at all times of the month.

We live in a society that still to a certain extent expects women to deny their needs for self-expression and growth. It seems to me that many female conditions are actually a language through which women's bodies are speaking of the wounds they carry from being treated with disrespect. Women's bodies are rebelling against being oppressed, and calling out against being dominated. Their healing requires the freedom to take control of their lives and express themselves as beings of wholeness and self-worth.

The medical profession, insofar as it views women's bodies as pathological and treats women as dependent, thus stands in the way of their healing. Padded stirrups and speculum warmers are worthwhile changes, but do not approach the depth of the real problem. Perhaps it is because orthodox medicine has been so patriarchal and dominating, and so consistently unresponsive to women's deeper needs, that the healing journey for many women today no longer automatically leads to the doctor's office or the hospital. **The longing for true healing is carrying many women away from wherever the female spirit is dishonored, and taking them instead on a path of increasing awareness of their bodies, appreciation for their feelings, and joy in their power to create.**

CONSCIOUSNESS AND THE PILL

There are women today who take birth control pills from puberty to menopause, at which time they start on hormone replacement therapy. Though few women would rely so relentlessly on pharmaceutical intervention, the extent to which women in our society take hormones concerns me. What happens when millions of women's bodies, instead of being in tune with the tides and responsive to their natural inner realities, are instead conforming to a schedule dictated by the products of pharmaceutical companies? What happens when women are more in tune with Monsanto than with the moon? Is it possible that oral contraceptives, while certainly a gift to the lives of many women, may nevertheless have removed the women who rely upon them from some aspect of their intuitive contact with nature and their inner sources of wisdom?

In her outstanding book *Women's Bodies, Women's Wisdom*, Christiane Northrup, M.D., tells of a colleague of hers, an obstetrician/gynecologist named Laurie, who was on the pill for nine years, during which time she considered it the optimum method of birth control and recommended it to all her patients. But a personal crisis around her sexuality forced Laurie to realize she had become separated from her body. "I felt sadness," Laurie says, "that I had taken for granted, drugged away, or labeled as a 'curse' all the wondrous workings of my brain, my hormones, my uterus, and my ovaries. No one ever celebrated my first period. No one had helped me to connect the power of giving birth to my sexuality. I longed to recapture some of that lost magic and mystery." When she decided to go off the pill, she said it was "something of an act of celebration and rebellion. . . . I threw away the last dial-pack and waited. I was pretty sure that after nine years of instruction from Ortho Pharmaceutical, my ovaries would be totally confused, so I was willing to be patient. I was prepared for swelling, irritability, wild emotions, and confusion. I was not prepared for what happened."

Two weeks after taking her last pill, Laurie was talking with a group of women about her feelings. "Suddenly, I was in tears and could hardly speak. I remember thinking, 'Now isn't this strange?'" Then it hit her. For years she had felt sadness about certain aspects of her life, and she had even told others about these feelings. But she had always done so, while she was on the pill, without any emotional or physiological reaction whatsoever. Now, for the first time in nine years, she was actually ovulating, and she suddenly discovered a greatly increased ability to feel and express her deepest emotions.

She soon found, in fact, that all her feelings were now more available to her, including her anger and her sexuality. "This body, that I had abused for so long and in so many ways, was suddenly talking to me again, giving me encouragement and reassurance. All was not lost."[23]

When Laurie found that birth control pills had impeded her access to the depth of her feelings and intuition, she wondered if they had also disrupted her sexual communication with her husband. This could well be. There is significant evidence that birth control pills reduce hormones that are vital to the ways women communicate sexually with men. Certain volatile fatty acids, known as copulins, are secreted in the vagina and stimulate male sexual interest and behavior. Women who take birth control pills, however, do not secrete copulins.[24]

WOMEN ARE NOT JUST TUBES AND WOMBS

To a medical establishment that often sees women primarily as reproductive units, the only test of a birth control method is whether or not women become pregnant. To a pharmaceutical establishment that sees women as customers, the matter is simply a business opportunity. But a perspective more sensitive to women's needs would understand that women's whole lives and spirits are involved in their sexuality and fertility. A medical profession more honoring of women would not overlook or fail to inform them about the dangers of certain drugs or devices, and would be concerned about the potential capacity of birth control pills or any other medication to deprive women of access to their feelings, intuition, and ability to express themselves fully. In conducting research and developing methods of birth control, it would be guided by respect for the lives of the women involved.

The Dalkon Shield, an intrauterine device (IUD) manufactured by the A. H. Robins company of Richmond, Virginia, was for many years hailed by the company as "absolutely safe." It wasn't. The device caused thousands of cases of life-threatening pelvic inflammatory disease, most of which left their victims unable to bear children. More than one-quarter of all users experienced severe cramps and bleeding. Of the estimated 110,000 women who conceived despite having the Dalkon Shield within their bodies, approximately 66,000 miscarried, and tens of thousands suffered septic spontaneous abortions. Hundreds of women gave birth to stillborn children, or children with serious birth defects including blindness, cerebral palsy, and mental retardation.[25]

In subsequent court cases, it became apparent that the manufacturer had systematically misled the public, and had withheld and destroyed crucial information about both the product's reliability and its safety. In trial after trial, however, the company sought to defend itself by shifting the blame to the women, and subjected them, whatever their age or background, to intense questioning about their sexual histories and practices.

One of the corporation's defense lawyers expressed the point of view in a manner that left little doubt where he wanted to find fault: "There is not a damn thing wrong with the Dalkon Shield. Ninety percent of these gals, Christ, you ought to read their histories. . . . It's unreal. The number of men they screw would knock you off your seat."[26]

On February 29, 1984, Judge Miles Lord had heard enough. After listening to some 400 Dalkon Shield cases in his federal courtroom in Minneapolis, Minnesota, he summoned the company president and two key vice presidents. In full public view, he told the executives that he was disgusted by the defense strategy. "Under your direction," he thundered, "your company has in fact continued to allow women, tens of thousands of them, to wear this device—a deadly charge in their wombs, ready to explode at any time. You have taken the bottom line as your guiding beacon and the low road as your route. . . . You inquired into their sexual practices. You exposed these women—and ruined families and reputations and careers—in order to intimidate those who would raise their voices against you."[27]

As the judge spoke, a number of the plaintiffs wept openly.

A. H. Robins ended up filing for bankruptcy in the effort to avoid paying the lawsuits against it. Women who were left infertile got minimal compensation. The average payment was only about $2,000.[28]

The Dalkon Shield has become the symbol of the defective IUD, but the Copper-7, manufactured by the G. D. Searle Company, may not be much better. And G. D. Searle has also been less than gracious to women who have brought suit against it. One gynecologist who was involved in a number of cases against the company explained: "The approach taken by the attorneys representing Searle was not usually focused upon proving that the Copper-7 did not cause pelvic infections, because they couldn't do that. Rather . . . they probed the plaintiff's sexual history. . . . Basically, the effect was to intimidate and assault the character of the woman involved, much as is done in the defense of rapists."[29]

The women's husbands, too, have been mercilessly attacked, in the attempt to suggest that the women's infections were the result of other sexual contacts the men might have had. If defense attorneys could get either partner to admit to any marital troubles, arguments, or separations, they then suggested to the jury that there had been infidelity, and the real problem was a venereal disease brought in from outside the marriage. In one case, the attorneys tried to make a case for this based on one sexual experience the husband had at the age of 17.[30] In another case, where the IUD had caused an infection so severe that it not only left the woman infertile, but required the removal of her uterus, fallopian tubes, and ovaries, the defense attorneys said that this had not really harmed her, but had in fact improved her life, because now she could not get cancer in those organs that had been removed.[31]

Although the Dalkon Shield has been taken off the market, and copper IUDs have been improved, the IUDs being used in the United States today are still associated with an increased risk of tubal pregnancy, with increased menstrual cramping and bleeding, and with increased risk of pelvic infection.

While corporate attorneys have become notorious for their willingness to be callous toward women, the medical industry seems also to be eminently capable of putting profits first. The original birth control pill was approved in 1960 based on the flimsiest of tests. Only 132 women had taken it for more than a year, and 718 women for less than a year. Five of the women had died during the course of the study, and yet the pill was declared safe.[32]

Obstetricians and gynecologists were given lengthy lists of potential complications, from dizziness to epilepsy, but women were given no such information. Why? Was there some problem with the idea of giving women the information about risks that they needed in order to make informed decisions? In 1970, the *Federal Register* explained that organized medicine, speaking through the AMA and other medical associations, opposed warning women about the risks of oral contraceptives with package inserts. In what was probably not the greatest moment for patient empowerment, the AMA declared that telling women of the risks would "confuse the patient," and "interfere with the physician-patient relationship."[33]

Although today's birth control pills are significantly different from the pills that caused the problems in the early studies, an important 1992 review of breast cancer in the *New England Journal of Medicine* found that the long-term use of oral contraceptives "appears to increase the risk of breast cancer by about 50 percent."[34] This is information that women considering their contraceptive options need to have. Yet today, when doctors place their patients on birth control pills, most do so without being aware of, or bothering to mention, the increased risk.

The Food and Drug Administration (FDA) has not exactly helped matters. Faced with lobbying pressure from the pharmaceutical industry, the FDA has repeatedly chosen not to require drug manufacturers to include package inserts that would advise women of the risk.

NATURAL AND NONTOXIC BIRTH CONTROL

There are, of course, other forms of birth control. One that has not received as much attention as it deserves (perhaps because there is little way to make money from selling it), is fertility awareness. By this I do not mean merely the "rhythm method," which is based on a woman's prior cycles, and is only about 70 percent effective. Fertility awareness involves a woman learning to read the natural physiological signs that occur in her body during her menstrual cycle, so she will know when she is ovulating and can avoid unprotected intercourse during the days each month when she could become pregnant. (Fertility awareness is also helpful for couples who do wish to become pregnant.)

There are several aspects to comprehensive fertility awareness: 1) By carefully checking her basal body temperature (the temperature of the body at rest, usually first thing in the morning), a woman can know with certainty when she has ovulated, because basal body temperature rises measurably after ovulation, and remains slightly elevated until menses. The unfertilized egg can only live 24 hours at most, so when a woman knows that a day has passed since she has ovulated, she can be sure that she is infertile from then until five days before her next ovulation (sperm can live a maximum of five days). 2) By observing and charting the cervical mucus, which changes noticeably and predictably during the monthly cycle, a woman can know when her ovulation is approaching, and thus when the fertile phase of her cycle is beginning.

The circular sequence of alterations in mucus are actually a beautiful expression of nature's cycles. Just as the seasons come and go, with winter giving birth to spring, which then reliably becomes summer, which then empties into fall, the mucus in a woman's body naturally flows through a succession of phases. And just as knowing what season it is lies at the heart of knowing when to plant seeds and sow crops in order to grow food and flowers, so too does understanding the menstrual cycle and observing the changes in cervical mucus allow a woman and her partner to take responsibility for whether or not they want to become pregnant.

Although few American women have heard of it, an additional level of fertility awareness can be obtained through the use of small microscopes such as the SR-44 and the PG/53 Fertility Testers. Through these devices, a woman can look at either her saliva or her cervical mucus to pinpoint the fertile phase of her cycle. During nonovulating times, the microscope reveals images that are shapeless. But as estrogen levels rise, ovulation approaches, and a woman becomes fertile, the images crystallize and form patterns that look like the fronds of ferns.

These microscopes are recommended by the World Health Organization, and are happily used today by women in more than 45 countries, including England, France, Mexico, Greece, Sweden, and Germany. They last indefinitely, and can also be a boon to women wanting to become pregnant who have not been able to do so.

A more expensive version is called the Natural Rhythm Fertility Tester. This instrument possesses a greater degree of magnification, an internal light, and better resolution and focus. (For information about obtaining an SR-44 or PG/53 Fertility Tester, the Natural Rhythm Fertility Tester and similar instruments, and for education in their use, see the resource guide at the back of this book.)

How effective is fertility awareness? According to at least one study, actually more effective than diaphragms, condoms, IUDs, spermicidal foams, cervical caps, contraceptive sponges, or the withdrawal methods.[35] The method does require couples to be motivated and conscientious, but when they are, fewer than 1 percent of them will ever become "accidentally" pregnant.

For the relatively brief period each month when a woman using this method is fertile, she and her partner have a number of options. They can abstain from sex, use a barrier method (condom, diaphragm, or cervical cap), or make love without intercourse. Couples relying on fertility awareness as their primary method of birth control share the responsibility for their capacity to reproduce, and in so doing are reminded of the awesome creative power of their sexuality. Most couples who use this method do not feel this to be a nuisance or an inconvenience, but a source of connection to themselves and each other.

If you are going to use this method, you will need more information than I'm able to give in this limited space. A splendid book on the subject is *A Cooperative Method of Birth Control*, by Margaret Nofziger, available from the Book Publishing Company (1-800-695-2241).

There are no side effects to this cooperative venture. Unlike other methods of family planning, neither the man nor the woman has to bear a health burden or take responsibility by themselves. As Nofziger points out: "Learning how to cooperate on this issue tends to draw a couple closer together." Having with my wife used this method successfully for almost all of the 30 years of our marriage, I agree.

(For those for whom fertility awareness might not be practical, and who want to evaluate the other birth control methods to see which would best suit their circumstances, I recommend the book *Women's Bodies, Women's Wisdom* by Christiane Northrup, M.D.)

RECLAIMING FERTILITY

I often find myself wondering what would happen if our medical system sought to help women take charge of their health, to trust themselves and value their own bodies. How would our world be different if organized medicine took seriously the rights of women to make informed choices, and if it helped them to reown their heritage as wise women and healers?

I think we'd be closer to finding out how beautiful, powerful, and strong women really are. We'd see women everywhere speaking their wisdom, reclaiming their worth, and creating healthy environments for themselves and their children.

We'd see young girls being introduced to the menstrual cycle in a way that helped them to understand and appreciate the wonders of their bodies. We'd see women creating rituals and ceremonies of celebration for themselves and their daughters.

We'd see more work like that of Tamara Slayton, founder of the Menstrual Health Foundation. In her workshops with adolescent girls, she helps them to understand and chart their monthly cycle. She provides differently colored wax which the blossoming young women use to mold a model of their reproductive systems, including the uterus, ovaries, and eggs.

One of Tamara Slayton's mentors, Jeannine Parvati Baker, helps prepare girls who are entering their fertility for the change in consciousness that lies ahead. Grandmothers, mothers, and daughters come together in her Family Vision Quests to share and deepen their understandings of what it means to be a woman.

While classes like these could be called "sex education," they are actually something far more profound, for they are teaching girls to understand and appreciate their own bodies, and uniting women across the generations.

Girls who are introduced to their menstrual cycles in a supportive way can more easily develop a sense of their cycles that is healthy, affirming, and natural. With a positive attitude toward their bodies and an understanding of their fertility, they can develop clearer boundaries, more self-esteem, and a greater ability to create meaningful intimate relationships. They become less prone to putting themselves at risk in order to feel loved, less likely to offer their bodies merely to accommodate men. With an enhanced appreciation for themselves, they become more capable of responsible, safe, and loving sexual behavior.

More respectful of their reproductive cycles, they are far less likely to become pregnant inappropriately, or to engage in activities that render them vulnerable to sexually transmitted diseases.

Knowing and cherishing their bodies, they are more able to take charge of their health.

Respecting themselves, they can grow into women of power.

7
When in Doubt, Take It Out

I have a right to decide what happens to my own body, not because I know more than anybody else, but simply because it is my body. And I have a right to acquire the information that can help me make those crucial decisions.
—Audre Lorde

If you are a woman living in the United States today, your chances of dying with your uterus intact are less than 50–50.[1]

More than 750,000 hysterectomies (the removal of the uterus) are performed in this country every year. Hysterectomies are the second most common major operation performed in the United States. (The only major surgery more common is also done only to women—cesarean sections.) About 20 million American women have had their uteruses removed.

The percentage of hysterectomies which are truly necessary is a subject of some debate. Stanley West, M.D., a gynecologist and the chief of reproductive endocrinology at St. Vincent's Hospital, one of New York city's most prestigious medical institutions, says "more than 90 percent are unnecessary."[2] Other authorities are more conservative, saying that somewhere between 50 to 90 percent should not have been done. All authorities agree, however, that 90 percent of the procedures are "elective," that there are alternatives in at least 90 percent of the cases, and that less than 10 percent of the operations are in fact medically imperative.

Why the rush to take out women's uteruses?

The prevailing medical wisdom has been that the uterus is a disposable organ that serves no useful purpose once a woman has had all the children she wants. Since there is a remote chance it might get cancer, they say, take it out.

124

The average age at which women have their uteruses taken from them is 42.[3] More than three-quarters of the hysterectomies performed are on women under the age of 49.[4]

Although perfectly healthy uteruses are removed less frequently in the United States today than they used to be, the practice is still quite common. One contemporary female gynecologist, seeing a physician remove yet another one needlessly, recently joked that it was obviously due to a case of "chronic persistent uterus."[5]

At a large teaching hospital in the Northeast a few years back, the head of the department of gynecology would typically perform two or three hysterectomies a day, every day of the week. Often assisting him was Stanley West, M.D., who reports: "I can assure you that most of the women we operated on had absolutely nothing wrong with them. One day when we were making the rounds, one patient asked [the chief] why she needed the operation. The residents were clustered around the woman's bed, and every head turned toward the chief. How would he answer her? I must say he had a masterful bedside manner. He smiled, took her hand, and shook his head as if addressing a not-too-bright child. 'You have your children now and a wonderful new life ahead of you. You will be much better off without your uterus.' He patted her hand, turned, and marched out of the room. As we followed him down the hall toward the next patient, he shook his head in exasperation. 'You see what you will have to contend with,' he asked us, as if it was unreasonable for his patient to inquire why she would soon be lying on the operating table."[6]

In 1971, when members of the American College of Obstetrics and Gynecology seriously debated whether every woman who is finished with childbearing should have a hysterectomy, gynecologist Ralph W. Wright, M.D., expressed the level of respect for the female womb that prevailed in the assembly by proclaiming: "It's a useless, bleeding, symptom-producing, potential cancer-bearing organ."[7]

Although it is the rare gynecologist who would speak that way today, most still view the uterus as having finished its usefulness when a woman's reproductive years are over. Very few would be likely to understand the viewpoint of Christiane Northrup, M.D.: "The uterus is related to a woman's innermost sense of self and her inner world. It is symbolic of her dreams and the selves to which she would like to give birth . . . [and] reflects her inner emotional reality and her belief in herself at the deepest level."[8]

Recently a female friend of mine told me of explaining to her doctor that although she wished to have no more children, she wanted to keep her uterus, and preferred an alternative way of dealing with the fibroids that were causing heavy menstrual bleeding. "I arrived in this world with these organs," she told him, "and I'd just as soon keep them."

Her physician's response, however, left a little bit to be desired. "I've heard that sort of thing before. Believe me, dear, it just doesn't make sense. The fact is it's a useless organ, now." He paused for effect. "Unless you want to get cancer."

"I'd still rather keep it. I'm sure there must be alternatives."

"If you were my wife, I'd advise you to have it out," he said with finality, obviously thinking that this utterance should take care of everything.

My friend would have none of it, though, and replied: "I'm not your wife. And I'd like you to explain to me the range of my options, so that I can make choices based on my own values and my own priorities. Maybe you make your wife's decisions, but if you don't mind I'd just as soon make the decisions about what happens to me."

Faced with an assertive and self-confident woman demanding that she be treated with respect, the doctor evidently did not have a clue how to respond. "Now there you go being emotional," he said, shaking his head in reprimand. "If you want to take the risk of getting cancer, that's certainly your choice. But you are never going to get very far if you don't trust your doctor."

As you might imagine, it was not very long before my friend was out the door.

A WOMB OF ONE'S OWN

While attitudes like this doctor's are becoming less common, it remains a fact today that in no other country in the world do doctors come close to matching the rate at which U.S. physicians perform hysterectomies.

While some of these surgeries are the result of women actively requesting them, many more occur because women simply look to their doctors for recommendations, and comply with their counsel. Unlike my friend, they believe that if a doctor says something it must be true. Most hysterectomies are performed by male physicians who were trained in a system which reinforced the idea that a doctor has every right to decide for a woman what she needs. The concept of giving her the knowledge and power to make decisions for herself was hardly in the curriculum.

Even when a woman is relatively self-empowered, she may consent to the surgery because she is anxious for relief from painful symptoms, and does not know that there are alternatives.

Why do doctors advocate so many hysterectomies? For one thing, it's a relatively easy operation to perform. For another, doctors are very well compensated for the surgeries by insurance companies, who know that as long as a woman has a uterus there remains a possibility that she might develop problems they would later have to cover. Indeed, some HMOs and insurance companies virtually prohibit doctors from performing more conservative procedures by refusing to pay for them.[9] If a woman has fibroids, for example, some HMOs and insurance carriers will pay for the healthy uterus to be removed (hysterectomy), but not for a procedure that removes the fibroids and repairs the uterus (myomectomy). If she's displeased with this arrangement, and tries to go to another insurance company, it becomes a "preexisting condition," and she's not covered.

It has not been pleasant for me to consider the possibility that a large number of unnecessary major surgeries are being performed on women in the United States for financial reasons. I know that many physicians are fine people, meaning only the best for their patients. But doctors are subject to financial pressures like the rest of us.

In 1994, Dr. Stanley West wrote of attending a seminar on medical economics: "The topic was how to care for women in order to maximize our fee. The experts who led the discussion reminded us that gynecologists make the most money by doing surgery and that the highest fees we can generate come from hysterectomy. With that in mind, we were urged to 'cultivate' our patients carefully. Initially their care would require advice on contraception. Then, in the normal course of events, we would supervise their pregnancies and deliver their babies. Once a patient had completed her family, we were advised to plant the idea that she might someday need a hysterectomy. The culmination of our years of care would be the hysterectomy. With proper planning, our advisors suggested, each year of practice would produce a lucrative 'crop' of women ripe for hysterectomy."[10]

THERE ARE CONSEQUENCES

Some women who have hysterectomies feel fine afterwards. They recover from the surgery, get on with their lives, and are glad to be rid of whatever difficulties prompted them to undergo the operation. But physical and

emotional problems occur frequently enough after the procedure that a
Lancet study named the concurrence of symptoms "the post-hysterectomy
syndrome."[11] Women talk about mood swings, lack of interest in their husbands and children, sexual difficulties, and abdominal pain. Some report
unrelenting depression.

Hysterectomy is a major surgery, and women typically must be hospitalized for several days. They are rarely told that many of the complications that arise can be serious, and may involve damage to their
bladders, bowels, or ureters. Nor are they usually told that postoperative bleeding can lead to fatal hemorrhaging, and one out of every 1,000
patients dies.[12]

Sometimes the ovaries and fallopian tubes are removed along with
the uterus (called a hysterectomy and bilateral salpingo-oopherectomy).
In most other Western countries, the ovaries are removed in 10 to 15 percent of hysterectomies. In the United States, however, women's ovaries are
removed along with their uteruses 42 percent of the time.[13]

What are the consequences to a woman of losing her ovaries? She
can't get ovarian cancer, which is the justification for the procedure. But
ovarian cancer is fairly rare, and is no more likely to occur in a woman
who has had a hysterectomy than in a woman who has not had the surgery.
Meanwhile, if she was premenopausal before the surgery (and most
women undergoing the surgery in the U.S. are) she will be thrust by the
sudden loss of estrogen into an abrupt menopause, with symptoms that are
more sudden, painful, and intense than she would have experienced in a
natural menopause.

One out of every four women in the United States today is thrown
into "surgical menopause" by the removal of her uterus and ovaries, rather
than transitioning gradually through a natural menopause.

The female body is an amazing and marvelous system, in which the
ebb and flow of a symphony of hormones enables life to unfold. Nature in
her genius has allotted approximately ten years for the gradual decline
in hormone production which precedes menopause. During this time,
vast numbers of exquisitely choreographed changes attest to the magnificent complexity of the body's intelligence as a woman makes the transition from one stage of life to another. Menopause does not arrive
overnight, but develops as the result of a long sequence of processes that
each in turn prepares the body for the next. Information is relayed
through a complex network of communication systems that are mar-

velously attuned to one another, maintaining the ever-changing delicate biochemical balance that underlies mental clarity and emotional equilibrium. When a woman's ovaries are removed, however, the entire process is abruptly short-circuited.

Doctors who see the ovaries as useless after menopause point out that in women's older years they grow smaller. But as women naturally age, the part of the ovary that shrinks is known as the theca, the outermost covering where the eggs grow and develop. The innermost part of the ovary, known as the inner stoma, actually becomes active at menopause for the first time in a woman's life.[14] With exquisite timing, one function starts up as the other winds down.

After menopause, the ovaries continue to function, working in concert with the skin, liver, and fat to produce hormones. Celso Ramon Garcia, M.D., director of surgery at the Hospital of the University of Pennsylvania, is one of many authorities saying that the hormones produced by the postmenopausal ovaries promote bone health and skin suppleness, support sexual functioning, protect against heart disease, and contribute to a woman's health and well-being.[15]

Ovaries are the female equivalent of men's testicles, and women whose ovaries are removed are, in effect, castrated. Unless there is a strong family history of ovarian cancer or other significant evidence of cancerous potential, the procedure is difficult to justify. Nevertheless, some hospitals require the removal of the ovaries with all hysterectomies for certain age groups. In 1994, the chief of gynecology at one of New York's major hospitals made it a requirement for all women 35 and older.[16] Other hospitals require patients to sign an authorization permitting the removal of their ovaries in the event of "suspicious findings." The result is that hundreds of thousands of women are having their ovaries removed to "prevent" a condition that only rarely would any of them ever develop.

Despite the efforts of many concerned gynecologists to bring about needed change, the prevailing belief in the medical profession today continues to be that after a woman's childbearing days are over, her uterus and ovaries no longer have any value. I can see why women might not feel respected by this point of view. A friend of mine who loves being a woman and has a healthy esteem for herself told me that this way of thinking, and the corresponding assault on women's uteruses and ovaries, brings to mind beliefs that she and many other women are refusing anymore to swallow — that women's only value lies in their sexual availability and capacity to reproduce, their self-worth merely a product of being someone else's lover, wife, or mother.

THERE ARE ALTERNATIVES

The removal of so many uteruses would be more understandable if there were no alternatives available to deal with the problems for which the operation is performed. But there are. In fact, it is stunning how often dietary approaches in particular can heal the problems without surgery.

Fibroids: Fibroids are the primary reason hysterectomies are performed in the United States. Extremely common, they occur to some degree in more than half of all women. They tend to run in families, and are particularly common in African-American and Jewish women. Although fibroids are benign growths and are never life-threatening, they can under certain circumstances become troublesome and painful. Most, however, cause no problems, and shrink at menopause when the level of estrogen drops. (Taking estrogen, however, stimulates fibroid growth.)

Some doctors say that a hysterectomy is indicated because a woman's fibroids could signify a cancer risk. Yet, a woman with fibroids is at no more risk for cancer than any other woman. Since the mortality rate for the hysterectomy itself is one in a 1,000, the risk of surgery is actually greater than the risk of the fibroid being malignant.[17]

Christiane Northrup, M.D., assistant clinical professor of obstetrics and gynecology at the University of Vermont College of Medicine, performs hysterectomies for fibroids if her patients so choose, but she provides and encourages other alternatives. Speaking from her experience treating fibroids with dietary changes, she writes: "A woman who . . . [adopts] a low-fat, high-fiber, mostly vegetarian diet will often experience decreased bleeding, bloating, and even a decrease in the size of her fibroids."[18] The diet she recommends eliminates dairy products, red meat, chicken, and refined sugar. Supplements include the lipotropic factors methionine, choline, and inositol (1,000 mg each per day), the vitamin B complex, and a multi-vitamin-mineral that contains at least 600 mg of magnesium. The results are impressive: "The vast majority of women who treat fibroids through diet get rid of their pain and heavy bleeding within three to six months."[19]

Surgery is usually only appropriate when women have heavy bleeding or pain that cannot be alleviated in any other way, if they want to become pregnant and the fibroids are a significant hindrance, or if the fibroids are interfering with the function of other organs. Even when surgery is required, however, there is usually a better choice than hysterectomy. Myomectomies, which remove the fibroids while leaving the uterus intact, do not cause the multitude of symptoms and problems associated with "post-hysterectomy syndrome."

Natural progesterone is another treatment alternative. It can shrink fibroids, or at least keep them from growing until menopause, when they will naturally atrophy.

Endometriosis: The second most common problem used to justify hysterectomies is endometriosis. This condition does not always cause problems, and when it does they usually go away naturally at menopause. But for some women the discomfort, which can include incapacitating menstrual cramps, heavy bleeding, nausea, and vomiting, is too great to bear in the meantime. There are drug treatments, but they have side effects, and do not always provide relief. Hysterectomies are often performed on women after the drugs have failed. Unfortunately, the surgery does not always alleviate the pain and difficulties.

The sadness is that doctors have not been taught how much can be accomplished with nutritional approaches. In fact, many women have obtained excellent results with dietary changes. Christiane Northrup, M.D., writes, "Endometriosis symptoms often disappear completely or lessen dramatically when women follow a low-fat, high-fiber diet free of all dairy products (even low-fat dairy products)."[20]

When dietary approaches are combined with attention to the role of the mind and consciousness, the results can be spectacular. A patient named Doris came to see Dr. Northrup, experiencing severe menstrual cramps, bloating, and extremely heavy bleeding due to fibroids and endometriosis. A previous doctor had strongly recommended hysterectomy. With her new doctor's support, Doris eliminated dairy products from her diet, and also undertook a healing regimen that included applying castor oil packs to her abdomen, and taking vitamin supplements. Doris had been through several miscarriages and abortions, and she now began writing letters to the unborn beings who had been in her body. She began to feel that in some way these beings "were still there in some form in my mind and had taken form as fibroids and maybe endometriosis in my body.

The most incredible experience occurred after I wrote the letters. I had been remembering my dreams with great regularity through visualization techniques. One night in a dream, I was fully aware of my body, and I dreamed that thousands of white doves were flying out of my uterus. An unbelievable feeling of lightness came over me, and I awoke crying with joy."[21]

Three months after Doris's dream experience, a physical examination revealed that many of her fibroids were gone, as was her uterine tenderness. Examinations have continued to indicate that her endometriosis is inactive.[22]

Pelvic Pain: Sometimes women experience chronic pelvic pain, but no diagnosable pathology such as fibroids or endometriosis can be found. Hysterectomies are often done under these circumstances, but they fail to relieve the pain 30 percent of the time. It is a shame that more women with pelvic pain don't try a combination of diet, exercise, and emotional exploration, for such an approach has none of the side effects of surgery, and often takes care of the problem.

Menstruation: There are unfortunately still doctors who consider menstruation to be something of a disease, and treat it by removing the uterus. As many of the gynecologists practicing today were preparing for a career in medicine, they were instructed by a textbook that was widely used in the late 1970s, *Novak's Textbook of Gynecology*. This leading text instructed them: "Menstruation is a nuisance to most women, and if this can be abolished without impairing ovarian function, it would probably be a blessing to not only the woman but to her husband. . . . Thus one can make a rather convincing case for the value of elective hysterectomy."[23]

I think I could make a better case for the value of a little consciousness-raising in the medical profession.

Cancer: Removal of the reproductive organs is clearly justified and has saved many lives when cancers have developed in these organs. Yet, precancerous changes in the uterus or cervix are often used to justify hysterectomies. This is unfortunate, because the vast majority of these changes can be arrested and reversed without major surgery, and without them becoming cancerous.

HONORING THE BODY, HONORING THE SELF

One patient who had developed cancer and needed to have a hysterectomy wanted to "let go" of her uterus in as conscious a way as possible. She chose to be awake for the procedure, so she was given a spinal anesthetic. Asking the staff to hold up a mirror so she could see her uterus, she began a spontaneous ceremony. She thanked it for providing her with three healthy children, blessed it, and then said good-bye.[24]

Her surgeon bore witness with respect to this woman's ritual. And when she was done, and she gave him permission, he removed her uterus so that she could have a healthier life.

If you are one of the more than 20 million women in the United States who have undergone hysterectomies, you may feel distress at realizing that the surgery may well have been unnecessary. Though nothing can bring back a uterus that has been removed, it can be healing, even years after such a surgery, to take a quiet moment, place your hands on your belly, thank your uterus for all it gave you, and say good-bye.

It is an act of self-honoring to appreciate yourself for the struggles and losses you've known, as well as for the accomplishments and joys. It is no crime to have learned something new, even when the learning leads you to question your past choices and actions. It is an act of love to forgive yourself for doing things that, knowing what you know now, you might do differently if you could do them over.

THE DEBATE OVER SEXUAL RESPONSE

Does a woman's experience of her sexuality change due to a hysterectomy? Many gynecologists have been taught to believe that the ovaries and uterus have absolutely nothing to do with female sexual desire or response. In the publication *Understanding Hysterectomy*, the American College of Obstetricians and Gynecologists recently stated: "Neither the production of hormones nor a woman's ability to have satisfying sexual relations is affected."[25]

In his book *A Woman Talks With Her Doctor: A Comprehensive Guide to Women's Health Care*, Charles E. Flowers, Jr., M.D., tries to help women understand the point: "Many women resist hysterectomy because they associate the loss of their uterus with the loss of their femininity. . . . The uterus has one single purpose: to carry and nourish the growing fetus.

The uterus has no relationship whatsoever to a woman's sexuality or her ability to make love."[26]

In *All About Hysterectomy*, Harry C. Huneycutt, M.D., takes the matter a step further, and casts a suspicious eye upon the women who oppose the medical dogma: "Women who claim their interest in sex has vanished after hysterectomy are subsequently proven by psychologists to have disliked their husbands for years."[27]

This statement seems to be a fairly masterful example of how to invalidate a woman's experience, but in that endeavor W. Gifford-Jones, M.D., is apparently no slouch himself. I must say that it strikes me as a bit odd for a male physician to write a book with the title of *On Being a Woman*, but this doctor has done exactly that.[28] He announces: "One of the most frequent old wives' tales concerns the operation causing some change in sexual function. The enjoyment of the sexual act is in no way dependent on whether the uterus or ovaries are present. . . . But of course the woman who has never really enjoyed sex, or who has fallen out of love with her husband, finds her hysterectomy represents an excellent excuse for pushing her husband away. . . . It is this type of woman who helps give the operation an unjustly bad name."[29]

Meanwhile, women who wander into gynecologists' offices may be handed an expensively produced brochure with the bright heading— "Don't be hysterical over hysterectomy." Having begun on such a bouncy note, the booklet maintains an upbeat tone, reassuring women that the "old wives' tale that hysterectomy makes you less of a woman is totally groundless. . . . Another old wives' tale, the most destructive of all, is that the woman is psychologically, in some unknown way, less of a sexual being. Yet the reproductive system is quite separate from her sexual apparatus. . . . Why do some women, even if they don't give voice to it, feel their sexual performance will be limited after hysterectomy? Obviously, only psychiatry can do justice to such a question!"[30]

Despite this formidable display of certainty on the issue from the profession, there have only been 14 studies published in the medical literature since 1944 on the sexual impact of hysterectomy. While the gynecological establishment ardently proclaims that the surgery does not alter a woman's sexual experience, all but one of these studies found evidence of diminished desire or lessened (or lack of) orgasm.[31]

The male medical establishment's appreciation of women as valid sexual beings, capable of pleasure in their own right, is not always apparent.

One gynecologist, when asked about the possible loss of sex drive after a hysterectomy, took male insensitivity to a new level: "You can't compare it with a man losing his testicles. After all a man has to be erect, he has to do something. All a woman has to do is lie there."[32]

"Sex may feel different after the operation," said another gynecologist, perhaps vying with him for chauvinist of the year, "but most happy, well-adjusted women don't even notice this."[33]

Don't even notice?

Eleanor Katzman, marriage counselor and sex therapist, reports that 98 percent of the patients in her clinic are women who have lost sexual desire following hysterectomy. "What women don't know about hysterectomy can hurt them irrevocably for the rest of their lives," she says.[34]

Niles Newton, M.D., professor of psychiatry at Northwestern Medical School, found reduced sexual drive in 60 percent of women who had their uterus and ovaries removed. Some 40 percent never resumed sexual intercourse.[35]

Naomi Miller Stokes interviewed 500 women from all walks of life and from all over the United States regarding their experiences in the aftermath of hysterectomy. "Of these 500 women, 51 did not know whether they still had their ovaries; 12 considered sex better after surgery; 477 did not care as much for sex after the surgery; 399 lost sexual appetite entirely. . . . Of the 477 who suffered from some degree of libido loss, all felt that had they been told beforehand that sexual dysfunction could occur, they and their mates would have been far more able to deal with it."[36]

There are some doctors who advise patients of the risk beforehand. Yet the American College of Obstetricians and Gynecologists to this day remains entrenched in denial.[37]

Women can be beautiful, glorious beings, whether or not they are sexual. Their love can work miracles, however it is expressed. But what kind of a medical establishment continues to deny that hysterectomies can decrease women's ability to enjoy sexual activity, when so many women who have undergone the procedure say that this is exactly what it has done?

I know who I believe.

8
Menopause
Naturally

The secret is to hear the music of the body. The body becomes, not a doomed machine, but a glorious composition.

—Larry Dossey, M.D.

FOR TENS OF THOUSANDS OF YEARS, all women who have lived long enough to reach menopause have passed naturally through this transition. They have known that their bodies will now produce no more children. They have sometimes been honored by their communities not only for all they have given, but also for all they have yet to give.

In some traditional societies, menopause is celebrated as a positive event in a woman's life. Her status, power, and freedom within the community increase. She is honored as an elder, and recognized as having attained a new level of leadership.

Marcha Flint, a professor of anthropology at Montclair State University, says that in India, menopausal women have few hot flashes or other symptoms, and the change is seen as something to be desired.[1] In some Muslim cultures, a woman is thought holier after menopause. In Indonesia, menopause is understood as the entrance into midlife, and is marked by ceremonies of celebration. Celtic cultures saw the girl as a flower, the mother as a fruit, the elder woman as a seed.[2] The elder woman was seen as the bearer of concentrated wisdom, a reservoir of experience, the product of many seasons of growth. She was revered.

In native cultures, according to Tamara Slayton, menopausal women "provided a voice of responsibility toward all children, both human and nonhuman, to the Earth and to the Laws of Good Relationship. These older women contained great power and scrutinized all tribal decisions. . . .

136

They also initiated and educated the younger women into this knowledge and responsibility."[3]

Among many other peoples, the elder woman is treasured as a source of wisdom. But in America today, where a woman who reaches the age of 50 is likely to live another 35 years, it's often a different story.

A 19 year-old friend of mine told me this morning that her mother has never mentioned a word about menopause to her. Unfortunately, her experience is all too typical. Most young women in the United States have a vague idea that they will someday cease being fertile, but as to how the process typically proceeds, what they can expect to experience, and when this might occur, they have little idea.

Is menopause a disease? You'd think so, based on the language found in many medical textbooks describing the passage: "deterioration," "estrogen starvation," "living decay."[4] The picture that is painted is not promising. Menopause marks the end of youth and beauty, and the beginning of uselessness and waste. Menopausal women have no future except irreversible physical and mental decline. Aging is a harrowing ordeal, not a hallowed opportunity.

David R. Reuben, M.D., gave voice to the bias against older women in his best-selling book, *Everything You Always Wanted to Know About Sex but Were Afraid to Ask*: "Having outlived their ovaries, they may have outlived their usefulness as human beings. The remaining years may just be marking time until they follow their glands into oblivion."[5] He said that menopausal women present "a tragic picture."

The possibility that the transition might be normal, healthy, and liberating seems hardly to have occurred to the American medical profession. Instead, the belief prevails that Mother Nature made a mistake in designing women, that she arranged it so that a woman's life after her fertile years has no purpose except to wither away and then finally die, that without medical intervention her remaining years will be a pathetic remnant of a life.

Welcome to the medicalization of menopause.

ESTROGEN

The medical profession's infatuation with estrogen began in 1938, when the world's first synthetic estrogen—diethylstilbestrol (DES)—was discovered by Dr. Charles Dodds. Dodds took out no patent on the drug.

He believed in it so strongly that he preferred to give it as a gift to the world.[6]

The motives of the pharmaceutical companies, however, were a shade more worldly. With visions of millions of postmenopausal women creating a billion-dollar estrogen replacement market, they pounced upon the gift, took out their own patents, and hurriedly began plans to market the drug.[7]

The AMA played right along, speaking of the "extraordinary clinical possibilities" offered by this "sensational drug" which could "mitigate suffering for millions of women over 40."[8] The *New York Times* said DES was capable of "pushing back the calendar an equivalent of 25 years."[9]

But why limit ourselves to older women as a market, thought the drug companies. Why not include pregnant women, too? Soon, they were advertising DES in leading medical journals, claiming the drug could do wonders for pregnant women. An ad in the *American Journal of Obstetrics and Gynecology* trumpeted: "Really? Yes . . . DES to prevent miscarriage, and premature labor. Recommended in ALL pregnancies."[10] The popular press dutifully forwarded the good news about the wonders of the new drug to the American public. A 1960 article in *Good Housekeeping* entitled "Why You Won't Lose Your Baby" heralded DES for pregnant women to prevent miscarriages. "Many obstetricians are convinced," the article said, that "hormonal treatments" are the answer.[11]

Answer, indeed. We now know that between 60 and 90 percent of daughters born to women who took DES during their pregnancies have abnormalities in their vagina or cervix. DES daughters, as they are called, stand at substantially higher risk than other women for miscarriage, stillbirth, ectopic pregnancies, and other poor pregnancy outcomes. About one in every thousand DES daughters develops a serious and otherwise unknown form of vaginal or cervical cancer.[12]

The miracle drug turned out to be something else. DES sons have highly increased rates of sterility and testicular abnormalities. DES mothers themselves have a 40 percent greater chance than nonexposed women of developing breast cancer. Approximately 60,000 American women will die of breast cancer due to taking DES.[13]

"Oops," said the drug companies, promising to do better next time.

In the 1960s, Wyeth-Ayerst, a company that made Estrogen Replacement Therapy (ERT) for menopausal women, financed the work of a Brooklyn gynecologist named Robert Wilson, M.D., who concluded that menopausal women needed ERT to prevent "being condemned to witness the death of their own womanhood."[14] In 1966, Wilson published the best-selling book *Feminine Forever,* in which he heralded ERT as the savior that would rescue women from the horrors of old age.[15]

A culture in which the first wrinkle or gray hair could be seen as a calamity was susceptible to Wilson's ideas. He wrote about "the staggering catastrophe" of menopause, which he said made women "no longer women."

The idea that estrogen might be some kind of fountain of eternal feminine youth caught on. By 1975, six million women (amounting to one-third of those over age 50) were taking the estrogen replacement drug Premarin, manufactured by Wyeth-Ayerst. It was one of the five best-selling prescription drugs in the United States.[16]

Then the bubble burst. In the late 1970s, women who took ERT were found to have increased their risk of uterine cancer more than tenfold.[17]

All the more reason to have a hysterectomy, said many doctors, and hundreds of thousands of women had their uteruses removed so that they could take ERT. Few of them were told that taking estrogen also increased their likelihood of breast cancer.

Of course some women were simply stubborn, and refused to give up their reproductive organs so they could take a drug for the rest of their lives, particularly when there was nothing wrong with them in the first place. The drug companies, never ones to give up when there was money to be made, found another way around the uterine cancer problem—by adding synthetic progesterone, known as progestins, to the estrogen, the incidence of uterine cancer was reduced. Accordingly, it has become general practice to add progestins to estrogen for women with a uterus.

There are a few problems with adding progestins, however. Women often don't care for the side effects, which in some cases include depression and continued monthly bleeding. One woman who was not entirely delighted with the experience reported, "Whenever I take Provera [the most common form of progestin], I have migraines, bloating, and breast tenderness."[18] Another woman called the experience "PMS Forever."

BRAINWASHING A GENERATION

Today, women are steadily confronted with a stream of advertisements touting the virtues of taking hormones. The strategy of the ads is to make women feel less confident in themselves, for the more alienated from herself a woman becomes, the more susceptible she is to the lure of the drugs. The ads insinuate, if not downright proclaim, that aging is to be feared; that it is impossible to remain strong, attractive, or lucid without the benefit of medical manipulation; and that the only way to avoid deteriorating with age is to take estrogen.

This is the mass marketing of self-estrangement.

If a woman today goes to her doctor seeking counsel on the subject of estrogen replacement, she has a right to expect impartial concern for her well-being. Some women benefit from the judicious use of estrogen, but today's physicians, having been taught to see menopause as a disease in need of treatment, frequently exaggerate the benefits of taking hormones and downplay the risks. They are continually deluged with materials and inducements from the pharmaceutical companies telling them that drugs are the answer. The studies they read on estrogen are usually directly funded or supported in other ways by the manufacturers. Their magazines and journals are full of ads for the hormones. On the cover of a recent magazine called *Menopause Medicine*, for example, a forlorn woman looks helplessly at dead trees and parched dry earth. The caption reads: "The Fate of the Untreated Menopause." The message is clear: Unless menopause is "medically managed," women will end up dry, brittle, parched, and devoid of life.[19]

It's hard to avoid the impression that the makers of the drugs seek to present an image of "the change" as a disease, with their products as the cure. In 1992, Wyeth-Ayerst spent more than $9 million advertising Premarin in women's magazines alone, while Ciba-Geigy spent $5 million on ads for its Estraderm patch.[20] Today, even more money is spent on ads in national magazines and medical journals, and a continuous stream of dollars is poured into sponsoring medical conferences. Since 1988, Ciba-Geigy has sponsored "educational" seminars around the country, led by local doctors and nurses. Some of these seminars have drawn 1,000 women eager for information. Of course, they leave with brochures touting ERT, generously donated by Ciba-Geigy.[21]

Ciba-Geigy also sends out direct mail solicitations promoting its estrogen patch. Cynthia Pearson, program director of the National Women's Health Network, told a congressional hearing what her organization thought of the practice. "We are outraged that a potentially risky drug is being promoted with the same techniques used by Publisher's Clearinghouse Sweepstakes."[22]

But the marketing has worked. In 1992, Premarin was the most widely prescribed drug in the United States. In 1995, *Time* reported that "doctors are handing out estrogen prescriptions with almost gleeful enthusiasm."[23]

In some areas of the country it is now considered the "standard of practice" to put all women on estrogen replacement at menopause. Increasingly, doctors warn women about the dangers of *not* using the drugs, implying that without medical intervention they will surely succumb to osteoporosis or heart disease. Many physicians today believe that all menopausal women should take estrogen for the rest of their lives.

A prominent gynecologist was asked in 1996 whether even women whose menopauses present no troubling symptoms should be put on estrogen. He answered: "Women who don't seem to have symptoms are at hidden risk. Those who have more severe symptoms are in a way fortunate, because they are forced to see their doctor, and get placed on estrogen. To get the full benefit, you've got to start ERT before menopausal symptoms become apparent, and stay with it indefinitely."[24]

If I understand this physician correctly, he's saying that regardless of whether there seems to be anything troubling a menopausal woman, she should immediately begin taking hormones, and continue to do so for the rest of her life.

"An entire generation of women is being brainwashed," says Christiane Northrup, M.D. "Most women's trust in their menopausal wisdom and their own bodies is almost nonexistent. . . . Yet if we lived according to our faith in our inner guidance and our bodily wisdom, menopause would be, for the majority of women, what it was meant to be—a safe transition into our wisdom years."[25]

TIME MAGAZINE ENTERS THE FRAY

A 1993 Gallup survey found that 84 percent of American physicians' discussions with their patients about menopausal symptoms centered on ERT. Fewer than 2 percent discussed natural approaches, such as diet, exercise, stress reduction, or smoking cessation[26]—approaches that can go a long way toward directing the body's hormone production in a balanced and healthy direction. Unfortunately, many physicians habitually prescribe hormones without even considering alternatives. They rarely (if ever) help women to understand and appreciate menopause as a natural journey, bringing gifts and opportunities as well as challenges.

In June 1995, *Time* featured a cover story titled "Estrogen—Every Woman's Dilemma."[27] While acknowledging many of the drawbacks to taking estrogen, including greatly heightened risk of both fatal ovarian and breast cancer, the article upheld a stereotyped, commercialized, and youth-fixated idealization of femininity. The magazine's cover contrasted two different hands. One had smooth skin and long polished nails. The other hand had wrinkled skin and short unpolished nails.

The "dilemma" was presented as the choice between: 1) Remaining young, though with monthly bleeding past age 60, a greatly increased risk of cancer, and a lifetime of drug taking, or 2) Withering on the vine before succumbing to heart disease or osteoporosis.

Some choice.

Explaining the many problems that menopausal women can encounter, and presenting estrogen as an answer, the *Time* article quoted women who "described their tribulations," barely mentioning in passing that they did so at a "discussion sponsored by Ciba-Geigy." The cover story was strangely silent about the fact that women who live healthier lifestyles and eat healthier diets have far fewer of these difficulties. The closest thing was a reference to "some lucky women," and the brief statement that "not every woman will feel the symptoms so intensely."

Similarly, virtually no mention was made of alternative approaches to resolving menopausal symptoms. **If indeed there were no viable alternatives, as the *Time* article certainly implied by omission, then estrogen replacement drugs would make more sense for menopausal women who encounter substantial difficulties. If there were no other options, our medical system might be pardoned for its fixation on drugs.**

But there are. And while estrogen can bring needed relief to some women, in most cases similar levels of relief can be obtained through natural means that do not carry the dangers and drawbacks of ERT.

THE ALTERNATIVES

Hot Flashes: In many women, the rapid decrease in estrogen levels that begins in their middle forties triggers sudden episodes of heat and sweating. At night, a woman may soak her sheets and bedclothes with perspiration. Night sweats that wake women up repeatedly can lead to insomnia.

Hot flashes are not usually visible to others, though the surface temperature of the skin in the area of the body involved increases measurably.

The experience can be intense, but hot flashes are harmless, and eventually cease.

Estrogen is usually effective in reducing or eliminating hot flashes. However, the hot flashes will return when estrogen is stopped, so they are only postponed by the drug. Some doctors prescribe estrogen indefinitely to avoid the experience.

Organized medicine sees hot flashes as a symptom of the disease of menopause, but there are other perspectives. Some women say that hot flashes are simply a release of energy they call "power surges." They speak of appreciating the experience, adding that they have learned to dress in layers and keep a sense of humor. Such women often enjoy a positive relationship to becoming elders.

Susan Weed, in her book *Menopausal Years*, explains: "I live in a country where . . . I am urged by both inner and outer voices to do whatever I can to appear young. . . . If I lived in a world safe for women, I would cherish my hot flashes and cherish myself as I experienced them. I would be taught to respect my flashes as part of the gestation of myself in the fiery womb of menopause/metamorphosis . . . I would *want* to be a wise old woman."[28]

In more natural settings and lifestyles throughout the world, many women do not have these problems in the first place. In some African tribes, where women's status increases after menopause, there is no word for "hot flash." Yewoubdar Beyene, an anthropologist at the University of California at San Francisco, studied the reproductive lives of Mayan village women, and of peasant women on the Greek island of Evia. She found that the menopausal women of these two cultures did not even know what she was talking about when she asked about hot flashes.[29]

When women experience hot flashes that are so intense or frequent that they want relief, there are proven methods besides estrogen:

• Women who exercise regularly, and women who eat a healthy vegetarian diet, have less frequent and less severe hot flashes. (My wife, Deo, is at this writing two-thirds of the way through menopause, and has never experienced anything remotely resembling a hot flash.)

• One controlled study of 94 women with hot flashes found that taking 200 mg of vitamin C along with 200 mg of bioflavonoids six times a day provided complete relief for 67 percent of the women, and partial relief for an additional 21 percent.[30]

- Studies at Wayne State University showed that a combination of progressive muscle relaxation and deep, slow breathing reduced women's hot flashes by about 50 percent.[31] Acupuncture, vitamin E, hypnosis, yoga, meditation, homeopathic remedies, ginseng, and other herbs, including black cohosh and chaste tree, have all been clinically shown to be effective in relieving hot flashes, sleep disturbances, and irritability associated with menopause.[32]

- In a double-blind placebo-controlled study, one group of women suffering from hot flashes and other menopausal symptoms were given two herbal capsules three times a day (made up of equal parts licorice root, burdock root, wild yam root, dong quai root, and motherwort) for three months. Another group received placebos that were identical in appearance. When the study was complete, it was found that 100 percent of the women who had received the herbs reported a reduction in the severity of their symptoms, compared to only 6 percent of those who received placebos.[33]

Osteoporosis: Bone is living tissue which is always changing. New bone is constantly being made, and old bone is constantly being taken up or reabsorbed. These two processes are normally in balance, but if more bone is lost than made, the bones become brittle and can break easily. ERT is widely used to slow bone reabsorption in menopausal women.

An ad for Premarin shows a healthy young woman, wearing an exercise leotard, with the words: "Aerobics every week, calcium every day, bone loss every year." The message is that, unless she takes the drug, this vibrant woman can exercise all she wants, and eat as consciously as she can, and yet her bones will crumble.

An ad for the Estraderm patch announces: "How to Keep the Change of Life From Changing Your Bones," implying that the best way a woman can prevent her bones from dissolving over the years is by taking the drug.

The trouble is that, to be effective, the hormones must be taken for many years. Stopping estrogen therapy, even after four years, causes a rebound effect, and the rate of bone loss can increase greatly. In 1992, the *New England Journal of Medicine* editorialized, "When estrogen therapy is begun, it is unclear how long it must be continued, because its discontinuation leads to a phase of accelerated bone loss. . . . Possibly 20 years or more is required."[34]

There are effective and natural alternatives:

• Worldwide, osteoporosis is only a problem among meat and dairy eating peoples.[35] In the United States, female meat-eaters at the age of 65 have lost an average of 35 percent of their bone mass. Female vegetarians of the same age have an average bone loss of 18 percent.[36]

• Despite the onslaught of advertising from the dairy industry, dairy products are not the best source of calcium, because the calcium they contain is accompanied by animal protein that leaches calcium from the bones.[37] The five countries in the world which consume the most dairy products are the five countries in the world with the highest rates of osteoporosis.[38] The best sources of calcium include green leafy vegetables, tahini, tofu (when made with calcium sulfate or calcium chloride), broccoli, and sunflower seeds.

• Exercise is extremely important. One study at the University of Wisconsin found that even 80-year-old women in a nursing home who exercised their arms and legs for 30 minutes three times a week while sitting in their chairs were able to increase bone mass.[39]

• Women who avoid smoking and excessive alcohol, salt, caffeine, cola drinks, and sugar have stronger bones.[40]

The pharmaceutical companies have been promoting estrogen therapy to prevent bone loss, but the combination of a healthy vegetarian diet and regular exercise accomplishes this goal without the side effects and dangers of the drugs. It also returns a sense of control to women, rather than placing them at the mercy of medical intervention.

Some menopausal women have already lost so much of their skeleton that additional support may be needed beyond adopting a healthy vegetarian diet and consistent exercise. It is fairly simple to evaluate bone density with the new methods now available in everyday office practice. (Osteomark measures bone collagen levels in urine, costs about $50, and shows results in a few hours.) If a significant amount of bone has already been lost, a better answer than ERT may be natural progesterone (not to be confused with the progestins, such as Provera). Unlike the progestins, natural progesterone has a molecular structure identical to the progesterone normally found in the female body, and none of the side effects of its synthetic relative.

Natural progesterone (which is typically derived from a type of wild yam) was not originally used because it is destroyed by stomach acids, and hence is ineffective when taken by mouth. In recent years, however, a new oral micronized form was developed, which has shown great promise. It has one drawback, however—it can cause drowsiness or sleepiness. Vaginal and rectal suppositories do not have that difficulty, but are far less convenient. Skin creams have none of these problems, and seem to provide the best of both worlds.

In 1990, John R. Lee, M.D., wrote in *Lancet* of his study of 100 post-menopausal women who applied a natural progesterone cream to their skin. Bone scans, he wrote, documented substantial increases in bone density. The amount of bone increase was proportional to the bone loss before treatment. Those women with the lowest bone density before the treatment gained the greatest amount of bone during the treatment. Of the 100 women, "97 of them showed 5 percent to 40 percent new bone formation within six to 48 months after using a wild yam progesterone cream. Some women attained as much as 105 percent of the average bone density of a 35 year old. . . . The occurrence of osteoporotic bone fractures dropped to zero."[41] Writing in *Clinical Nutrition Review*, Dr. Lee reported that osteoporosis had been reversed in patients as much as 16 years past menopause using natural progesterone, exercise, and diet. Bone density increased significantly, and the incidence of fracture decreased considerably.[42]

Although I am not aware of any long-term studies demonstrating the safety of natural progesterone, it appears to be a promising nontoxic alternative when additional steps are required beyond lifestyle changes. I would suggest, however, that women using natural progesterone on an ongoing basis do so with the aid of a health professional familiar with hormones.

A number of women have asked me whether I can recommend such a clinician who could work with them over the phone and via mail. I can: Anna Keck, R.N, F.N.P., the founder of Wellcare Associates (Soquel Therapy Center, 5030 Soquel Drive, Soquel, CA 95073; 408-685-1636). A knowledgeable and caring clinician, she can provide a comprehensive assessment of midlife issues, and help fine-tune hormone and other treatment choices in a holistic way. She teaches women how to safely monitor their own bodies as they go through menopause. The service she offers is especially useful to women who do not wish to overly medicalize menopause, and want support in making informed choices that will optimize bone, breast, and heart health.

Heart Disease: Women who take estrogen for long periods of time have been shown to have lower rates of heart disease. Apparently, estrogen provides some of the same benefits more naturally gained through a low fat diet and exercise—it lowers the amount of cholesterol in the blood, and raises high density lipoproteins (the "good" cholesterol). But these benefits disappear as soon as these women stop taking the drugs. Women who eat a low-fat, high-fiber vegetarian-type diet, and who do not smoke or have high blood pressure, obtain these same benefits without drugs, and have little risk of heart disease.

The outstanding work of Dean Ornish, M.D., has helped to make the connection between heart disease, diet, and lifestyle well known. He has documented that even severely disabled patients with extremely serious cardiovascular problems can substantially reverse their difficulties with a low-fat vegetarian diet, moderate exercise, stress reduction practices, and positive attention to their emotional and spiritual lives.[43]

Vaginal Dryness: As hormone levels drop, the vaginal lining becomes thinner, drier, and less elastic. The vagina is then more likely to become sore or irritated by sexual intercourse. The situation can be alleviated by estrogen, taken either as tablets, the patch, or applied topically to the vagina as a cream.

A small amount of estrogen cream applied periodically is usually sufficient to keep the vaginal area from becoming dry and overly sensitive. Women who use the cream on a regular basis, however, increase their danger of uterine cancer, because the hormone is absorbed into the bloodstream.

Fortunately, there are other answers. Simple lubricants such as castor oil and vitamin E, or water soluble jellies such as KY Jelly may be all that is needed to achieve comfort. Natural progesterone cream can be obtained through a licensed health practitioner, and may help not only with vaginal dryness, but with a host of other menopausal symptoms. Many drug stores sell a variety of creams and other over-the-counter products specifically designed as personal lubricants, such as Astro-Glide and Super-Lube. Some of these also lower the pH of the vagina, and help provide relief from itching by preventing the overgrowth of bacteria. Remaining sexually active has also been shown to help alleviate vaginal dryness.

Sexuality: An ad for one form of ERT shows an attractive middle-aged woman leaning against a handsome gentleman on a sailboat. "I feel like a woman again," she says, perhaps implying that before taking the drug she had some uncertainty to which sex she belonged.

A Premarin ad shows an attractive middle-aged woman smiling while a man kisses her. For this, the ad suggests, she has the drug to thank.

Many women and doctors believe that without estrogen, sexual attractiveness, desire and activity decline significantly after menopause, and they look to estrogen to prevent this occurrence. "Without it [estrogen], you may soon have no sex life at all," contends Lila Nachtigall, M.D., coauthor of a popular handbook on the subject.[44] Such thoughts often frighten women into taking hormones. I am aware of no studies in the medical literature, however, to support this belief.

How is it, then, that so many menopausal women have become convinced that in order to remain attractive they must masquerade as younger women? Could this be an extension of the many other ways in which women in our culture have learned to devalue their bodies as they are? How many women in our society have subjected themselves to merciless scrutiny in the cause of being attractive? Forced their feet into shoes that deformed their posture and damaged the health of their feet, knees, hips, and spine? Worn skirts so tight they couldn't take a full stride, or dresses that buttoned in the back and held them prisoners in their own clothes? Subjected their hair to a never-ending parade of toxic dyes, bleaches, and perms? Counted calories and undertaken diets so ascetic they might make a yogi cringe? Continued to smoke in order to remain thin? Even developed serious eating disorders in the effort to force their bodies to reach unattainable and culturally contrived ideals of feminine beauty?

It is both thrilling and heartwarming to see how often, after a natural menopause, many middle-aged women stop viewing their appearance as the primary measure of their self-worth. This is not because they have become less feminine or beautiful; it is because they have become more whole, dignified, and complete. They finally feel permission to be themselves. Energy that had been bound up in obsessing over appearance can become freed, and the woman who was buried underneath layers of eye shadow and rouge and the effort to look a certain way can begin to emerge. No longer striving so hard to please or impress others, she can live more for her own purposes. No longer fretting over the surface of things, she can discover the springs of inner beauty from which love and joy naturally bubble into life.

Germaine Greer writes: "The older woman's love is a feeling of tenderness so still and deep and warm that it gilds every grass-blade and blesses every fly. It includes the ones who have a claim on it, and a great deal besides."[45]

In *A Gift of Joy,* Helen Hayes adds: "There is nothing more beautiful than an unadorned old face with the lines that tell a story, a story of a life that has been lived with some fullness."[46]

Mood Swings and Depression: The estrogen industry claims that without estrogen, women will be subject to mood swings and depression. There are some women for whom this is the case, and for whom ERT can be useful, but they are hardly the majority. In fact, studies show that menopausal women aged 45 to 64 actually have a significantly lower rate of depression than younger women.[47] And those who do have problems can often gain substantial help through improved nutrition and exercise, and by using herbs such as blue cohosh, vitex, dong quai, and blessed thistle.

Most doctors only see women who are seeking medical advice, and so get a distorted picture of how women handle the transition. Like a car mechanic who never works on a car that actually runs, they may come to believe that menopause is inherently problematic.[48] When Dr. Sonja McKinlay of Brown University researched menopausal women who were not seeking medical advice, she arrived at a different conclusion. "For the majority of women," she says, "menopause is not the major negative event it has been typified as." Fewer than 3 percent of the women in her study expressed any regret about the process.[49]

There are some women, of course, for whom menopause is a difficult time, but not necessarily because of hormonal imbalances. If a woman is caring for an aging parent or a sick spouse, or having difficulties in her marriage or other relationships, or experiencing serious financial pressures, her body will reflect the stress. If she is trying to meet intense emotional challenges, there will be physical consequences. It is no crime for this to show.

Drug companies trivialize women's lives when they imply that the answer for any problems they might experience around the time of their menopause is estrogen. One ad shows a white-haired lady holding tightly to the arm of a distinguished looking gentleman, with the headline "Menrium treats the menopausal symptoms that bother him the most."

The ads say that women on estrogen "make better wives." Leaving aside the issue of whether a woman's purpose is to be a better wife in the first place, it turns out that the touted "personality improvements" are sometimes only skin deep. A study of estrogen's effects on personality was not reassuring to women who take the drugs in order to feel more upbeat and become more peaceful and happier human beings. The study found that women taking the drug often "become less outwardly aggressive, but more inwardly hostile."[50]

THE DARK SIDE OF ESTROGEN REPLACEMENT

Of course, you would not expect drug ads to discuss the drawbacks to estrogen. But this is all the more reason for the medical community to thoroughly inform women about the risks.

• If estrogen is taken for a short time, it probably does not raise the risk of breast cancer. But to obtain any benefits for osteoporosis or heart disease, it must be taken for many years, which significantly raises breast cancer risk. There is no doubt that long-term ERT raises the risk of breast cancer; the only controversy is how much. In 1995, the *New England Journal of Medicine* reported that women who take estrogen for five years or more have a 30 to 40 percent increase in breast cancer.[51] Women who take estrogen for 25 years, a "goal" toward which many doctors are pushing their patients, are at greatly heightened risk. Long-term use of estrogen also heightens the risk of fatal ovarian cancer.[52]

• After the discovery that unopposed estrogen increased the rate of uterine cancer dramatically, it became uncommon for estrogen to be prescribed to women who still had their uteruses without the addition of progestins. Because of the unpleasant side effects of the progestins, however, some women insist on taking only estrogen, placing themselves at greatly heightened risk for uterine cancer.

• When progestins are added to estrogen for 12 to 14 days of the month, as is common, 90 percent of women experience monthly bleeding, requiring the continued use of pads or tampons. When progestins are taken along with estrogen every day, the bleeding usually stops within a few months; however, the other side effects from the progestins are usually worse.

• Women taking estrogen (with or without progestins) are at increased risk for liver and gallbladder disease. They require surgical removal of their gallbladders more than twice as often as other women.[53]

• Uterine fibroids and endometriosis are usually alleviated by menopause. When ERT is taken, however, this benefit does not occur.

• In one recent ad, a woman says defiantly: "I don't intend to grow old gracefully. I'm going to fight it every step of the way." Women who take estrogen in an attempt to assert control of their bodies and their lives may be disappointed. Their attempt to obtain this control by taking hormones typically leads to higher medical expenses and greater dependence on the medical system.

• The most commonly prescribed estrogen in the United States today (conjugated equine estrogen) is sold under the brand name Premarin. Touted as "natural," it probably wouldn't sell as well if it were called "Pregnant-mare-urine," but that, in essence, is what it is.

The drug is manufactured by a process that causes great suffering to the horses from whose urine it is derived. These animals—confined on hundreds of factory farms in North Dakota and Canada—are impregnated, then hooked up by surgical tubing to a catheter-like device to extract their urine. The mares are kept dehydrated, in order to concentrate their urine, and forced to stand constantly on hard, cold, concrete floors, unable to take more than a couple of steps, and unable to lie down comfortably, for 7 of the 11 months of their pregnancy. Each year, 90,000 foals are "disposed of" as an unwanted "by-product."[54] (Not all ERT drugs stem from such cruelty—those made from plant-derived estrogens include Estrace, Estraderm, Estratab, Menest, and Ogen.[55])

In addition to containing two types of estrogen that are found in humans, estradiol and estrone, Premarin also contains large amounts of equilin, a horse estrogen not found in humans. When I asked a pharmaceutical company representative who was touting the product whether equilin might have any negative effects on women, he replied that women who develop a tendency to rear up on their hind legs and whinny should probably discontinue the hormone. He assumed, I gather, that his little joke was a satisfactory answer to the question.

• Hormones can have profound effects on consciousness. We know that it is when estrogen levels are highest during menstrual cycles that women's emotions and behavior are directed toward the outer world. Estrogen appears to focus attention "outward" rather than "inward." Could it be that a degree of insight and inner depth might be lost to women who keep their bodies stimulated with estrogen past the natural time? If the natural hormonal balances associated with menopause are disrupted, is it possible that women are hindered in accomplishing what Germaine Greer called "the difficult transition from reproductive animal to reflective animal?"[56]

When some women successfully accomplish this transition, they bloom with strength and courage. The poet Audre Lorde spoke of passing through the years of menopause: "Contrary to the media picture, I find myself as a woman of insight ascending into my highest powers, my greatest psychic strengths, and my fullest satisfactions. I am freer of the constraints and fears and indecisions of my younger years, and survival throughout these years has taught me how to value my own beauty, and how to look closely into the beauty of others."[57]

Gail Sheehy, author of *The Silent Passage*, says women who pass through the transition naturally emerge with "a greater sense of well-being than any other stage of their lives."[58]

The Nobel Peace Prize has been awarded on four separate occasions in recent years to female elders:[59] Alva Myrdal of Sweden for her efforts toward disarmament; Mother Teresa of Calcutta for her humble and loving efforts on behalf of the poor; Mairead Corrigan and Betty Williams of Northern Ireland for their work to bring peace to their country; and Aung San Suu Kyi of Myanmar (formerly Burma) for her labors and sacrifices on behalf of human rights and social justice. None of these extraordinary women, who inspire so many with their courage and accomplishment, made hormones a part of her daily routine.

Although, frankly, I find it hard to picture someone like Mother Teresa taking estrogen, I know there are some women for whom ERT does bring genuine help. Recently I met with a wonderful female elder who is accomplishing extraordinary things and who has derived benefit from taking very small amounts of the hormone. But millions of women are today taking these drugs, unaware of their darker side, and equally unaware that there are natural alternatives. Part of the reason is that our medical establishment has joined with the drug companies in downplaying the dangers of ERT, ignoring the many viable natural alternatives, and looking at this natural life transition as if it were a disease.

I like to think it possible that someday our society will come to an appreciation of women's bodies that would enable us all to honor the words of Michele Robbins: "The female body, at any age, speaks of the beauty, the mystery, and the miracle of the universe."

RECLAIMING MENOPAUSE

There are increasing numbers of heroines today, women who are finding their voices and taking stands for life. While some of them are winning Nobel prizes, others are relatively anonymous. But all are raising the consciousness and upholding the spirit of our time.

One of these women, who continually inspires me with her beauty and courage, is my partner and wife, Deo Robbins. I am indescribably blessed to share my life with her, and to have done so for more than three decades. She has shown me that when a woman learns to respect, listen to, and care for herself, she grows in inner strength, in health, and in connection and love with all of life. Now moving gracefully through menopause, Deo is increasingly coming to trust the power and wisdom she has gained through her years of experience.

In many traditional cultures, women cannot become shamans, or healers, until after they pass through menopause. "Menopause," writes Tamara Slayton, "when understood and supported, provides the next level of initiation into personal power for women."[60]

What would happen if we had ceremonies and public rites of passage for women ending their reproductive years? What if we had rituals that honored these women and celebrated their lives?

Some women create their own rites of passage, to demonstrate to themselves and the world that their power has not left them, as the pharmaceutical companies would imply, but has in fact become more their own. Not about to throw in the towel simply because she was 52, Helen Thayer skied to the North Pole with her dog. Pulling a 160-pound sled for 27 days and 345 miles, she survived seven polar bear confrontations, three blizzards, near starvation, and several days of snow blindness.[61]

Others are not quite so physical or dramatic. Some women rent a cabin and spend time alone, reading and writing. Others take time to be in nature, or create gifts for friends and loved ones. One woman gathered her grown children together, and affirmed that she was becoming more playful than ever. To celebrate, they made head wreaths, and put on a puppet show.

One woman created a ceremony renouncing her addictions. For her, giving up meat, sugar, tobacco, coffee, and a few other things that had been aggravating her menopausal symptoms was an act of self-care as well as a relief to her body. "I've been using my addiction to these substances to stay out of touch with my pain," she said, "pain that comes from deny-ing my needs for self-expression and intimacy. I've abused my body with judgments that it is ugly and not worth loving. I'm ready now to acknowl-edge and release this pain. I want to love and care for myself."

It is common for women to bring their friends and extended family together to witness and support their excitement about the years to come. Some paint pictures or create other art objects to use in healing rituals. One woman, determined to express her artistic side more, created a song that symbolized life as she had lived it, another song to show her deeper feelings that had not been fully expressed, and yet a third to represent how she wanted to live in the future. Another woman made a lengthy list of all the things she was waiting for in order to be happy, then went to the seashore and waded out into the water where she tore her list into tiny pieces and cast them into the ocean.

In *The Fountain of Age*, Betty Friedan writes: "Through our actions, we will create a new image of age—free and joyous . . . saying what we really think and feel at last—knowing more than we ever knew we knew, not afraid of what anyone thinks of us any more, moving with wonder into that unknown future we have helped shape for the generations coming after us."[62]

It seems that Margaret Mead, one of history's great anthropologists, was on to something when she said, "The most creative force in the world is the menopausal woman with zest."

WOMEN OF POWER

Though the medical profession is not exactly leading the way, many women today are reclaiming the wisdom of their bodies. They are taking back their power and their lives. They are climbing out of the insanity of a culture that denigrates their natural bodily processes, and moving for-ward into balance and self-trust.

Marianne Williamson writes, "When a woman rises up in glory, her energy is magnetic and her sense of possibility is contagious. We have all seen glorious women, full of integrity and joy, aware of it, proud of it, over-flowing with love. They shine. I have known this state in other women and, at moments, in myself. But it could be a stronger statement, a col-lective beat."[63]

It is becoming so. Women today are learning to trust their inner sources of guidance and inspiration. Despite centuries of oppression, they are finding that their bodies can be instruments of truth and healing. Despite a culture that still sometimes views them as second-rate, they are rediscovering the wisdom that has been hidden, buried in their cells, for centuries.

Something is happening today. There is a choir of women and it is growing. Every day another voice is added. They are singing of joy, and of the return to a world grounded in love.

Part Three

9
Hugs,
Not Drugs

*There is no single effort more radical in its potential for saving the world
than a transformation of the way we raise our children.*

— Marianne Williamson

L IKE BIRTH, MENSTRUATION, AND MENOPAUSE, the unfolding of childhood is an inherently natural process. Nevertheless, every morning
before going to school, 3 to 5 percent of American schoolchildren take a
mind- and behavior-altering prescription drug called Ritalin (methylphenidate).[1] They do so because they have been diagnosed as having "Attention Deficit Hyperactivity Disorder" (ADHD).

It may seem paradoxical to give stimulants to children who are hyperactive in order to calm them down. But this is done because these drugs
often have the reverse effect on children than they do on adults. Although
the actual impact of Ritalin and similar substances on the brain and mind
of young people is poorly understood, children diagnosed with ADHD
often continue to take it for years.

What happens to the youngsters who take this medication? Their actions tend to be more goal-directed and "on task" than before. They often
become less distracted by things going on around them, and better able to
stay focused on their schoolwork. They tend to become less aggressive, less
apt to get into trouble, and generally more docile and compliant. They follow rules better.

These changes make them easier for adults to manage. Psychiatrists,
parents, and teachers are often pleased with the changes they see in a child
who is put on Ritalin, who may appear to be "finally settling down."

I have been dismayed to learn, however, that the drug usually does
nothing to enhance learning or improve actual academic achievement

beyond the short term.[2] Actively seeking to find evidence for enhanced learning in children on Ritalin, psychiatrists Russell Barkley and Charles Cunningham analyzed 17 studies on the subject, and called the results "uniformly discouraging."[3]

In 1995, a school board member from Litchfield City, Connecticut named Patrice Fitch publicly described her daughter's response to Ritalin: "In the classroom, she became more likely to pay attention or do what the teacher instructed. Yet, while she may have had her pencil poised over the work assignment, closer inspection revealed that she was not actually forming the answers but instead imitating the stance. While Ritalin made it possible for Amanda to sit more or less calmly in her chair, it did not help her to learn."[4]

CONSEQUENCES

Approximately one-third of the children diagnosed as hyperactive do not become less restless on Ritalin. Some actually become more agitated. At best, the drug can help those children who have been accurately diagnosed to focus their minds so they can temporarily absorb information better. But others become withdrawn and stare off into space, not responding to much of anything. While these children no longer make trouble for their teachers or get into fights, they begin to exist in a state of disconnected social isolation.[5]

Even for those children whose behavior does respond as intended, the effect is only a temporary suppression of symptoms, not a cure. When children stop taking Ritalin, they are back where they started, only now they may also have to deal with a rebound effect from the medication, which may make them more distraught than ever.

And then, as with any drug, there are inevitably adverse side effects.[6] Many children crash when their dose wears off, behaving even more uncontrollably than they did before. The *Physicians' Desk Reference* lists more than 25 symptoms—ranging from anxiety to hair loss to convulsions—that have been observed in Ritalin users having no preexisting conditions. Reactions include nausea, insomnia, headaches, weight loss, and a slowing of growth. Some children develop bizarre compulsive behaviors, such as insistent biting of their fingers and nails until they bleed. Other reactions include elevated heart rate, increased blood pressure, and a serious disorder known as Tourette's Syndrome, characterized by repetitive involuntary movements or tics.

Are there long-term side effects from the drug? This is an important question, because children are often placed on this medication for many years. It is also a frightening question, because to date no adequate long-term studies have been performed.[7]

Although more difficult to quantify than physical side effects, there are emotional and psychological consequences to labeling a child as having ADHD and putting the youngster on drugs. Having this kind of a diagnosis and treatment become a permanent part of a child's health files and educational records hardly helps her or him build self-esteem and self-respect. In 1993, pediatric neurologist Fred Baughman, M.D., asked in the AMA *Journal*, "What is the danger of having these children believe they have something wrong with their brains that makes it impossible for them to control themselves without a pill? What is the danger of having the most important adults in their lives, their parents and teachers, believe this as well?"[8]

Others have asked what the implications are of telling a child, "Say no to drugs, but don't forget to take your behavior-controlling, consciousness-altering medication before lunch." **What happens to children when the full weight and authority of the medical profession tells them to take drugs to control their behavior? How will children learn to understand their emotions and deal with them constructively if they are told to take a drug to make them go away?**[9]

When *Clinical Psychiatry News* discussed the heavy use of illicit drugs among adolescents, the journal lamented the increasing numbers of young people falling prey to substance abuse. Ironically, right next to the article, and visually overpowering it, was a prominent ad for Ritalin.[10]

Ciba-Geigy, the company which manufactures Ritalin, says that the drug is not addictive if used as directed. But like cocaine and amphetamines, it is classified by the Drug Enforcement Agency as a Schedule II drug, meaning that among those substances regarded as having medical use, it is considered to have the highest potential for abuse. And even Ciba-Geigy acknowledges that some youngsters buy or steal the drug from classmates, sniffing and injecting it to get high.

In England, physicians simply do not prescribe Ritalin or other stimulant medications for children.[11] They are far more cautious than we are about drug use in children to begin with, and particularly so for drugs with pervasive central nervous system effects. Throughout western Europe children almost never receive medication for hyperactivity.

In the United States, however, it's a different story. Although the *Physicians' Desk Reference* specifically states Ritalin "should not be used in children under six years [of age]," that did not stop U.S. physicians from writing 200,000 prescriptions for Ritalin and similar stimulants in 1993 for children ages five and younger.[12] In the U.S., Ritalin has been prescribed to children as young as 18 months old.

The 1980s saw a dramatic increase in Ritalin use among children in the United States which coincided with publication of influential work by the University of Pittsburgh's Stephen Breuning. His research was believed to have proven that stimulants such as Ritalin were effective answers to hyperactivity. But evidently Dr. Breuning was somewhat lacking in the noble spirit of open-minded scientific inquiry. In 1988, it was discovered that much of his data had been completely fabricated. It turned out that he had reported studies that had never been performed.[13]

Breuning was sentenced to prison for this fraud, and articles condemning his actions appeared in major medical journals. Yet many teachers, pediatricians, psychiatrists, and parents are still influenced by the pro-Ritalin wave that washed across the country during the years when his "research" was believed to be genuine.

In the years immediately following Breuning's exploits, there was an exponential increase in the use of medication for children diagnosed with ADHD. A 1987 study found that 6 percent of all schoolchildren in Baltimore were on medically prescribed stimulant drugs.[14] An outraged public response in that city caused Ritalin use there to decline in the following few years, but in the rest of the nation, the number of children being dosed with this and other medically prescribed stimulants continued to increase.

By 1995, more than 6 million psychiatric prescriptions were being written every year for Americans under the age of 18.[15] And in 1996, the World Health Organization estimated that nearly 5 percent of all elementary schoolchildren in the United States were on Ritalin.[16]

WHICH KIDS ARE PUT ON RITALIN?

The assumption is that these children have a brain dysfunction or disease. Yet doctors prescribing Ritalin rarely, if ever, perform neurological tests.[17] Instead, they take the word of parents or teachers, whose judgments are invariably subjective. The scores that are obtained from the various scales used to diagnosis ADHD give the appearance of scientific precision, as though they were measuring something tangible, like blood sugar levels. But in reality, ADHD is defined entirely in behavioral, nonmedical terms. The numbers merely sum up a particular teacher or physician's subjective impressions. In fact, a number of studies have shown that when parents, teachers, and clinicians rate the same child, they frequently come up with wildly differing scores.[18]

Who, then, are the children who get diagnosed with ADHD?

Some, who may be so unruly that they can completely disrupt an entire class, or who are impossible for their parents to handle, may benefit from the drug, at least in the short term. But many are simply children who have a strong sense of their own inner rhythms and timing. These youngsters often feel frustrated in authoritarian situations, and conforming to the rules of a classroom or of autocratic parents can be difficult for them. Such children are potential recipients of an ADHD diagnosis, because the American Psychiatric Association's criteria for ADHD officially points the finger at children who "interrupt others, and have difficulty following instructions."

Children who are especially intelligent are often bored in today's schools, and will sometimes try to answer their teacher's questions as quickly as possible, in the manner of game show contestant "whiz kids" eager to display their knowledge. This behavior, while hardly evidence of pathological brain chemistry, may nevertheless lead to a diagnosis of ADHD, because another of the official criteria targets kids who "often blurt out answers to questions before they have been completed."

Children who are assertive by nature may also receive the diagnosis. One of the scales that is most widely used by parents and teachers to assess for ADHD is the Revised Conner's Questionnaire.[19] According to this scale, children are suspected of being hyperactive if they are "sassy," and guilty of "wanting to run things."

Then again, those children who happen to be especially sensitive or timid aren't exempt, because other criteria include being "shy," and having their "feelings easily hurt."

Kids who come from difficult family situations are also likely candidates for the diagnosis. Being "basically an unhappy child," and "feeling cheated in the family circle" are considered symptoms of ADHD.

It's hard to avoid the suspicion that just about any kid who doesn't fit easily into the school or family system might fall prey to the diagnosis and consequently be treated with Ritalin. The Revised Conner's Questionnaire actually goes so far as to state that children who behave in a "childish" way are displaying a symptom of ADHD. And here all along I had thought that behaving in a childish way was a natural part of childhood.

In fact, the more I've looked at the diagnostic criteria by which children are labeled as having ADHD, the more I've begun to suspect that the only children who are completely safe from a diagnosis of ADHD are those who are so frightened to disobey that they are compulsively dutiful and obedient.

ARE OUR SCHOOLS FOR COMPLIANCE OR FOR LEARNING?

Not being a particularly big fan of either Ritalin or our mass production school system, educator John Holt told Congress plainly that we give kids this drug so that "we can run our schools as we do, like maximum security prisons, for the comfort and the convenience of the teachers and administrators who work in them."[20]

I would have to agree that America's public schools are not particularly shining examples of how to bring out the best in young people. Although thousands of humane, caring people work in schools as teachers, aides, and administrators, a good number of schools end up teaching little more than obedience and conformity. Research by the Carnegie Council on Adolescent Development concluded, "Many large middle grade schools function as mills that contain and process endless streams of students. Within them are masses of anonymous youth. . . . Such settings virtually guarantee that the intellectual and emotional needs of youth will go unmet."[21]

One of the most penetrating critics of contemporary schooling is New York State's 1991 teacher of the year, John Gatto. "The school bell rings," he says, "and the young man in the middle of writing a poem must close his notebook and move to a different cell, where he learns that man and monkeys derive from a common ancestor. . . . It is absurd and anti-life to be part of a system that compels you to sit in confinement with people of exactly the same age and social class. . . . It is absurd and anti-life to be part of a system that compels you to listen to a stranger reading poetry when you want to learn to construct buildings, or to sit with a stranger discussing the construction of buildings when you want to read poetry. It is absurd and anti-life to move from cell to cell at the sound of a gong for every day of your youth, in an institution that allows you no privacy."[22]

For the entire school day, students are under constant surveillance. They have no private time or private space. Many teachers do their best to be humane, but pupils are typically expected to sit still for hour upon hour, and to do whatever they are told. This is not only totally unnatural, and profoundly frustrating for children; it also inhibits learning. Human beings are programmed by millions of years of evolution to develop by moving, touching, and being involved in life's tasks.

There are alternative approaches to learning which involve children as active participants and do not produce boredom and restlessness. An example is the classroom of Wendy Borton, an elementary school teacher in the Shoreline District's Room Nine Program in Seattle, Washington. To teach her ten- to twelve-year-old youngsters about government, she got them involved with an issue that was relevant to their lives. In September 1992, when a bill to ban corporal punishment in the state's public schools was to be introduced (for the ninth year in a row), the students began researching the issue, reading and discussing articles both in support of corporal punishment and opposed to it.[23]

They learned that it was legal to inflict physical punishment on schoolchildren that would be considered too severe for prisoners in the state penitentiary. They learned that when an adult hits another adult, it is usually called "assault" and is a crime, but when an adult hits a child, it is usually called "discipline" and is often considered acceptable. They learned that the spanking of pupils by teachers is illegal in every European country, and that in Sweden, television spots advise children of their right not to be spanked. They learned that among the world's industrialized countries, only the United States and South Africa have persevered in the practice.[24]

The surgeon general has pleaded for a reduction in spanking as a matter of public health, saying such a shift would decrease the cultural acceptance of violence. Yet in 1993, a poll of primary-care doctors published in the AMA *Journal* found that 70 percent of family practitioners and 59 percent of pediatricians still supported corporal punishment.[25]

After thorough discussions and many heated debates, during which their teacher remained steadfastly neutral and allowed the youngsters to come to their own conclusions, the class decided that corporal punishment should not be allowed in schools.

On February 2, 1993, four students from the class traveled to Olympia to testify before the state House Education Committee. Saying that "schools are for learning, not hitting," the youngsters urged that the bill be passed. At the conclusion of the children's testimony, the committee's chairperson congratulated them on their excellent presentation.

The bill passed the House, but faced a much tougher battle in the Senate, where it had been soundly defeated in previous years. On March 19, 1993, four different students made the trip to Olympia, this time to testify before the Senate Education Committee. When the senators asked them what teachers could do to maintain order if the option of corporal punishment were removed, the kids showed they had done their homework. One observer recalls: "The students presented several productive, nonviolent ways in which their school deals with behavior problems, including behavior contracts based on agreements among teachers, students, and parents; loss of privileges when contracts are broken, and rewards for achieving contract goals; instruction in creative conflict resolution; and allowing students to help set classroom policy by establishing rules and the consequences for breaking them."

On April 6, 1993, the Senate passed the measure abolishing corporal punishment. Governor Mike Lowry subsequently signed it into law.

EVERY CHILD IS SPECIAL—EVERY CHILD IS UNIQUE

Some pupils who are labeled as "hyperactive" may simply have a different learning style than the one dictated by the school environment. Thomas Armstrong, author of *Awakening Your Child's Natural Genius*, notes: "Research has found that most of the children at risk for ADHD labeling are actually quite good at paying attention. . . . They often possess superior 'incidental attention' abilities. They pay attention to everything except what they are 'supposed to be' paying attention to. In the classroom, they hear Joey tell Suzy about what happened to Billy during recess. They see the funny drawings that Ed made on the chalkboard before the beginning of class—drawings the teacher has not yet noticed. They observe their own inner thoughts, including daydreams. . . . Is this sort of attentional style truly a disorder? Probably not. After all, infants and toddlers engage in some of the most powerful learning they will ever experience in their lives. They master the complex tasks of walking and talking by letting their attention be drawn to points of interest and by absorbing knowledge in incidental ways. Millions of years of evolution may have endowed the human being with this inborn drive toward spontaneous exploration, curiosity, and the need for variety and novelty, so that a person would have the lifelong capacity to search out new possibilities—a decided asset when outer conditions change and new forms of adaptation are required. And children labeled ADHD may be carriers of this special trait."[26]

Some children labeled hyperactive are multiscanners. These children are adept at what anthropologist Jules Henry called polyphasic learning—absorbing information through several channels at once.[27] Paying attention to many things at the same time is natural for them, and in many environments would be a great asset. But not in a classroom where "central-task" learning requires them to pay attention to one thing at a time. Their natural learning styles do not involve organizing their experience in a linear way, and they can easily feel bewildered when asked to do so. Yet, when exposed to integrated thematic instruction programs (including the use of art, music, field trips, and other multisensory approaches), these children often emerge as not only capable, but brilliant, imaginative, and creative.[28]

A dreamy child may be destined to a career as an artist or inventor. Asking such a child to be as detail oriented as someone whose future lies in accounting is like asking everyone to wear the same size shoes.

In this regard, a particular child comes to mind, by the name of Alva. His teacher was a minister, and an observer left us this record of their interaction: "The minister, of course, taught by rote, a method from which Alva was inclined to disassociate himself. He alternated between letting his mind travel to distant places and putting his body in perpetual motion in his seat. The Reverend, finding him inattentive and unruly, swished his cane. Alva, afraid and out of place, held up a few weeks, and then ran away from school."[29]

It is fortunate that young Alva lived some years ago, before the medicalization of childhood was under way. His full name, by the way, was Thomas Alva Edison, and today, he would almost certainly be diagnosed with ADHD and given Ritalin. If he had been, we might still be reading by kerosene lamps.

Ritalin helps children to conform to externally imposed rules and regulations. But I have serious questions about drugging children to make them more obedient to authority. What happens to those young people whose special destiny lies in being innovators, who carry it within themselves to challenge abuses of power in order to help create a better world?

What if young Martin Luther King, Jr., had been drugged as a child? Would the world have ever been touched by his dream, and had the opportunity to make it come true? What if young Rosa Parks had been subjected to such treatment? Would she have grown into the woman who had the courage to keep her seat on the bus that auspicious day in Alabama? Young Thomas Paine was quite a rebel as a child. If he had been subjected to Ritalin, there might not even be a United States. If a young William Shakespeare had found himself in the hands of modern medicine, I doubt that the world would ever have heard him remind us, "To thine own self be true."

I'm not saying that the children diagnosed ADHD are all potential Thoreaus, marching to a different and higher drummer. I recognize that some of these children may benefit from medication, and I sympathize with teachers who must cope with certain young people who seem preternaturally gifted at bringing chaos into a classroom. But I also know that some of these youngsters come from very difficult home situations, and act out at school the pain they carry. Tragically, some of these children are the very ones the U.S. Advisory Board on Child Abuse and Neglect was referring to in the recent statement, "Every year, hundreds of thousands of children are starved, abandoned, burned and severely beaten, raped, and sodomized, berated and belittled."

Some children are rebellious because within them there is creative genius that has yet to find its expression. Others misbehave because they have been badly ill treated. And others who have difficulties in school are simply youngsters whose unique neurological functioning and natural learning styles are incompatible with an authoritarian school system. For one reason or another, many of the children who are diagnosed as having ADHD are poorly suited to the mass production assembly line system of education. When these youngsters are permitted to make more choices about their learning activities, and to feel a sense of control over their learning processes, the results can be stunning.[30]

"The wildest colts," said the Greek philosopher Themistocles, "make the best horses."

ALTERNATIVES TO DRUGS

I see great importance in respecting young people and providing them an environment in which they can express themselves as they learn, because I believe that is the best way to raise them to be self-reliant and self-respecting. **We awaken in our children the same attitude toward themselves that we hold toward them.**

When my son, Ocean, was five, we moved to Victoria, British Columbia, so that he could attend an experimental alternative public school called Sundance Elementary School. There, the school day was divided into periods, during each of which the students could choose from six different activities ranging from physical play to art to a range of academics. Instead of grading the students, the teachers had ongoing discussions and dialogues with the children to help them set their own goals and evaluate themselves. Parental involvement was high. Remarkably, there seemed to be no drop-off in academic achievement among the youngsters, though not all learned at the same pace.

I remember one young friend of my son's, an extremely high energy boy named Ricky Walker. He had been diagnosed as hyperactive, and was a real problem at his former school. His teacher there said that the only way Ricky could continue in her class was if he took medication.

Ricky's mother recalls those days all too vividly. "We were at our wit's ends, but didn't like the idea of starting Ricky on drugs. He said he hated school, and always dreamed up the most bizarre excuses so he wouldn't have to go. He was often sick, and many times I wasn't sure whether he was really sick or just trying to stay home.

"Sundance sounded a little impractical to me. But I visited the school, and was struck by the bright faces and spirit of cooperation I saw. The kids actually seemed to be enjoying themselves. With some apprehension, we enrolled Ricky. And at the same time we made the decision to clean up his diet, to get rid of the junk food, the sugared cereals, the soda pop and hot dogs and donuts.

"At first, he didn't like any of this. He didn't want to eat whole wheat bread and he didn't want to go to Sundance, but within two weeks he was saying how much better he felt, and that he liked being able to choose his own activities. After that, Ricky became much happier, and actually got to the point that he was eager to go to school. One sign that this was the right direction was that Ricky was hardly ever sick after we made the changes. Even more important, though, was the change in his attitude. He became a positive person."

Today, Ricky is a successful teacher of martial arts and skiing. I recently asked his mom whether she thought it was the change in school or the change in diet that had made the most difference. "We made both changes at the same time," she answered, "so I can't separate them. They were both important—two good things that multiplied each other's benefits."[31]

IF YOU LOVE ME, DON'T FEED ME JUNK FOOD

Among the many factors that shape the lives of children, nutrition often plays a critical role. What children eat exerts a profound influence over the molecular environment and neurochemical functioning of their brains, governing the way they process information, and influencing the way they think, learn, and act. Many studies have found, for example, that children with higher intakes of B vitamins and other brain-active micronutrients do better in school than those children whose diets are lower in these nutrients. Others studies have found that children who are exposed to heavy metals (such as lead, cadmium, or mercury) through their food, air, or water have reduced learning and memory, and impaired functioning of the central nervous system.[32]

A landmark 1990 study concluded that lead poisoning in childhood is the single most important predictor of criminality among adults, far outweighing poverty, the absence of a father in the household, and other major social factors commonly cited by criminologists. In 1996, Dr. Herbert Needleman and his colleagues at the University of Pittsburgh School of Medicine reported in the AMA *Journal* that even nominal doses of lead, well below those associated with poisoning, can lead to antisocial behavior and delinquency in young boys.[33]

If exposure to even minute amounts of lead can disturb children's brain chemistry and behavior so dramatically, is it possible that other forms of chemical pollution, such as artificial food additives, might underlie some cases of ADHD? It was just this sort of question that led to the remarkable work of Ben Feingold, M.D., of the Kaiser-Permanente Medical Center in San Francisco.

In 1973, this distinguished pediatric allergist told a meeting of the AMA that food additives were responsible for 40 to 50 percent of the hyperactivity he had seen in his practice. He had found that a substantial number of hyperactive children improved dramatically when they stopped eating foods that contained artificial colorings, flavors, and certain preservatives.[34] Additionally, he found that a variety of childhood learning disabilities and other behavioral problems were reduced by the same diet changes.

The Feingold program is based on the fact that although most human beings have the ability to tolerate a certain amount of exposure to harmful substances, some of us are more reactive biochemically than others. Some of us are not having an easy time coping with a world where neither our water nor our air is pure, where we are exposed to countless chemicals every day that have never been known in nature until the last few decades, and where our food has been subjected to processing and refining that removes essential nutrients and adds a plethora of artificial chemicals. For children who happen to be especially sensitive, the three most troublesome chemicals—synthetic food dyes, artificial flavorings, and preservatives—can cause a host of physical, emotional, and mental reactions, and lead to being diagnosed as hyperactive.

Unfortunately, many parents, educators, and physicians believe that the Feingold program has been disproven. This erroneous idea stems from a series of studies undertaken during the late 1970s which purported to find Feingold's methods wanting, and which were widely quoted.[35] But serious questions have been raised about the validity of these studies.[36]

One study, for example, eliminated only eight of the more than 3,000 additives in our food supply, and when children did not show major improvement, wrote the program off as worthless. Others were undertaken by the Nutrition Foundation, an organization funded by the makers of Coca Cola, Fruit Loops, C & H Sugar, and other junk food manufacturers.[37] The studies took hyperactive kids, gave them doses of either additives or placebos, and then noted very little difference in response. But an analysis of the controversy, published in the journal *Science* in 1980, disclosed that the researchers had used doses of the additives that were far too small to produce a noticeable effect.[38] In fact, when the amounts were raised to a level commensurate with children's actual eating habits, the hyperactivity/food additive link was confirmed. Some 85 percent of the hyperactive children reacted adversely when they were exposed to realistic levels of artificial colorings, flavorings, preservatives, and other synthetic food additives.

In 1985, *Lancet* published the most convincing evidence to date. In an extremely well designed study, 79 percent of hyperactive children improved when suspect foods were eliminated from their diets, only to become worse again when the foods were reintroduced. Artificial colorings and flavorings were the most serious culprits; sugar was also found to have a noticeable effect.[39]

When parents are willing to try the Feingold approach, the results can be extraordinary. One such mother, Gayle Giza, described a long history of disappointment and frustration with her son, Mark. Finally, she tried the Feingold program. Mark was willing, she says, because he "had become so unhappy with his life by the time he was ten years old, he welcomed a chance to change things. . . . After we began the program he no longer had problems which we hadn't even identified as problems! He could come to the dinner table and sit down without spilling everything, could go to sleep without rocking, and stopped talking out in his sleep. He stopped incessantly teasing his sister, being argumentative, and could now turn off the TV without a confrontation. I soon received a letter from his teacher, which said, 'Mark is a pleasure to have in class.' After ten years of worry and searching, I can't describe the feelings this brought. Needless to say, I still have the letter. Mark had no problems with reading or spelling after that, and sixth grade was a real success story. . . . The day our ten-year old told us, 'I really like me the way I am *now*,' I knew no amount of effort would have been too much."[40]

Of course, a program can generate marvelous anecdotal success stories without being grounded in scientific testing. It may work for a few kids here and there without being of any use to the vast majority. Do programs that improve nutrition and remove chemical additives in children's diets actually have value on a large scale? I have found that the scientific literature supporting such programs, though not widely known to the general public, is impressive.

A series of studies in the 1980s removed chemical additives and reduced sugar in the diets of juvenile delinquents. Overall, 8,076 young people in 12 juvenile correctional facilities were involved. The result? Deviant behavior fell 47 percent.[41]

In Virginia, 276 juvenile delinquents at a detention facility housing particularly hardened adolescents were put on the diet for two years. During that time, the incidence of theft dropped 77 percent, insubordination dropped 55 percent, and hyperactivity dropped 65 percent.[42] In Los Angeles County probation detention halls, 1,382 youths were put on the diet. Again, the results were excellent. There was a 44 percent reduction in problem behavior and suicide attempts.[43]

These and other studies have found that when troubled youngsters are put on a healthy diet based on nutrient dense foods like whole grains, vegetables, and fruits, and avoid sugar and artificial colors, flavors, and preservatives, the results are predictably outstanding.

Supplementary vitamins and other essential nutrients also often help. A number of double-blind placebo-controlled studies have found that the frequency of antisocial behavior in juveniles is lowered significantly by appropriate supplementation.[44]

One remarkable double-blind, placebo-controlled study actually compared Ritalin directly with vitamin B6. Published in 1979 in the *Journal of Biological Psychiatry*, this study found that high doses of vitamin B6 actually did a better job than Ritalin at reducing hyperactivity.[45] Vitamin B6 is, of course, far cheaper (Ritalin prescriptions cost $30 to $60 per month), and far safer than the drug, and the study's protocol was outstanding.

In 1992, Jane Hersey, executive director of the Feingold Association of the United States, explained why she and others work as volunteers for the organization:

"I hear some chilling stories from parents of troubled children. They are told that their children are abnormal and have a deficiency that can be corrected by Ritalin. Some doctors call it 'replacement therapy,' as though the drug were a naturally occurring substance. We hear about teachers and counselors telling parents—'If you really loved him, you'd agree to give him the medication.' We hear of doctors prescribing Ritalin or Valium to two-year-olds. We know of parents coerced by treatment centers to agree to multiple medications, and of families facing bankruptcy as a result of these expensive yet unsuccessful therapies. We know of ADHD groups run by professionals with a vested interest in the choice of treatment, and of pharmaceutical industries supplying money to such groups. The trend appears to be growing, and with frightening speed."[46]

(The Feingold Association of the U.S. can be contacted at: P.O. Box 6550, Alexandria, VA 22306.)

ONE MILLION AMERICAN SCHOOLCHILDREN CHANGE THEIR DIETS

Perhaps the most amazing study of all those ever undertaken regarding the Feingold diet and children occurred when no less than 803 public schools in New York city were put on the diet for four years.[47] Dr. Elizabeth Cagan (the chief administrator of the Office of School Food and Nutrition Services for the New York City Public School System Board of Education) and Barbara Freidlander Meyer (city-wide nutrition education supervisor) decided to test what effect, if any, the Feingold diet would have on academic performance. Over a period of several years, they gradually eliminated all artificial colors and flavors, and the preservatives BHA and BHT, from the schools' cafeterias, while also reducing the amount of sugar available.

It was an extremely large-scale, ambitious, and ingenious experiment. The dietary modifications were introduced in a series of steps that took place simultaneously in all 803 schools. The alterations took place in the school years 1979–1980, 1980–1981, and 1982–1983. The reason no changes were made in 1981–1982 was to insure that any results that might be obtained during the course of the experiment would in fact be due to the dietary improvements, and not due to some other unknown occurrence that might be taking place simultaneously.

The schoolchildren were tested each year using the standard California Achievement Test. The testing began several years before the dietary modifications commenced, and continued throughout.

The results were spectacular. In the three years before the experiment began, the schools had placed in the 41st percentile, the 43rd percentile, and the 39th percentile, compared to other schools in the country. After the first year of dietary improvement, during which the Feingold program was partially implemented, the schools advanced to the 47th percentile. The second year, when the program was implemented further, the schools jumped to the 51st percentile. Interestingly, the next year, when no further dietary improvements were made, no increase in academic performance was found. The schools simply held steady in the 51st percentile. The following year, when the program was implemented further, the schools advanced again—this time to the 55th percentile.

When the study was published in the *International Journal of Biosocial Research*, the authors wrote, "In short, New York City Public Schools raised their mean national academic performance percentile rating from 39.2 percent to 54.9 percent in four years, with the gains occurring in the first, second and fourth years [precisely when the dietary improvements were made]."[48]

This was the largest such gain ever measured in any comparable period of time in any metropolitan school district in the country. But that's not all. The researchers added: "In 1979 [before the dietary changes], 12.4 percent of the one million student sample were performing two or more grades below the proper level. Yet, by the end of the 1983 year, the

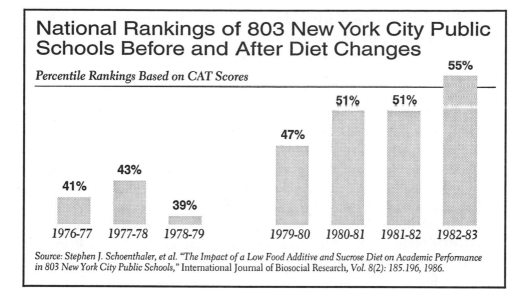

National Rankings of 803 New York City Public Schools Before and After Diet Changes

Percentile Rankings Based on CAT Scores

55%
51% 51%
47%
43%
41%
39%

1976-77   1977-78   1978-79   1979-80   1980-81   1981-82   1982-83

Source: Stephen J. Schoenthaler, et al. "The Impact of a Low Food Additive and Sucrose Diet on Academic Performance in 803 New York City Public Schools," International Journal of Biosocial Research, Vol. 8(2): 185.196, 1986.

rate had dropped to 4.9 percent. Again, all gains were found in 1980, 1981, and 1983 [corresponding exactly to the dietary improvements]."[49]

Such stunning results were obtained even though only at-school meals were modified. No attempt was made to alter what children ate at home. Since these children only ate a relatively small percentage of their daily diet at school, we can only imagine how great the benefits would be if children's entire diets were improved.

When foods containing artificial additives are eliminated and foods high in sugar are dramatically reduced, the resulting benefits are not simply due to the elimination and reduction of offending substances. This kind of dietary change inevitably involves a corresponding shift to more whole and natural foods. Diets become higher in fresh fruits and vegetables, whole grains, and more plant-based proteins. They become lower in fat, and lower in adulterated, refined, and highly processed foods.

The Healthy School Lunch Program, a project of EarthSave International, is today working to change the food served in schools in a healthier direction. Parents and teachers throughout the country who would like to see these kinds of changes implemented in their local schools are invited to contact EarthSave at P.O. Box 68, Santa Cruz, CA 95062 (1-800-362-3648). School districts consistently find that when they improve the food available to their students, the young people become healthier, the rates of ADHD and antisocial behavior plummet, and there are substantial gains in academic achievement.

SOMETIMES MIRACLES DO HAPPEN

Doris Rapp, M.D., clinical assistant professor of pediatrics at the State University of New York, is quite familiar with the importance of diet in children's lives. One of the world's foremost experts on food and environmental allergies, she became well known to the general public after her appearances on the Donahue show in 1987 and 1988. Her presentations, along with those of the children she had treated and their parents who appeared with her on the show, generated more than 140,000 letters. In her outstanding book *Is This Your Child?*, she shows parents how to identify the common foods, chemicals, or allergenic substances that can be the culprits behind a wide range of problems in children (and adults). She tells the poignant story of a young boy named Paul.[50]

When Paul's mother was advised, three days after the boy started kindergarten, to see a doctor for his hyperactivity, she was not surprised. The lad had exhausted his entire family for years. He was constantly jumping around, and was known to roller-skate through the living room at 3:00 A.M. To say he was "out of control" was an understatement.

His mother had feared there might be trouble when Paul started school. She understood when the kindergarten teacher said the boy was "too much" to handle. He was, well, the word *exuberant* was a polite way of putting it. There was no doubt about it, he could be a problem.

Paul's mother took the five-year-old boy to a neurologist, who didn't take very long to start him on Ritalin. The doctor warned her, "Don't believe what you read about the drug having side effects. It's best just to not read that stuff."

Ritalin made Paul calmer, which was at first a welcome relief. But he soon became depressed and crabby. His mother called the neurologist, who reassured her that the boy would be fine in a little while. After a time, however, the school psychologist called, saying that she was concerned because the boy would stand out on the playground, just staring at the other children. She suggested that the boy be taken off the drug.

Disturbed, Paul's mother took him back to the neurologist. She told the doctor that each time Paul took the medication, he became very withdrawn, and then became overwhelmingly sad. The doctor advised her not to worry, and made some adjustments in the dosage.

When Paul entered first grade, he had been on Ritalin for a year. His new teacher commented that the boy "acted like a zombie, and never smiled." Paul's mother was becoming increasingly alarmed.

She knew the medication had relieved Paul's overactivity, but now at times he refused to eat or drink. The school nurse said she could barely get him to drink enough water to swallow his Ritalin tablet. Socially, the boy was not doing well. He was gradually becoming more and more moody, nasty, and morose. What had happened, his mother wondered painfully, to the spirited rascal he once had been? Now when he came home from school, he slammed the door and went angrily to his room. When she tried to talk to him, he would yell, "Why can't everyone just leave me alone." He seemed to have forgotten how to play, laugh, or even smile. Every day he complained that no one liked him. His mother would hear him alone in his room moaning bitterly, "Everyone hates me." He had no friends, and had to be forced to get on the school bus every morning. The other children pushed him around, refused to let him sit next to them, and made fun of him.

Paul told his mother he wished he could go to heaven because he'd be happy up there. He asked her repeatedly, if people killed themselves, could they go to heaven? At night when he said his prayers, he would beg God to please let him die before morning so that he could go to heaven and be happy. His mother listened helplessly as he lay in bed for hours crying before finally falling asleep. Sometimes she cried, too. She thought she must be an awful mother because he was so troubled and she couldn't help him. She began to think seriously that maybe she should give him away.

She made an appointment with Paul's pediatrician, and told him Paul had become severely depressed. She was told to continue giving him the drug.

Then Paul tried to kill himself. He took the screen off his bedroom window and tried to jump out. After that, his mother decided that she must take him off the Ritalin. After checking with the neurologist, who assured her that an abrupt, complete withdrawal from the drug could not harm Paul because Ritalin "was not addictive," she stopped giving him the medication. Within days, Paul became hysterical. His mother found him crying uncontrollably, thrashing about, kicking his feet, and holding a pillow over his head as tightly as he could. As he tried to suffocate himself, he moaned, "I wish I was dead, I wish I was dead."

Paul's mother took him to a psychologist who told her that the boy's behavior problems were her fault because he had not been disciplined correctly, and she was letting him manipulate her.

She asked another doctor whether it was possible that Paul might have allergies that were behind the problems, but he scoffed at the idea and told her not to waste her money with that sort of thing. In spite of his advice, however, she took the boy to a board-certified allergist. He told her that diets were not helpful in treating hyperactivity. He said all that had been disproven. He was adamant that the boy's behavior was unrelated to additives or foods. "There's nothing you can do," he declared. "He's never going to have any friends. He'll have to be put away someday."

Paul's mother took the boy to yet another pediatrician, who told her he was learning disabled.

The turning point in this six-and-a-half-year-old child's life began when his mother saw the Donahue show that featured Doris Rapp's work with hyperactive children and allergies. She heard another mother tell of her experience with a hyperactive child who "sounded just like Paul." With the help of Doris Rapp's book, she immediately put Paul on a Multiple Food Elimination Diet, and within three weeks he was transformed into a happy, contented child. She says she knew for certain that they were on the right track the day his teacher remarked how nice it was to see him smile. The teacher had never seen the boy smile before.

The final confirmation of Paul's improvement was dramatic and heartrending. He came home from school one day, and rang his own doorbell. His mother opened the door and there was Paul, all smiles, tightly clutching a little boy's hand. Bursting with happiness, he said, "Mommy, I have a friend."

RECLAIMING CHILDHOOD

In the first five years of the 1990s, Ritalin use among children in the United States nearly tripled.[51]

For most of the kids taking Ritalin today, none of the many alternatives have been tried before resorting to drugs. Their classroom environments are mass production assembly lines, and no effort has been made to discover what or how they want to learn. Their diets are full of artificial chemicals, and no responsible attempt has been made to discover any food allergies that they—like Paul—might have.

There are so many alternatives to Ritalin that have proven helpful for countless children that it seems a shame to put a child on the drug without first trying these other approaches. To my eyes, the best strategy often turns out to be a combination of enhanced nutritional support, the creation of a more nurturing atmosphere at home, and a more responsive learning situation at school. The human body and spirit are designed with a basic intelligence, and often respond exquisitely to loving attention and a healthy lifestyle. Human beings can be beautiful, creative, and powerful, but need support and the opportunity for self-expression. When we provide a nurturing environment and diet for children, many of the problems that otherwise tend to be treated by pharmaceutical interventions simply disappear.

I have a hard time seeing so many children drugged, and yet it is certainly not my intention to condemn the many parents or teachers who mean well for their youngsters and have given them Ritalin. Often they have been directed to do so by medical authorities, whom they have been taught to trust. Often they have known no other course to take.

One uncontrollable child can so disrupt a whole class that learning becomes impossible for everyone involved. There are parents and teachers who are at their wit's end, and many who do not have the time, information, or financial resources to make adequate positive changes. And there are certainly some children for whom the judicious and temporary use of Ritalin has value, bringing at least a semblance of normalcy and unwinding vicious cycles in which they have become caught.

But given the outstanding results that have so very often been obtained when life-affirming and drug-free approaches are used, what can be said about the medical and psychiatric establishments who have so far simply ignored them? **Unlike drugs, the alternative approaches typically enhance learning, build self-esteem, promote overall health, encourage self-reliance, and have no side effects. They do not so much seek to make children more "manageable," as to make it easier for children to manage the challenges and opportunities life brings them.**

When I called the American Dietetic Association's National Center for Nutrition and Disease in late 1995 to ask about the Feingold program, I was greeted by a recorded voice cheerfully telling me: "This month, the nutrition hotline is supported in part by grants from Kellogg Company, Glaxo-Wellcome [pharmaceuticals], Meade-Johnson, and Quaker." Not overly impressed with the organization's impartiality, I plodded forward and soon found myself being told by a spokesperson for the organization that there is no reason to worry about chemical food additives in children's diets.

The American Dietetic Association does promote a consumer fact sheet on diet and health that focuses on ADHD, and an accompanying booklet titled "Questions Most Frequently Asked About Hyperactivity."[52] After asking—"Is there a dietary relationship to hyperactivity? Should I restrict certain foods from my child's diet?"—the material responds: "The answer to both questions is 'No.'" As if this were not enough, the fact sheet adds: "Sugar has a mildly quieting effect on some children," and then goes out of its way to find fault with the Feingold program. I find it troubling that these materials, promoted by the American Dietetic Association, were written and produced by the Sugar Association.[53]

Similarly, in 1995 the American Academy of Pediatrics (AAP) accepted $50,000 from the Sugar Association and $70,000 from the Meat Board to fund a nutrition video for children.[54] The AAP's position paper on ADHD thoroughly endorses medication and drug treatment, and contains not a single word about diet or nutrition.[55]

What would happen if instead of cozying up to the junk food industry, our medical authorities stood up and demanded that our children be fed a healthy, natural, and uncontaminated diet? Our children might have a better chance to grow up calm and clear. We might see fewer of them becoming trapped in substance abuse, and more of them becoming balanced and capable human beings.

What would happen if organized medicine became an advocate for the creation of healthy learning environments for our children? Our schools might begin to become places of learning that nurture the wholeness and well-being of young people.

What would happen if instead of resisting and ignoring the use of proven alternatives, the medical establishment offered its support? Perhaps fewer of our children who are having difficulties would be pathologized and drugged, and more would grow into competent people with joy to share and a contribution to make.

What would happen if the American Psychiatric Association, the National Institutes of Health, the American Medical Association, the American Academy of Pediatrics, and other representatives of organized medicine threw their considerable weight behind safer, more effective ways of responding to children's problems?

Our youngsters would be healthier and happier. Their lives would be blessed with greater opportunity for fulfillment and meaning. They would become increasingly centered and self-reliant, and better able to learn.

The future would look a lot brighter for all of us.

10

Medical Monopoly: The Game Nobody Wins

Unless we put medical freedom into the Constitution, the time will come when medicine will organize itself into an undercover dictatorship.
— Dr. Benjamin Rush, a signer of the Declaration of Independence

IN DISCUSSING THE COURSE OF HEALTH CARE in the United States, the noted Princeton medical economist Uwe E. Reinhardt once said: "What the head of the American Medical Association thinks in the shower in the morning is much more important than the aspirations of millions of Americans."[1]

The AMA is indeed the most powerful medical organization on the planet. The *Journal of the American Medical Association* has a circulation of 700,000, making it the world's largest medical journal. The AMA also publishes ten medical specialty publications, numerous books on health for the public, as well as its weekly newspaper, the *American Medical News*. Each week, its public relations department sends news releases to 4,000 medical and science journalists, and dispatches video news releases via satellite to 340 TV outlets. Every day, the AMA sends one-minute medical reports to 5,000 radio stations. The information it dispenses is presented to the public by the major networks, newspapers and magazines as objective and reliable, and is in fact often incorporated verbatim into news stories, or directly presented to the public as the news.

In their outstanding 1994 review of the AMA titled *The Serpent on the Staff*, Howard Wolinsky and Tom Brune describe the AMA's enormous influence over what's taught in medical schools, over physicians' continuing education, and indeed over every aspect of the practice of medicine today. "If you are admitted into the hospital to have a baby or to undergo a bypass operation, or into a nursing home to recover from a stroke, or into a hospice to live out your days, the AMA is there. . . . The AMA determines the very language of medical practice; when the doctor submits your bill to the insurance company or government program for reimbursement, he or she writes down a code number for whatever the problem may be from a book written by the AMA."[2]

Not content merely to supervise and control the practice of medicine, the AMA spends more money than any comparable group in the world to influence public policy. Since 1975, the AMA has spent more than $100 million for such purposes, most of which has been channeled through the organization's political action committee, the American Medical Political Action Committee (AMPAC).[3]

The activities of the roughly 4,000 political action committees in the country are regulated and monitored by the Federal Election Commission (FEC), whose job it is to oversee political campaign contributions, and make sure that the PACs play by the rules. Every day, scores of reporters and consumer activists use the vast resources of the FEC building at 999 E Street, NW, in Washington.[4] The building that houses the FEC's national offices is impressive and formidable.

There is only one small problem. The AMA literally owns the building. The AMA, which completely controls the second largest spending PAC in the nation, is the FEC's landlord.

When the AMA wants to elect, or defeat, a particular political candidate, they do not appear to be overly concerned with the FEC's regulations. Witness what happened in 1986, for example. The AMA was not pleased with the performance of Representative Pete Stark, a California Democrat who had recently taken over as chair of a congressional committee that dealt with health issues. In July, the AMA flooded Stark's district with billboards promoting the Republican challenger for his seat, David M. Williams.

No one else gave Williams, a virtually unknown owner of a local package engineering firm, the slightest chance to win. The California Republican Party didn't give his campaign a dime, and the National Republican Congressional Committee contributed a grand total of $16. Williams loaned $14,000 of his own money to his campaign, which was about all it had to spend until AMPAC appeared on the scene, sinking in more than $250,000 dollars. It came to be called "the most expensive and controversial 'shadow' campaign ever conducted in a Congressional race."[5]

When Congressperson Stark went to the FEC to report serious improprieties by AMPAC in the campaign, FEC commissioner Lee Ann Elliott, a former top officer of the AMA, saw no reason to remove herself from the proceedings, even though she still received an annual pension from the AMA. Elliot was not only present; she cast the deciding vote as the FEC determined not to investigate AMPAC's spending on the campaign.

The AMA's candidate, however, lost the election.

NOT ALWAYS THE FIRST TO SUPPORT ALTERNATIVES

When it comes to treating patients, the AMA has never been a fan of alternatives to drugs or surgery. Whether dealing with menopausal women or hyperactive children, high cholesterol or high blood pressure, the organization's allegiance seems always to be to pharmaceuticals. Throughout its history, the AMA has displayed a seemingly ever-present willingness not only to ignore, but to actively denounce alternative forms of healing.

In the AMA's early days, the practice of homeopathy was extremely popular in the United States, thanks to its impressive success in treating many of the epidemics of the 19th century. Death rates from cholera, typhoid, and scarlet fever in homeopathic hospitals were between one-half and one-eighth those in conventional hospitals.[6]

Homeopaths were highly trained medical doctors who had a completely different approach from the new medical profession, and tended to be critical of an overreliance on drugs. They believed that drugs often simply masked and suppressed the person's symptoms, creating deeper, more serious diseases.

At the AMA's founding, however, a clause was placed in its code of ethics which stated that any AMA member would be kicked out if he ever so much as "consulted" with a homeopath. The results were remarkable.

One Connecticut physician was expelled from his local medical society for consulting with a homeopath—his wife.[7]

On the night that President Abraham Lincoln was shot and Secretary of State William Seward was stabbed, Joseph K. Barnes, the surgeon general of the United States, rushed to the statesmen's aid. For this, however, he was loudly denounced—because in so doing he "consulted with" Seward's personal physician, who was a homeopath.[8]

One of the AMA's top physicians eventually acknowledged the organization's motives: "We never fought the homeopaths on matters of principle; we fought them because they got our business."

CHIROPRACTIC

From homeopaths to midwives, the history of the AMA is resplendent with a long, illustrious, and unbroken tradition of trying to do away with its competition. In each case, the AMA appears to have been motivated more by the desire to monopolize the medical market than by wanting to help people or protect them from frauds. How else, for example, can we explain the organization's war on chiropractic?

In 1993, the Ontario Ministry of Health funded a comprehensive study on chiropractic that generated a great deal of international attention. It is known as "The Manga Study," after its principal author. Professor Pran Manga is an internationally renowned health economist and Director of the Health Administration Program at the University of Ottawa.[9]

The study began by noting that low-back pain has become one of the most costly causes of illness and disability in Canada, and the leading cause of disability in middle-aged persons, as well as the most expensive source of worker's compensation costs.

The study also noted that there was an alternative to conventional medical management of low-back pain—chiropractic.

The Manga Study then proceeded to systematically compare these two modes of care for low-back pain. Based upon "the most scientifically valid clinical studies," the report concluded, "spinal manipulation applied by chiropractors is shown to be more effective."

The report answered many of the questions about chiropractic held in the public mind.

Is chiropractic safe? "There is no . . . study that even implies that chiropractic spinal manipulation is unsafe in the treatment of low-back pain. . . . Chiropractic manipulation is safer than medical management."

How about cost? "There is an overwhelming body of evidence indicating chiropractic management of low-back pain is more cost-effective than medical management." The report estimated savings of "many hundreds of millions of dollars annually" if even some of the management of lower-back pain in Canada were transferred from physicians to chiropractors.

How about public acceptance? "There is good evidence that patients are very satisfied with chiropractic management of lower-back pain and considerably less satisfied with physician management." The Manga report further noted that the public's use of chiropractic had grown steadily over the years, despite the disapproval of orthodox medicine, and despite higher out-of-pocket costs since it was not fully covered by health insurance.

The Manga Report concluded by finding "an overwhelming case in favor of much greater use of chiropractic services in the management of low-back pain." The study called for chiropractic services to be fully insured under the Ontario Health Insurance Plan, and to be fully integrated into the health-care system.

Many health analysts hailed the Manga Study as a step toward a higher quality, safer, and less expensive health care system. Chiropractors, they said, should be applauded for frequently encouraging their patients in self-care. More often than conventional physicians, they provide nutritional guidance, and promote activities that promote health and prevent disease, including exercise, massage therapy, yoga, and healthy lifestyles.

At the same time, studies in other nations were also finding increasing value in chiropractic. In the early 1990s, readers of the *British Medical Journal* were presented with a report that found chiropractic more effective than medical treatment for lower back pain.[10] In 1992, the *British Medical Journal* published a corroborating Dutch study that came to a similar conclusion in the treatment of persistent back and neck complaints.[11] Meanwhile, an Australian study comparing chiropractic and medical management in 2,000 cases of lower-back pain found chiropractic to be four times as effective at one-quarter the cost.[12]

Yet in the United States, chiropractic has been fighting an uphill battle for decades, mostly, it turns out, due to the persistent efforts of the American Medical Association.

THE AMA DECIDES TO DO AWAY WITH CHIROPRACTIC

In 1963, the AMA hired Robert B. Throckmorton as its general counsel. Throckmorton was an attorney from Iowa, who had caught the eye of the AMA a few months before at a meeting in Minneapolis, where he had given a rousing speech calling for an end to "the menace of chiropractic."[13] The public, he proclaimed, looks "to the medical profession for unbiased and authoritative information on the subject."[14] The medical profession, he demanded, should oppose chiropractic efforts to be covered by health insurance and worker's compensation; oppose chiropractic efforts to get hospital privileges; and encourage complaints against chiropractors.

The hiring of Throckmorton was the beginning of a remarkable saga, ably recounted by Wolinsky and Brune in *The Serpent on the Staff*, and also by a man who came to be centrally involved in the entire drama, Chester Wilk.

Throckmorton was aware, of course, that it would not look good if the public became aware that the AMA was behind a campaign to destroy its competition. He repeatedly emphasized that "action taken by the medical profession should be . . . behind the scenes whenever possible."[15]

Throckmorton proposed forming a "Committee on Chiropractic" to organize and oversee the campaign. In November 1963, the AMA Board agreed. They made one change, however—they thought that a focus specific to chiropractic was too limited in scope. Why stop with chiropractic, when they could undermine or eliminate the whole flock of pesky alternative holistic healing practices? **The board renamed the panel the "Committee on Quackery," and determined that its first goal was to "contain and eliminate chiropractic."**[16]

Of course, this goal was never expressed in public. The Committee on Quackery publicly said its purpose was to eliminate charlatans and snake-oil salesmen who would prey upon the public for financial gain. In this endeavor, the word *quack* proved particularly useful. The AMA delighted in using it to besmirch the reputation of chiropractors and other alternative healers they wanted to discredit.

Shortly after the committee was formed, Throckmorton brought in another Iowa attorney, Doyl Taylor, to head the campaign. Taylor's qualifications for the job included knowing absolutely nothing about chiropractic. "I didn't know a chiropractor from an antelope," he later confessed.[17] But within weeks he was publicly proclaiming that chiropractors were "the greatest hazard to public health."[18]

Why would he speak this way? Had he perhaps rapidly scrutinized the major studies done on chiropractic? Had he interviewed disgruntled chiropractic patients? No, there was another explanation: "I opposed what I was ordered to oppose."[19]

Taylor was soon working full time alongside Throckmorton to create a climate of opinion hostile to chiropractic. In 1966, the AMA's House of Delegates officially adopted a position statement Taylor helped write. Unbothered by little things like accuracy, the AMA humbly called itself "the medical profession," and then proceeded to declare: "It is the position of the medical profession that chiropractic is an unscientific cult whose practitioners . . . constitute a hazard to health care in the United States."[20]

Soon, Taylor was contacting hundreds of medical groups and societies, encouraging them to deem it unethical for a physician to refer patients to chiropractors or to consult with chiropractors professionally or personally. In order to further sabotage and undermine chiropractors' activities, Taylor created a team of agents who took assumed names, pretended to be chiropractors, spied on chiropractic conventions, and did what they could to generate divisiveness and dissension.[21]

Meanwhile, the AMA purchased and distributed 10,000 copies of Ralph Smith's savagely anti-chiropractic book *At Your Own Risk: The Case Against Chiropractic*. Repeatedly using words like *fraud, hoax,* and *cult,* the book all but said that chiropractic was a form of organized crime. In a haunting and eerily reminiscent phrase, it announced that: "According to the unanimous voice of science, chiropractic theory has about the same medical validity as witchcraft."[22]

THE CAMPAIGN CONTINUES, AND
THE TENSION MOUNTS

Despite the AMA campaign, however, chiropractic was becoming increasingly popular, and even Americans who knew little about chiropractic were becoming curious. In 1967, Congress instructed the Department of Health, Education and Welfare (HEW) to appoint a panel to study and make a recommendation on whether chiropractors should be reimbursed by Medicare. Knowing that reimbursement would be a major blow to their campaign, the AMA immediately set about attempting to persuade the members of the panel that it was critical to the health of the nation that chiropractic not be covered.

Some of the panelists, however, were offended by the pressure. One, Dr. John McMillan Mennell, from Jefferson Medical College in Philadelphia, complained of receiving phone calls "clearly inspired by the AMA, suggesting what the tenor of my paper should be."[23] He said the AMA showed a "bitter bias" against chiropractic, which was completely uncalled for, because "there is substantial evidence that manipulative therapy brings relief to sufferers from [certain kinds] of pain."[24]

After the vote went against providing Medicare coverage for chiropractic, the AMA took the campaign to a new level of intensity. The AMA's consumer magazines began printing articles that repeatedly called chiropractic "quackery," and greatly exaggerated its dangers. Caught up in the excitement, the officials of the Committee on Quackery went about the country making speeches about chiropractic that were increasingly malicious. The chairperson of the committee, Dr. Joseph A. Sabatier, told a gathering of medical society officials that "rabid dogs and chiropractors fit into the same category. . . . Chiropractors are nice [but] they kill people."[25]

The chiropractors who were being subjected to these attacks were attempting to conduct a business and provide a healing service that was legal and licensed. They had undergone extensive training, but now were beset by the officials of a highly esteemed organization who were calling them killers. One chiropractor described the experience: "The repeated attacks were like a hammer being pounded against all of us. You couldn't get away from it. I was proud of what I did. I spent time with my patients, and my goal was to get them back on their own feet. I didn't need that much income to be happy, and never wanted my patients to become dependent on me. I had a wonderful practice, and got excellent results for most of my patients. But as the attacks continued, I had to spend more and more of my time defending myself and my profession. It took a toll. Eventually I had to close my practice. Such a waste. The AMA didn't care who they hurt."[26]

The Committee on Quackery, however, was delighted with the way things were going. In 1971, the committee wrote a memo to the AMA Board of Trustees, saying that it was "moving toward the ultimate goal" of eliminating the chiropractic profession. The memo also explained that the committee did not usually submit reports on its activities and progress because "to make public some of [our] activities would be unwise."[27]

THE CAMPAIGN EXPLODES IN THE AMA'S FACE

Much to the AMA's horror, someone spilled the beans.

In the early 1970s, the new executive vice president of the International Chiropractors Association, a man named Dr. Jerome McAndrews, received at his office in Davenport, Iowa a parcel containing a book titled *In the Public Interest*, by an unknown author named William Trevor. The book stated that the AMA was working to eradicate chiropractic, and that its war on quackery was a front for its real purpose, which was to eliminate competing healing professions. It described the project in detail, and included what purported to be reproductions of internal documents and memos from the AMA campaign. These internal documents were graphic, and if authentic, would be extraordinarily damaging to the AMA. They supposedly had been obtained from an anonymous source within the AMA itself.[28]

McAndrews did not know if the material was genuine, and had no way to check. He couldn't exactly call up the AMA, and say, "Excuse me, but are you illegally conspiring to destroy your competition?" But sensing truth, his group quietly printed copies to distribute among chiropractors.

One copy found its way to the office of a Chicago chiropractor named Chester A. Wilk. An extremely principled man who had a copy of the Bill of Rights conspicuously displayed in his living room, he had long sensed that the AMA was trying to destroy chiropractic, and had written a book on the subject called *Chiropractic Speaks Out: A Reply to Medical Propaganda, Bigotry, and Ignorance.*[29] In his book and frequent public speeches, Wilk pleaded with the AMA to stop trying to destroy alternative healing systems, and instead to join forces toward the common goal of helping patients. When Wilk saw the documents, he felt the ring of truth. Though he could not be sure, he strongly suspected that they were legitimate. And if they were, they were explosive.

In 1975, an anonymous individual who came to be called "Sore Throat" sent a draft of what he or she said were internal AMA documents to reporters at most of the major newspapers in the country, as well as to congressional committees and consumer activist groups. If these documents were to be believed, they revealed a flock of illegal and sinister activities by the AMA, including postal and income tax abuses, unethical use of the AMA *Journal*, AMA control of congressional leaders, and the campaign to destroy chiropractic. Some of these documents were identical to those that had appeared in *In The Public Interest*. Sore Throat claimed to be a disgruntled AMA staff member, seeking to expose the organization's seedy side so that reform could be brought.

Headlines in major newspapers began appearing, such as "Secret Memos Show AMA Deeply Involved in Politics," "Drug Firms Gave AMA $851,000," and "Secret AMA Link to Nixon Disclosed."

The AMA claimed the documents were fabricated, but its actions were not exactly those of one with nothing to hide. The AMA immediately began buying paper shredders to destroy documents, hiring private detectives, and setting up elaborate camera surveillance systems—with cameras in hallways, in lobbies, in the parking lots, and even in the alleyways near the building. Employees found their briefcases and purses being searched.

They were asked to submit to body checks, and to take lie detector tests. Individuals suspected of copying documents were put under constant surveillance.

Meanwhile, an AMA spokesperson told the press that Sore Throat was just "a fruity chiropractor in Georgetown whose hobby is hairdressing."[30]

While all this was happening, Chester Wilk began to consider an antitrust suit against the AMA. An attorney named George McAndrews agreed to take on the case, and to do so without pay for his time or his out-of-pocket expenses if donations and/or settlements did not come in to cover them. Why would George McAndrews, who was not that wealthy, take the case on these terms? George's father had suffered terribly for many years from severe asthma, and merely to survive had had to take a form of adrenaline. He had to take the drug, which was normally administered every four hours, every fifteen minutes. Close to death, he had been taken as a last resort to a chiropractor, and after several sessions, never had another attack of asthma.

On a historic day in October 1976, Chester Wilk and three other chiropractors filed suit against the AMA, naming 11 of the nation's other most prominent medical groups along with them as codefendants. According to the suit, the American Hospital Association, the American College of Surgeons, the American College of Physicians, the American College of Orthopedic Surgeons, the American College of Radiology, and the Joint Commission on Accreditation of Hospitals, among others had all taken part, in various ways, in an illegal conspiracy to destroy chiropractic.

In preparing for the trial, George McAndrews visited 34 states and collected over a million pages and 164 depositions.[31] And the more he learned, the more committed he became.

By this point, the AMA was backpedaling as fast as it could. Trying to avoid the appearance of conspiring against chiropractic, the AMA House of Delegates in 1979 adopted a new position statement, saying that not everything the chiropractors did was without therapeutic value.[32] Not all chiropractors were cultists.

If they thought that would get Wilk and McAndrews to call off the suit, they were sorely mistaken.

Meanwhile, AMA members were confused. Here all along they had been told that chiropractors were practically the scum of the earth, and now their leadership was telling them to cool it. Dr. William S. Hotchkiss, a member of the AMA Board who had also been a member of the Committee on Quackery, probably knew better than anyone how embarrassed the AMA would be if everything came out. He proposed buying off the chiropractors. "If we could settle it all for a . . . sum," he told the other doctors, "this would not be surrender, but would represent good common sense."[33]

But McAndrews and Wilk weren't buying.

The AMA made further attempts to head off the lawsuit. The House of Delegates now eliminated the section from their ethical code banning consultation with "unscientific practitioners," such as chiropractors.

But the chiropractors had come too far and knew too much to stop now. In December 1980 the case of *Wilk et al. vs. AMA et al.* went to trial. In one of the epic court battles in U.S. history, the adversaries fought bitterly in court for the next ten years. There were verdicts and appeals, new trials and more verdicts and more appeals.

The AMA tried to show that chiropractic was "unscientific," that it was not based on sound biological principles, but instead believed in some kind of vague healing spirit or power that resided in the body and which purportedly could be released by chiropractic intervention. One of the AMA's witnesses was a man named William Jarvis, cofounder of the National Council Against Health Fraud, and a faculty member at Loma Linda University. He summarized the AMA's position that there was nothing to chiropractic: "As I see it," he told the court, "the major problem is a substitution of the chiropractic philosophy for science."[34]

In response, the chiropractors pointed out that much of what conventional medicine does has no basis at all. Doctors did not yet know even how aspirin worked. And a report by the Congressional Office of Technology Assessment had said that, other than emergency medicine, 80 percent of what conventional medicine did had never been proven to be effective.[35]

As the battle continued, the AMA repeatedly hammered at chiropractic's alleged weaknesses. Chiropractors were accused of promising more than they could deliver, of pretending to know more than they actually did, of using too many X-rays, and of being more interested in making money than helping people. Again and again, the chiropractors fought back, pointing out that doctors were equally vulnerable to the same allegations, and worse.

During closing arguments, AMA trial lawyer Douglas R. Carlson tried to explain why the AMA had softened its positions on chiropractic in recent years. It had not been done, he claimed, in the attempt to fend off the lawsuit. No, he said, the AMA was now speaking more kindly of chiropractic because the alternative healers had finally begun to improve themselves. Mustering his full chutzpah, he then added that these positive changes had come about as a result of the AMA's criticisms that had let the alternative healers know where they were going wrong. In other words, if the court was discovering that chiropractic wasn't as bad as the AMA had always said, well, that was only because the chiropractors had smartened up thanks to the AMA attacks. The AMA, he concluded, should be given the credit for any progress the chiropractors had made.[36]

George McAndrews, the chiropractors' attorney, was not overly impressed by such logic. In his closing statement, he said that Carlson's statement reminded him of a German U-boat captain who "took credit for the American Olympic team being so good because . . . by sinking their ships, he taught them how to swim."[37]

JUSTICE AT LAST

When the trial ended, there were 3,624 pages of transcripts, 1,265 exhibits, and 73 depositions. **On August 24, 1987, U.S. District Court Judge Susan Getzendanner ruled that the AMA and its officials were guilty of attempting to eliminate the chiropractic profession.** This conduct, she said, "constituted a conspiracy among the AMA and its members . . . in violation of Section 1 of the Sherman Act."[38]

She ordered the AMA to admit the "lawlessness of its conduct," to change its course, and to publish her entire order in the AMA *Journal*.[39]

The AMA appealed, but in February 1990, the Appellate Court upheld the ruling. And in November 1990 the U.S. Supreme Court let the ruling stand.

By this time, all the other codefendants had reached settlements with the chiropractors. But the AMA continued to bicker. Finally, in December, 1991, 15 bitter years after Chester Wilk and the McAndrews brothers had filed suit, the AMA agreed to make a $3.5 million payment for the chiropractors' legal costs, and to revise its position.

Things finally began to change. Mainstream medicine began to reluctantly acknowledge that there actually might be something to chiropractic and other alternative methods of healing. Encouraging studies of chiropractic began to appear in prestigious American medical journals.

In 1994, the federal Agency for Health Care Policy and Research (a division of the Public Health Service) declared that most conventional therapies, including prescription painkillers and surgery, were rarely helpful for back pain. Instead, the agency recommended simple, over-the-counter anti-inflammatory medications, and spinal manipulation.[40] It was quite a switch from the days when chiropractic was constantly flogged as quackery.

At about the same time, chiropractors were made eligible to become commissioned health-care officers in the U.S. Armed Forces. And a military advisory panel, the Chiropractic Care Demonstration Project, was formed to implement chiropractic health care for military personnel.

By 1995, chiropractors had gained hospital privileges at more than 100 hospitals. Nearly 20 million Americans were visiting chiropractors annually, and many of their visits were being paid for by state, federal, and private insurance sources.

GOING UNDERCOVER AT AMA HEADQUARTERS

Meanwhile, the AMA was left wondering how in blazes its internal documents had ever become so embarrassingly public. At least part of the answer may have been publicly revealed for the first time in 1994, when a man named P. Joseph Lisa published a book titled *The Assault on Medical Freedom.*

Lisa's discoveries began when, as an undercover investigator operating under an assumed name and credentials, he found himself face to face with some of the AMA's darkest secrets:

"My introduction to the seedy world of medical politics began at the American Medical Association's headquarters in Chicago in April, 1969. . . . I was not prepared for what I was confronted with once I entered into the halls of orthodox medicine. . . .

"The first thing I noticed were the security surveillance cameras pointing at the entrance. . . . A uniformed security guard looked up from his paperwork and suspiciously asked who I was there to see and if I could produce identification. I could feel his steel-cold stare as he stood measuring me up and down, making judgments about this outsider standing before him. It was as if I were some trespasser infringing upon the turf which he had been entrusted to guard. . . . I stated my purpose, which was an appointment with the head of the AMA's Department of Investigation, Doyl Taylor. . . .

"A few minutes later, a tall lanky man dressed in a dark pin-striped suit stepped authoritatively toward me. With a stern expression on his face, he droned, 'I'm Doyl Taylor.' I introduced myself, we shook hands, and he turned around without saying a word. . . .

"I walked behind Taylor through a maze of offices, hallways, and partitions, [and into] a huge room that contained hundreds of file cabinets. . . . These filing cabinets contained the most comprehensive collection of misinformation, correspondence, propaganda, and reports of 'quackery' in the world. ('Quackery,' I was later to find out, was a label that orthodox medicine attached to anything they wanted to discredit in the public's eye.)

"At first he was very leery of me, and checked out my background with phone calls. He made it a point to tell me that if it were not for my impeccable credentials he never would have allowed me access to his records. . . .

"After the first few hours of talking with him, I won his confidence by playing on his ego. I deliberately positioned myself in the subordinate position of a neophyte having to rely on his expertise and direction in my quest to expose 'quackery.' He hoped to use me as a medium to spread AMA propaganda about 'quackery' to the general public. . . .

"Taylor was so proud of his files that he quickly pointed out that the FBI, the FDA, the IRS, and even foreign countries came to him to extract data and collect information on 'quacks.'

"I was given access to targets of the AMA's propaganda campaigns . . . psychic healing, faith healing, acupuncture, cancer and arthritis 'cures,' chiropractic, homeopathy, naturopathy, vitamins, herbs, and more. . . . I found that there was a major campaign against every single aspect of alternative medicine . . . an organized campaign to discredit alternative forms of healing as 'quackery.'

"I [later] found myself confronting thousands of documents that [I] copied from their files on 'quackery.' I 'lived and breathed' AMA documents for almost a full year. I knew what they were doing better than some of their own staff. . . .

"These documents were then used by William Trever to write an expose on the AMA's propaganda campaign against chiropractic. The book was self-published and titled *In the Public Interest*."[41]

If P. Joseph Lisa is to be believed, and there are indications his statements are valid, then the AMA's war against chiropractic was simply the tip of a rather ugly iceberg. In his 1994 book, he presents evidence that after the Wilk case, the war against alternatives went underground, and continues to this day. A wide variety of drugless healing methods, he says, are being branded as "quackery" or "health fraud," not because they've been tested and found not to work, but because they threaten the power of the AMA, as well as the monopoly, ideology, and profits of the pharmaceutical-medical complex.

At this point I can't but wonder how much of the outrageously high cost of American medical care stems from the AMA's tradition of seeking to eliminate competition. It's hard not to think of the countless people who have suffered because alternative therapies that could have helped them have been the victim of an aggressive campaign to discredit them as quackery.

There was a time that when I thought of the AMA, I'd picture a group of silver-haired, knowledgeable leaders of the medical community. I wasn't so naive as to think that the actions they took were always wise, but I thought they had integrity and principles. I believed they worked for what they believed to be the common good, and tried, in their perhaps stodgy way, to uphold the highest values of the medical profession.

But while more sensible voices have asked the medical profession to make the wisest use of both worlds, to allow valid holistic approaches to complement and reinforce the best uses of conventional medicine, the AMA has taken a different approach.

In 1993, the AMA published a book titled *Alternative Health Methods*, which none-too-open-mindedly characterized holistic medicine as "a melange of banalities, truisms, exaggerations, and falsehoods, overlaid with disparagement . . . of logical reasoning itself."[42] In 1996, the AMA featured the book in its catalogue, touting it as an authoritative source of information on "unproven, disproven, controversial, fraudulent, and/or otherwise questionable approaches [such as] acupuncture, faith healing, biofeedback, homeopathy, naturopathy, colonic irrigation, and more!"[43]

HERE COME THE NURSES

The AMA's none-too-welcoming attitude toward chiropractic and other alternative approaches to healing is consistent with its longstanding attitude toward women. Whether seeking to eliminate chiropractic, midwifery, or homeopathy, the organization has never been a fan of the more feminine healing methods, those that seek to nurture the natural healing forces of the body. This is the organization, after all, that originally launched itself into the marketplace by destroying the network of female community healers.

The original nursing schools, conceived by Florence Nightingale and Dorothy Dix, trained women to be absolutely obedient to doctors. According to Barbara Ehrenreich and Deirdre English: "At first, male doctors were a little skeptical about the new Nightingale nurses—perhaps suspecting that this was just one more feminine attempt to infiltrate medicine. But they were soon won over by the nurses' unflagging obedience. (Nightingale was a little obsessive on this point. When she arrived in the Crimea with her newly trained nurses, the doctors at first ignored them all. Nightingale refused to let her women lift a finger to help the thousands of sick and wounded soldiers until the doctors gave an order. Impressed, the doctors finally relented and set the nurses to cleaning up the hospital.)"[44]

At that time, nursing was mostly low-paid heavy-duty housework. The 1888 rule book for the School of Nursing at Lenox Hill Hospital in New York provides a glimpse of the profession in its early days. Among the many duties nurses were expected to perform that year were mopping floors, cleaning chimneys, and fetching coal. The hours were 7:00 A.M. to 8:00 P.M., seven days a week.

Not that it was all work, with no pay. Nurses who performed faultlessly for five years became eligible for an increase in pay of five cents a day—providing, of course, that the hospital budget could handle it.

Despite such not-entirely-auspicious beginnings, however, the nursing profession came to produce some of the most important advances in health care. As physicians were taking over childbirth from the midwives, pregnant women were receiving little attention until they went into labor. Poor women typically worked long hours in sweatshops right up until delivery, and went back to work almost immediately. Alarmed that mother and child death rates were rising, a group of nurses in Boston in 1901 developed the concept of prenatal care.[45]

Nurses began visiting pregnant women and learning how to care for them. By 1912, they were performing physical exams, checking blood pressure, taking urine samples, encouraging healthier eating patterns, and educating women about pregnancy and childbirth. The idea made sense, and soon spread through the nursing networks, with the result that wherever nurses provided prenatal care, both maternal and infant mortality rates began to decrease.

It was a nurse and midwife, Margaret Sanger, who led the campaign for access to contraception. Despite violent opposition from the AMA, she forged ahead, educating women about family planning, and coining the term *birth control*. In 1917, while AMA officials were making speeches denouncing birth control and attacking Margaret Sanger as "insubordinate," she founded the National Birth Control League, the organization that later became the Planned Parenthood Federation of America.

NURSES TO THE RESCUE

Today, nurses have once again come forward with a number of ideas that could rejuvenate and revolutionize health care. One suggestion they are making responds to a problem the doctors have not been able to solve. Increasing numbers of doctors are shunning primary care medicine in favor of higher paid specialties. Fewer and fewer physicians are becoming family doctors, pediatricians, and internists—the kinds of doctors who treat common ailments and practice preventive medicine. Even fewer doctors are making themselves available to provide care in rural areas and to the poor.

Nurses say they could be the answer.

Over the years, studies have repeatedly found that advanced practice nurses (registered nurses with additional training) can provide most of the basic care currently provided by physicians, at a far lower cost. Study after study has found that nurses with advanced training—including nurse-midwives, nurse practitioners, clinical nurse specialists, and registered nurse anesthetists—can do this with no drop in quality, and at half the expense.[46]

A 1986 study by the Office of Technology Assessment found that nurse practitioners could provide quality basic health care "as good as or better than physicians." The report noted that nurse practitioners have "better communication, counseling, and interviewing skills than physicians."[47]

The American Nurses Association says that using nurses in this way could be the key to shifting the health-care system from a *medical model*, based on expensive, acute, and high-tech equipment, to a less expensive *health model* that promotes wellness and prevention.

Many nurses are already providing primary care. They spend far more time with their patients, getting to know them and gaining understanding of their lives. Physicians usually have only a few minutes with each patient, and must tick off assembly line diagnoses. But these nurses ask their patients more questions, and listen to their answers. They find out what they eat, how they live, and what pressures are in their lives. They take time to understand who their patients are, to get to know their families, and to understand their values.

Patients appreciate the kind of basic care advanced practice nurses can provide. They respond to the emphasis on health promotion and disease prevention, and the feeling they get of being listened to and valued.

Today, nurse practitioners are running public health clinics, establishing school health services, and teaching preventive medicine. And they are often in the forefront of the battle to create a health-care system that respects and honors people.

How, you may wonder, has the AMA responded to all this? Well, let's just say that the AMA's treatment of nurses, while not identical to its treatment of midwives, chiropractors, and other alternative healers, seems to fall a little short of the organization's stated goal of "forging partnerships in healing."

In a 1994 AMA report on the "question" of nurses providing primary care, the chairman of the AMA's Board (and soon to be its president), Lonnie Bristow, M.D., berated the very idea that nurses could function without constant supervision from doctors: "It's illogical and potentially dangerous to have this type of activity performed independently of the oversight and coordination of a physician."[48]

The speaker of the AMA's House of Delegates, Daniel Johnson, Jr., M.D., was also not overly enthusiastic about the concept. The problem, he said, is that "Some of these nurses are going to overstep their boundaries. Medicine ought to be practiced by physicians, and nursing ought to be practiced by nurses."[49]

Another AMA spokesperson chipped in, "Nurses ought to go to medical school if they want to be doctors."[50]

In late 1995, one physician tried to explain the reasoning behind the AMA position. His statement, however, did not entirely convince me that the AMA respects the nursing profession. "Sometimes a doctor needs an assistant at his side, someone who is not too full of herself to obediently perform menial tasks, and who is willing to follow orders. The role of a nurse is to fulfill that function."[51]

Why do I get the impression that the AMA is not composed of the humblest people who ever walked the Earth?

The president of the American Nurses Association, Virginia Trotter Betts, has not been thrilled with the AMA stance. "The issue," she says, "is control. The AMA wants physician supervision because then the physician gets the first dollar." She adds that the AMA "has opposed autonomy for any practitioner, whether that be nurse, podiatrist, psychologist, social worker, or chiropractor."[52]

THERAPEUTIC TOUCH

Although doctors have typically occupied a superior status to nurses in the medical pecking order, it has in fact been nurses who have provided most of the direct person-to-person patient care over the years. It's often been nurses who have touched patients with love and kindness, who have made hospitals a little more humane, and who have provided a compassionate presence for people in pain.

Today, it is a group of nurses who are responsible for a remarkable new development in health care. Dora Kunz and Dolores Krieger, professor of nursing at New York University, have developed a new and systematic version of the ancient art of laying on of hands, called Therapeutic Touch.

Every healing tradition in the world has long held that human touch can be a healing force, and that the energies that radiate from human beings influence others in their vicinity. Therapeutic Touch attempts to direct this energy for healing. Dolores Krieger believes that anyone can learn to do it. "It's a natural potential in all human beings, and this potential can be developed."

Unlike therapeutic massage, the process is done without actually making physical contact. It normally takes about 15 minutes.

When I first learned of Therapeutic Touch, I was skeptical. I knew that massage can be deeply relaxing, and greatly assist the body's natural healing forces. But could healing reliably occur without actual physical contact? Evidently having similar questions, Daniel Wirth, J.D., president of Healing Sciences International in Orinda, California, designed an ingenious method to test the efficacy of Therapeutic Touch.[53]

The study went as follows: A group of willing college students had substantial experimental wounds made in their arms. They then placed their wounded arms through a hole in a wall that had been specially made for this purpose. They could not see what took place, if anything, on the other side of the wall, where their injured arms now lay. By random lot, some of them received Therapeutic Touch, and some of them did not. There was no way they could know whether or not they had received the "healing."

It turned out that the wounds in the group receiving Therapeutic Touch healed substantially faster than the wounds in the group that did not, and the results were highly significant statistically. Furthermore, each time the experiment was repeated, the results were confirmed.[54]

Other studies have found Therapeutic Touch to be effective in reducing pain, promoting relaxation, and supporting the healing process across a wide spectrum of situations.[55] In childbirth, it leads to less pain in labor, easier births, and more peaceful babies.[56] In premature infants, it has been found to reduce stress.[57] In hospitalized cardiovascular patients, it has been shown to decrease anxiety.[58]

The practice of Therapeutic Touch is now used by tens of thousands of nurses in major medical centers, hospices, and in home care throughout the world. Impressive scientific studies validating its efficacy have been made by researchers including Janet F. Quinn, associate professor at the Center for Human Caring at the University of Colorado School of Nursing, and Theresa Connell Meehan, associate director of Nursing at New York University Medical Center.[59]

Even the Department of Defense has been impressed. It has allocated $355,000 to University of Alabama scientists to investigate Therapeutic Touch's ability to help burn victims.[60]

There have, however, been certain factions in the medical establishment who have not been entirely delighted with all this. Perhaps the most colorful example of such attitudes appeared in the newsletter of an organization calling itself the National Council Against Health Fraud. The group's president and cofounder, Dr. William Jarvis, was an AMA witness in the court battle against chiropractic, and author of the AMA's 1993 book *Alternative Health Methods*. In 1994, the organization expressed its displeasure with the Colorado Nursing Board for allowing Therapeutic Touch to spread throughout the nursing profession: "The clique of highly-placed nursing politicos responsible for Therapeutic Touch's proliferation looks like a coven of Shirley Maclaine wannabees. Some critics say that underlying Therapeutic Touch is a kind of ecofeminism that extols women's intuition and mysticism as superior to male-dominated medical science."[61]

Somehow I get the impression that not everyone in the health-care world is excited by the possibility that women might have some role to play besides that of smiling handmaidens.

Larry Dossey, M.D., tells of an event that took place recently in a large hospital. Several nurses became interested in learning Therapeutic Touch, and went away to take a weekend course in the technique. The hospital authorities were apparently not pleased. "When the nurses returned to work on Monday morning, fresh from the course, they were met by a large sign on the bulletin board in the nursing department: THERE WILL BE NO HEALING IN THIS HOSPITAL!"[62]

While defenders of the AMA mentality are busy attacking alternative approaches to healing, Therapeutic Touch is being used with cancer patients throughout the country to relieve nausea and pain, and to enhance the quality and duration of sleep. The president of the Commonweal Cancer Help Program in Bolinas, California, Michael Lerner reports: "For the vast majority of participants, the experience [of Therapeutic Touch] is a profoundly positive one. It often induces deep feelings of mental, emotional, and spiritual healing, and sometimes has significant effects on physical symptoms as well."[63]

The nurses who devised and who are performing Therapeutic Touch are doing something praiseworthy. I do have concern for them, though. Given the AMA's attitudes, I hope they don't get arrested for practicing love without a license.

11
Dedicated to the Health of America?

Resistance to change is likely to reach its peak when significant change is imminent.

—George Leonard

THE STATISTICAL EVIDENCE demonstrating the harmful effects of tobacco is so strong, and so often expressed, that a tobacco industry spokesperson recently said, "Smoking is the leading cause of statistics."

He could be right. According to the Centers for Disease Control, cigarettes kill 434,000 Americans every year.[1] That's more than automobile accidents, fires, alcohol-related deaths, murder, suicide, AIDS, cocaine, and heroin combined.[2]

Cigarettes cause lung cancer. They also cause heart disease, emphysema, bronchitis, miscarriages, and cancer of the uterus, cervix, mouth, esophagus, bladder, kidney, and pancreas.[3]

You don't even have to smoke. Secondhand smoke causes 50,000 deaths among nonsmokers each year in the United States.[4] It also aggravates a million cases of asthma, and creates 25,000 new ones.[5] Tobacco kills more *nonsmokers* each year than die from AIDS, illegal drugs, and teenage drinking combined.[6]

The children of smokers have far more asthma and other respiratory diseases than those of nonsmokers. Babies born to smoking mothers have more than double the risk of dying of sudden infant death syndrome.[7] Smoking in pregnancy is the primary cause of low-birth-weight babies, who have a much higher death rate than normal-weight babies.[8] And smokers have a miscarriage rate that is twice as high as nonsmokers.[9]

The tobacco industry says smoking is a personal choice, an adult habit, an issue of individual freedom.

Others say it is an addiction, pointing to the fact that every year 20 million Americans try to stop smoking, and only 3 percent have long-term success.[10] Even among smokers who have lost a lung to cancer or undergone major cardiovascular surgery, only half can manage to stop smoking for more than a few weeks.[11]

No wonder former Surgeon General Dr. C. Everett Koop said: "Cigarette smoking is the chief, single, avoidable cause of death in our society and the most important public health issue of our time."

WE'VE KNOWN FOR A WHILE

The evidence proving that cigarettes kill has been around for quite a while. In 1925, cigarette "tar" was shown to cause cancer.[12] In 1938, a professor of biology at Johns Hopkins Medical School presented a major study to the New York Academy of Medicine, showing that smoking reduces life expectancy. He found that even moderate smokers died younger than nonsmokers, and that the more people smoked, the shorter their lives.[13] His study caused quite a stir. *Time* magazine reported it was enough to "make tobacco users' flesh creep."[14]

In 1941, the *Reader's Digest* began a long history of standing up to the tobacco industry (for many years they were the only major U.S. magazine that did not accept tobacco advertising) by publishing former heavyweight boxing champion Gene Tunney's emotional article titled: "Nicotine Knockout."[15]

As Wolinsky and Brune have shown clearly in *The Serpent on the Staff*, the AMA was far from eager to inform people of the dangers of smoking. Instead, the AMA *Journal* continued to regularly run cigarette ads, and the AMA even helped develop advertising campaigns that implied cigarettes were endorsed by physicians.[16]

"More doctors smoke Camels than any other cigarette," trumpeted one ad. Another popular brand, L&M cigarettes, said it was "just what the doctor ordered." Philip Morris joined in the chorus, saying that its cigarettes were "recognized by eminent medical authorities."

The eminent medical authorities at the AMA saw no problem with these and other ads presenting smoking as a healthy thing to do. Some of the most popular ads implied that you should smoke, if for no other reason, for your health's sake. "For Digestion's Sake, Smoke Camels," said one ad brightly, adding that cigarettes would "stimulate the flow of digestive fluids." Another company's ad appealed to people's desire to be healthy by proclaiming: "Chesterfield Is Best for You."

Former Senator Maurine B. Neuberger (D-Ore.) sensed what was happening. "The cigarette smoker," he said, "could have been forgiven for confusing his favorite brand of cigarettes with the latest wonder drug."[17]

THE AMA AND THE TOBACCO INDUSTRY— A SPECIAL RELATIONSHIP, INDEED

Meanwhile, Dr. Morris Fishbein, editor of the AMA *Journal* for a quarter century, and the single individual most identified with the organization throughout its history, was helping Philip Morris design a sales strategy to target doctors. The company wanted to promote one of the chemicals that it added to its cigarettes, diethylene glycol, as providing a health benefit.

Following Morris Fishbein's instructions, company scientists poured diethylene glycol into rabbits' eyes, and found that the damage was less than occurred when they poured another chemical additive, used by other cigarette companies, into the creatures' eyes.[18] Based upon this master-piece of comprehensive scientific inquiry, Philip Morris then turned around and, with Dr. Fishbein's blessing, used this research as the basis for ad campaigns that ran regularly in the AMA *Journal* and other medical journals for nearly 20 years. The ads offered doctors free packs of Philip Morris cigarettes; and the company sent representatives to doctors' offices to give them free samples and talk to them about the health advantages of the company's products.[19]

The campaign was a great success, propelling Philip Morris on its way to eventually becoming the largest producer of cigarettes in the world. As a token of their gratitude, the company offered Fishbein an annual retainer, having in mind a modest amount that happened to be greater than Fishbein's annual AMA salary.[20]

When more than 100 people were killed because a new antibiotic was contaminated, and it was discovered that it was none other than diethylene glycol that had been the culprit, Fishbein found another way to be helpful. The AMA *Journal* quickly ran an editorial reassuring everyone that the chemical was perfectly safe as an ingredient in cigarettes.[21]

In 1950, it was learned that no less than 96.5 percent of patients with lung cancer had been smokers.[22] In 1957, Surgeon General Dr. Leroy Burney told a major televised news conference that the evidence was conclusive and irrefutable: Cigarettes caused lung cancer. In the face of information like this, some smokers were getting worried. But to Philip Morris, the health concerns about smoking were simply another opportunity to promote their brands. Diethylene glycol, trumpeted the company's ads, "took the fear out of smoking."[23]

About this time, the *Reader's Digest* began running a powerful series of articles on the dangers of smoking. One outstanding piece was titled "Cancer by the Carton." Another article revealed how little protection was afforded by filters. The tar and nicotine levels for filtered Pall Mall, Chesterfield, and Lucky Strike were actually higher than the unfiltered versions of the same brands.[24]

The AMA *Journal* responded with a small study on the effectiveness of cigarette filters. None of them were found to do much good, but the benefits from one type, the Kent Micronite filter, were not quite as negligible as the others.[25]

The P. Lorillard Company, manufacturer of Kent cigarettes, knew an opportunity when presented with one. The company sent letters to every physician in America, telling them Micronite filters offered "health protection," and suggesting doctors prescribe these cigarettes to smokers with sore throats or other problems from smoking. Enclosed with the letters, of course, were free samples.

Lorillard milked its connection with the AMA for all it was worth, running ads in the AMA *Journal* and presenting displays and exhibits at the AMA convention. At the same time, the company ran ads in *Life*, *Time*, and other popular magazines, declaring that, according to AMA tests, "Kent offers the greatest health protection in cigarette history."[26]

At this point, everybody started complaining to the AMA. Physicians didn't like the organization appearing to endorse a particular brand. Other cigarette companies threatened to pull their ads from the AMA *Journal*. And pharmaceutical companies were worried that the cigarette ads would discredit the drug ads they ran in the *Journal*. Under increasing pressure, the AMA tried to distance itself from the Kent ad campaign, printing an editorial criticizing what it called an unacceptable "commercial exploitation of the American medical profession."[27]

But it wasn't as easy as the AMA would have liked to disentangle themselves. For it had been none other than Dr. Morris Fishbein who had helped design the experiments that were the basis for the advertising campaign. Fishbein, meanwhile, was receiving a retainer as a "research consultant" to Lorillard that was only slightly smaller than the salary of the president of the United States.[28]

The P. Lorillard Company continued to run ads based on the AMA study. Further, they boasted that the substance from which their Micronite filters were made was a "pure, dust-free, completely harmless material that is so safe, so effective, it is actually used to help filter the air in hospital operating rooms."[29] Very few smokers knew that the primary ingredient in Micronite was asbestos—a poisonous substance that researchers had already linked with a host of serious respiratory diseases, including lung cancer. And neither the P. Lorillard Company, nor the AMA, bothered to tell them.

THE SURGEON GENERAL TAKES A STAND

In late 1963, the AMA learned that Surgeon General Dr. Luther Terry was preparing to release a landmark report that would forever change America's relationship to tobacco. The surgeon general, along with virtually every other health group in the country, had by now become convinced that smoking not only caused lung cancer, but heart disease and emphysema, and was costing the country tens of billions of dollars a year in health-care costs.

In early January 1964, AMA president Edward R. Annis warned the state legislature in Kentucky of what lay ahead. He said that the federal government would soon be presenting "insurmountable evidence that smoking causes cancer." But he was quick to reassure the legislators of this tobacco-growing state: "The AMA is not opposed to smoking and tobacco."[30]

On January 11, 1964, the surgeon general released his report. He considered it so potent that he deliberately presented it on a Saturday, when the stock market was closed.

It was indeed a blockbuster, stating that the health damage from tobacco was so enormous that warning labels on cigarettes and control of cigarette advertising should be federally mandated. The American Cancer Society said the report "produced shock waves" throughout the country.[31]

The tobacco companies, however, predictably argued that there was not enough evidence and more research was needed. And guess who joined them in throwing cold water on the surgeon general? None other than AMA president Annis, who insisted that more research was needed to discover "how tobacco smoke affects health." Accordingly, he said, the AMA was launching a study to determine "whether" smoking caused disease.[32]

Launch it they did, but not quite the way one might expect of an organization that called itself "The Voice of American Medicine." The AMA put $500,000 of its own money into the hopper, and a few weeks later, on February 7, 1964, the six major tobacco companies chipped in a few more dollars, ten million of them to be exact.[33] **The study was named the American Medical Association Education and Research Foundation (AMA-ERF) study, and the AMA pointed to it for more than a decade as proof that the organization was working on the tobacco issue. The study just happened to be more than 95 percent funded by tobacco companies.**

When some physicians complained that it didn't look all that good for the AMA to be accepting $10 million from the tobacco industry less than a month after the surgeon general's report, the organization decided this was a fine time to launch an educational campaign. In May 1964 the AMA published a six-page brochure titled *Smoking: Facts You Should Know*.[34] The booklet, however, was a little short on what anticancer activists might have wanted. It did warn of the dangers of burns from smoking in bed, and about the damage cigarettes could do to sofas, rugs, and clothing. But as far as other health hazards, the best it could do was to mention that some researchers were of the opinion that smoking "shortens life expectancy" and that smoking was "alleged to cause cancer of the lungs and bladder." The AMA's consumer education booklet reminded its readers not to get carried away with all this, because after all, "some equally competent physicians and research personnel are less sure of the effect of cigarette smoking on health." Its conclusion? "Smoke if you feel you should, but be moderate."[35]

The tobacco companies were evidently not terribly unhappy with the AMA brochure. They soon contributed another $8 million to the ongoing AMA-ERF research study.[36]

The American Cancer Society, the Public Health Service, and many physician groups had by this time almost grown hoarse calling for health warnings on cigarette packages. When the Federal Trade Commission finally agreed to move in that direction, however, it found its way blocked by none other than the AMA. FTC commissioner A. Everett MacIntyre was horrified. "Thousands of doctors and many individual medical societies favor the proposed warnings" he declared, "but the AMA . . . [says] there is no further need for educational statements to the youth. This is precisely the position of the tobacco industry."[37]

The FTC commissioner wasn't the only one who was outraged. Dr. Alton Ochsner, an eminent chest surgeon from Tulane University School of Medicine and one of the world's leading authorities on smoking and cancer, made headlines when he accused the AMA of being "derelict" as a health leader.[38]

The pressure on the AMA to explain its opposition to the health warnings was mounting. The media was demanding an explanation. The time had come for AMA president F. J. L. Blasingame to speak out. He rose to the occasion, but his remarks were not widely seen as the battle cry of the ultimate antitobacco warrior. "It seems to me," he announced, "that Dr. Ochsner and those who share his opinion are really advocating that an agency of the federal government be granted the power to destroy an $8 billion industry on the extreme theory that the American people need to be protected from themselves in the matter of smoking."[39]

THE AMA'S INVESTMENT IN TOBACCO

Why, you might ask, was the AMA being so relentlessly spineless? The answer, according to almost all observers, was that they wanted the votes of congresspeople from the tobacco states on issues that affected their pocketbooks. Nationally syndicated columnists Drew Pearson and Jack Anderson explained: "The doctors were more concerned about Medicare, which they fancied to be a threat to their fees, than about the threat to the nation's lungs."[40]

Of course, the AMA denied that anything of the kind was happening. But the man who was president of the AMA in 1981–1982, Dr. Daniel T. Cloud, later admitted the truth. There was, he acknowledged, "a tacit understanding . . . between the tobacco-state lawmakers and the AMA that the AMA would lay off, if the tobacco people would support us in the fight against the government. . . . We did have support [from the southern states] and we got the support because of our laying off the tobacco issue."[41]

And what ever happened to the AMA-ERF study to which the tobacco companies had been so exceedingly generous? Well, for more than a decade the AMA just kept saying things weren't conclusive yet, and more research was needed. The tobacco companies understood the message. On cue, they would pitch in more money.

That way, everyone was kept happy. The AMA had funds and the votes of the tobacco-state congresspeople to help them fend off proposals for national health insurance; the researchers had employment; and the tobacco companies had the AMA's silence.

On the other hand, millions of Americans were dying of lung cancer.

The situation couldn't last forever. In 1978, some 14 years after the study had begun, the AMA learned that the surgeon general was once again preparing to present a devastating report on tobacco that would not only confirm the 1964 report, but go further yet in describing it as a health menace. Concerned about being caught with its pants down, the AMA quietly released the concluding report of the AMA-ERF study. It said only that not much had been found to "alter the conclusions of the 1964 report of the surgeon general."[42]

Shortly thereafter the surgeon general's 1979 report indeed came forth, and in dramatic contrast to the AMA-ERF tobacco-funded report, said that cigarettes were even more hazardous than had been thought in 1964. In the report's introduction, Health Secretary Joseph Califano wrote that the report "demolishes the claims made by cigarette manufacturers and a few others 15 years ago that the scientific evidence was sketchy, that no link between smoking and cancer was 'proven.' These claims, empty then, are utterly vacuous now."[43]

As a result of the new surgeon general's report, Congress found itself considering no less than 12 different bills aimed at reducing smoking. When AMA student delegates, led by Ronald M. Davis, discovered that the AMA had not testified or even written a single letter in support of any of the bills, they presented a resolution at the AMA annual meeting calling for the organization to lobby actively for antismoking bills. But the AMA did not greet the students' proposal all that warmly. Its reference committee said that the AMA had "already done its bit to fight tobacco."[44]

The AMA evidently thought it acceptable that, at that time, 30 percent of the American public did not know that smoking shortened life expectancy, and almost 60 percent did not know that smoking was connected to emphysema.[45]

But the AMA was coming under increasing pressure from many physicians to change its ways. Alan Blum, M.D., founded an activist antismoking group of doctors and medical students, "Doctors Ought to Care (DOC)," which pioneered the use of ads to undermine tobacco ads. When a cigarette company put up billboards in Houston advertising Dakota cigarettes, Dr. Blum's group came back with ads that read: "Dakota, DaCough, DaCancer, DaCoffin." When the Virginia Slims tennis tournament was gaining notoriety, they made public appearances, calling the tournament "Emphysema Slims." And as the Philip Morris "Marlboro" van traveled around the country making smoking seem cool, Doctors Ought to Care came along in their own "Barfboro" van, telling the not-so-cool truth about tobacco.

Now Dr. Blum learned that the AMA's Member Retirement Fund owned $1.4 million in tobacco securities. He tried to get the AMA to divest, but AMA president James H. Sammons argued that the point of the investments was to make money, and it was not appropriate for the AMA to "inject itself into the investment field" by telling its fund managers what stocks to buy.[46] Infuriated, Blum went public with the fact that the AMA, supposedly dedicated to protecting the public health, had invested its members' financial security in tobacco stocks. Replying on behalf of the AMA, Dr. John J. Coury, chairman of the AMA Board's Finance Committee, explained that the purpose of the retirement fund was "to make the biggest buck," not to make a social statement.[47] Newspapers had a field day with this. A 1981 editorial cartoon showed a doctor speaking to a patient about smoking. "I can't say this strongly enough. . . . If your cigarettes are made by anybody other than Philip Morris or Reynolds Industries, you've got to stop smoking!"[48]

The publicity was embarrassing for the AMA. Observers agreed that its decision to quietly sell the tobacco stock did not stem from an upsurge of ethical conscience prompted by the controversy, but rather from the awareness that they were being presented in the media as a laughingstock.

If the AMA had realized that its position on tobacco was a betrayal of the public trust, it was not particularly apparent. In 1983, *Newsweek* published a special supplement on personal health that the AMA had written for the occasion. The stated goal was to "help [readers] avoid self-induced illnesses," but the supplement never even mentioned the health hazards of tobacco. The only reference to smoking was: "If you smoke, you should discuss the risks with your doctor."[49]

The AMA's public relations difficulties continued when, in 1985, Howard Wolinsky of the *Chicago Sun-Times* disclosed that two AMA Board members, including the AMA's president-elect, Dr. Harrison L. Rogers, owned a farm on which tobacco was grown.[50] The AMA management defended the officers' right to invest as they pleased, but newspapers once again had a field day, and the whole thing became so embarrassing that Rogers sold his portion of the farm rather than put up with it anymore.

The person who bought it from him, however, was another AMA Board member, Dr. F. William Dowda.[51]

It was evidently a little difficult for these gentlemen to understand why they were being ridiculed. At the time, when AMA officials were in Washington they would stay at a posh townhouse in Georgetown owned by the AMA (the Needham House), where their favorite cigarette brands were always available on the house. And at AMA headquarters in Chicago, cigarettes had always been available from vending machines in the lobbies and bathrooms.

TURNING OVER A NEW (TOBACCO) LEAF

Today, the AMA likes to say that all that is history, and it is true that in the last few years the AMA has finally begun to speak out against tobacco, and to pass various resolutions calling for measures to combat smoking. But when push has come to shove on tobacco issues in Congress, the AMA has not contributed much to the fight.

In 1989, the Durbin bill was passed, effectively banning smoking on almost all commercial domestic airplane flights. The AMA claimed credit for the legislation, and sent out letters boasting about the role it had played. But the lobbyists who had fought for the bill did not see it quite that way. Congressman Richard J. Durbin graciously thanked the Association of Flight Attendants for playing an active role in the victory, and also a number of other groups. How about the AMA? "There was no evidence," he said, "of any strong support for our effort from the American Medical Association."[52]

After smoking was banned on airflights, Congress began considering H.R. 5041, the most comprehensive bill in U.S. history to fight smoking. It was a bill with real teeth, and it stood a good chance of passage. Called the Tobacco Control and Health Protection Act, it terrified the tobacco industry and would have greatly reduced the advertising and promotion of cigarettes. Cigarettes are the most heavily advertised consumer product in the United States. The tobacco companies spend $11 million a *day* to promote cigarettes. That is more than the U.S. Federal Office on Smoking and Health spends to prevent smoking in an entire year.

When it became clear that the vote was going to be very close, the activists who were fighting for the bill realized that one particular congressperson, J. Roy Rowland, M.D., was poised to play a crucial role. One of only two physicians in Congress, he was a great friend of the AMA, and regularly the recipient of major financial donations from AMPAC, the AMA's lobbying arm. Aware of what was at stake, the antismoking activists went to the AMA, and pleaded for help in getting Rowland's support for the bill.[53]

The AMA smiled and promised they'd help, but Dr. Rowland ended up playing a key role in the bill's narrow defeat. According to medical journalists Howard Wolinsky and Tom Brune: "When the subcommittee voted on the proposed advertising and promotion ban in September, 1990, Rowland was involved in maneuvers to cripple and then euthanize the legislation."[54]

The American Lung Association, appalled by Dr. Rowland's activities, expressed their opinion of his behavior in no uncertain terms: "Dr. Rowland has consistently championed the interests of the tobacco industry. He has actively opposed measures designed to protect children from tobacco addiction and even voted against legislation to eliminate smoking on airplanes."[55]

The AMA, however, did not seem to mind. Each year it bestows the Nathan Davis awards, named for the AMA's founder, for outstanding contributions to the betterment of public health. In recent years it has gone to people like Dr. C. Everett Koop. In 1993, however, shortly after Rowland helped sabotage what would have been the most important piece of antismoking legislation in American history, the AMA saw fit to present him with this prestigious award.

Subsequent years did not find the AMA seeking to distance itself from Dr. Rowland. In fact, when the Nathan Davis awards were presented in 1996, the panel of judges deciding who received the awards included the AMA's president and executive vice president—and Dr. J. Roy Rowland.

THE AMA AND TOBACCO —
WHAT'S CHANGED AND WHAT HASN'T

The AMA knows that it is now to its advantage to project a public image of deep concern over the tobacco issue. In 1993, the organization ran a major ad in the *Washington Post*, with a headline that included the statement, "Stopping Tobacco Deaths Is Our First Priority."[56] The ad listed a toll-free number to call for more information. When physicians called the number, however, their call was answered by an employee in the AMA's membership-recruitment office who knew nothing about any plans to fight tobacco.[57]

There are signs, however, that the AMA is finally beginning to take antitobacco stands. Most significantly, in July 1995 the AMA *Journal* ran an article analyzing Brown and Williamson Tobacco Corporation internal documents that had been anonymously sent to Dr. Stanton A. Glantz of the Institute for Health Policy Studies at the University of California, San Francisco.[58] The documents indicated that as early as the 1960s, Brown and Williamson had proven in its own labs that cigarettes are addictive and cause cancer, and yet the company deliberately chose to ignore the evidence and to claim publicly that cigarettes were neither dangerous nor addictive. The article, written by Glantz, was powerful. It labeled the cigarette "a drug-delivery vehicle," called for the elimination of tobacco advertising, and for withholding federal funds from cancer research organizations that accept money from the tobacco industry. An accompanying editorial said that the AMA's Board of Trustees joined the journal's editors in taking the stand.

There is no doubt that, of late, the AMA has become more antitobacco than it was only a few years ago. In May 1996, the organization called on all investors to divest themselves of tobacco stocks, and on all the mutual funds traded in the U.S. to do likewise. But I will believe the AMA is seriously committed to fighting tobacco when it finally begins to lobby effectively for higher taxes on cigarettes. And when its political action committee (AMPAC) stops giving money to people in Congress who support the tobacco industry. To date, this has not occurred.

This last point deserves some elaboration. In 1994, the *New England Journal of Medicine* published a special article analyzing the campaign contributions made by the AMA to congressional candidates between 1989 and 1992.[59] The study sought to determine whether the AMA had given more money to legislators supporting or opposing tobacco export promotion.

Under pressure from tobacco lobbyists, U.S. trade representatives had helped to force open the markets of Japan, South Korea, Taiwan, Thailand, and other countries for U.S. tobacco companies, protesting these countries' antismoking health measures as unfair barriers to trade. The result had been a tremendous rise in tobacco use in these and similar countries, especially among young people. The year after Korea was forced to lift import restrictions on U.S. made cigarettes, smoking among teenage girls rose by more than 300 percent.[60]

The United States Has One of the Lowest Cigarette Taxes in the Developed World.

Average Tax Per Pack of Cigarettes

Norway	$3.93
Denmark	$3.64
Canada	$3.25
England/Wales	$3.09
Ireland	$2.84
New Zealand	$2.02
Germany	$1.95
Belgium	$1.67
Hong Kong	$1.45
Holland	$1.30
France	$1.29
Italy	$1.12
Luxembourg	$1.01
Japan	$0.95
Portugal	$0.80
Greece	$0.53
UNITED STATES	$0.51

Source: WorldWatch,
Sept.–Oct. 1992, 5(5), 9.

Cigarette taxes not only raise money, they also reduce smoking, and thus health-care costs. In New Zealand, when the price of a pack of cigarettes nearly doubled between 1980 and 1991 due to a tax increase of $1.97, cigarette consumption dropped more than 60%. The United Kingdom achieved similar reductions in smoking rates through cigarette tax hikes until 1987, when it reversed itself and lowered taxes. Between 1987 and 1990, the country cut cigarette taxes 15%, with the result that smoking rates rose 25% among teenagers.

The activities of American tobacco companies in these countries can seem a little excessive. In Taiwan, RJR Nabisco organized a rock concert with a local teen idol. The only acceptable "ticket" for admittance was five empty packs of Winstons.[61] At a high school in Buenos Aires, a woman wearing safari gear and driving a Jeep with a yellow Camel logo passed out free cigarettes to 15- and 16-year-olds at their lunch recess.[62]

The 1994 *New England Journal of Medicine* study found that the AMA "gave significantly larger average contributions to House members who favored tobacco-export promotion than to those who opposed it."[63]

In 1995, Representative Thomas J. Bliley, Jr., of Virginia became the new head of the Health and Environment subcommittee. A pro-tobacco mortician, Bliley was now uniquely placed to uphold his pledge to end

Congress's investigation of the tobacco industry. As he put it, "I don't think we need any more legislation regulating tobacco."[64] A systematic analysis of the money AMPAC had invested in the 1995 Congress revealed that Bliley was a highly favored recipient of AMA money, receiving more funds than 92 percent of the other legislators. Even as Bliley was being called "the congressman from Philip Morris," the AMA was continuing to make direct contributions totaling more than $50,000 to his campaigns.[65]

NOT A LOT OF CREDIBILITY LEFT

What, I've wondered, do AMA members think about all this? Do the 275,000 physicians who belong to the AMA feel well represented? Do they think that their annual dues of $420, and the organization's annual budget of $180 million, are being well spent?

When an AMA official introduced First Lady Hillary Clinton to an AMA meeting, he stated that the organization represented 100 percent of American patients. But on virtually every social issue of significance to public health, it is hard to avoid the impression that the AMA functions more as a trade lobby seeking financial advantage than as a guardian of the common good. When criticized for owning tobacco stock, the AMA said it was not trying to make a social statement with its investments. Frankly, I don't see much evidence that the organization has ever tried to make much of a social statement anywhere, except, of course, for public relations purposes. When it comes to issues of social responsibility, the AMA seems to be more or less permanently out to lunch.

In its defense, the AMA points to programs such as the one it produced in 1992 for CNBC, dealing with diet and cholesterol. But the program was funded by the National Livestock and Meat Board, the Beef Board, and the Pork Board.[66] The AMA also points to its recent educational programs on alcohol. But these were funded by $600,000 from the liquor industry.[67]

There was once a time when I thought of the AMA as a reliable authority to which we could look for medical guidance. I thought they were a group of medical elders who looked after us and saw to our welfare. There was a time when I believed them when they said they were protecting us from charlatans and snake oil salespeople. Their name, the American Medical Association, gave them a ring of authority, and made me think they were here to serve the people of this country. I once assumed, in fact, that they were some kind of governmental organization.

But now that innocence is gone. It is hard to give the AMA credibility, when the organization so often seems more devoted to the elimination of its competition and the advancement of its members' financial interests than to serving the health of the American people.

It is hard not to feel betrayed.

OTHER VOICES

Fortunately, there are other voices in medicine, including those of the many physicians who are motivated by the desire to relieve suffering and help people.

In 1988, the people of California made it clear that they wanted to see smoking decrease by passing Proposition 99 to fund smoking prevention programs, particularly for children and teenagers. (The average new smoker is an 11-year-old girl.)

Due to the efforts of the California Medical Association, however, more than $100 million of the money was diverted to experiments intending to determine "whether" tobacco is really addictive and harmful. How did researchers ever expect to achieve such a radical breakthrough in scientific understanding? By spending $418,000 to determine the effect of tobacco smoke on the lining of rats' lungs; by addicting primates to tobacco smoke and watching them develop bronchitis; and by spending $333,000 to study racial differences in menthol cigarette selection.[68]

Not all physicians were impressed with the overwhelming necessity for such research. Members of a group called Physicians' Committee for Responsible Medicine campaigned to redirect the money, and succeeded in reducing the future budget for such experiments by more than 80 percent, thus making more of the money available for its intended purposes.

In 1995, this same group published a stunning analysis of the health costs from tobacco and meat consumption in the peer-reviewed journal *Preventive Medicine.* Their conclusion? "The combined medical costs attributable to smoking and meat consumption exceed the predicted costs of providing health coverage for all currently uninsured Americans." Not surprisingly, an AMA spokesperson said he had "very serious reservations" about the report.[69]

Over the years, other physicians' organizations have also come forth to speak as the conscience of American medicine. Recognizing the extraordinary power that is bestowed on the medical profession by the American people, they have called for this trust to be used to improve health and quality of life for all members of society.

In a historic 1962 issue of the *New England Journal of Medicine*, three of the founders of Physicians for Social Responsibility openly discussed the hideous medical consequences of a nuclear attack on the United States, and the role of physicians in a postattack aftermath. Exposing the horrors that would ensue from a nuclear war, they made people aware of the critical importance of preventing such a war. Over the years thereafter, the organization emphasized that if nuclear war were to be prevented, physicians would have to play a crucial role. Year after year, in city after city, they educated and mobilized the medical community.

It was after one of the organization's conferences on the medical consequences of nuclear war that the videographers and social activists Ian and Eric Thiermann created the monumental documentary film *The Last Epidemic*. This film enabled millions of people to see that a nuclear war would not simply be a more powerful kind of war than had existed previously, but an entirely new situation in which the survivors would literally envy the dead. Immensely motivating, the documentary activated large segments of society to take action to prevent nuclear war from ever occurring.

Meanwhile, Physicians for Social Responsibility was continuing to document the devastating health and environmental risks of open-air nuclear testing. By exposing the increasing presence of strontium-90 in children's teeth, a by-product of nuclear testing, the organization helped stop U.S. atmospheric testing and achieve a Limited Test Ban Treaty.

Since that victory, Physicians for Social Responsibility has continued to work to protect the public from the health hazards of weapons of mass destruction and environmental poisons. Recently, for example, the organization exposed and publicized the health and environmental problems stemming from the activities of America's worst polluter—the military. Pointing out that the armed forces have produced vast amounts of toxic and radioactive waste, and are exempt from most federal environmental laws and regulations, Physicians for Social Responsibility won the public release of secret government data on radioactive emissions and other toxic substances at 2,000 military bases across the country. Thanks to the work of these dedicated doctors, environmental officials are now able to levy fines against military violators.

And yet the group has also been doing something that may in the long run actually be even more important than getting the military to clean up its activities and reduce its pollution. Physicians for Social Responsibility has undertaken a sustained effort to create a world where greater peace prevails, a world where fewer resources are needed for military activities, and where more are devoted to enhancing life and health for all people.

While the AMA has been waging its war on midwifery, the chiropractic profession, and many other alternative modes of healing, and has busied itself befriending the tobacco industry, Physicians for Social Responsibility has been accountable to the public good. Though comparatively small in size, the group has been educating medical professionals, legislators, and the public about environmental health hazards and solutions. It has been working for the peace, safety, and health of the whole earth community. It has been undertaking projects to reduce the level of violence in people's lives, and sponsoring creative ways of managing conflict at the level of the family, the nation, and the global community.

The world community has recognized the work of this outstanding organization. In 1985, as the U.S. affiliate of International Physicians for the Prevention of Nuclear War (a network of 200,000 physicians in 80 countries), Physicians for Social Responsibility shared in winning the Nobel Peace Prize.

TIME FOR A CHANGE

Although it is still true that no other group in health care can come close to matching the AMA in terms of its economic clout, or in terms of its influence over policy makers, increasing numbers of U.S. doctors are speaking out against the AMA's self-serving performance. They know that with power comes responsibility. They are tired of watching the AMA squelch alternatives, and tired of watching this organization wield its enormous budget in the pursuit of selfish, greedy, and even ruthless purposes. Though most doctors are not fully aware of the extent to which the organization has betrayed the public trust, many of them sense that there is something slimy going on. The number of American doctors who pay full dues to the AMA has been shrinking rapidly, and is now less than half of what it was only 20 years ago.

Across the country, not only doctors, but also legislators and millions of other citizens are realizing that the most prominent voice in medicine has not lived up to its social responsibility. People are sick of the greed and patriarchal closed-mindedness that have tainted medicine. They know the American people place a sacred trust in their physicians, and deserve better.

At the same time, the American people are becoming increasingly dissatisfied with the care they receive from physicians who know little about prevention, and who rely primarily on expensive medical technology and writing prescriptions for drugs. Many doctors, in turn, are becoming equally frustrated because that's all they have been trained to do, and in many cases that's about all they are allowed to do according to the strict "standards of care" established by state medical boards.

The level of indignation in America is surging. Increasing numbers of people are calling for an end to the monopolization of American medicine, and for the creation of a medical system that includes the alternative and drugless modes of healing in a true partnership.

On December 14, 1993, U.S. Congressperson Berkley Bedell delivered a series of stirring remarks to the New York State Assembly that served as a rallying cry in the struggle for freedom of health care. He had contracted Lyme disease, and spent $26,000 and many months pursuing pharmaceutical treatments. Strong antibiotics had been injected into his veins every day for periods of three, four, and six weeks. But that hadn't worked, and he had eventually been forced to try an alternative approach, which to his surprise had brought him complete healing. The congressperson had also been diagnosed with prostate cancer. In this case, too, he went the conventional route, this time spending over $10,000 and undergoing radiation, but the cancer had returned. Justifiably fearing for his life, he underwent an unconventional approach that was shunned by the AMA and the American Cancer Society. "That was four years ago," he told the Assembly, "and all tests indicate that I no longer have cancer."

Congressman Bedell did not blame doctors for believing that everything except pharmaceutical drug treatments was quackery. That, he explained, is the only point of view they receive. "At medical school, students are taught to use pharmaceutical drugs. For continuing education, doctors go to seminars put on by pharmaceutical companies. Salespeople from pharmaceutical firms are constantly calling on doctors to inform them about new pharmaceutical drugs, and give out free samples. Medical journals depend upon advertising revenues from pharmaceutical companies, and their editorial content reflects that fact. And colleges and universities get grants from pharmaceutical firms for research on drugs. . . . But the sad fact is that whereas pharmaceutical drugs such as antibiotics are very effective for some communicable infectious diseases, they have not proven to be similarly effective for degenerative diseases."

As a young man, Congressperson Bedell had, with $50 saved from his newspaper route, started a fishing tackle manufacturing business. Over the years, it had become one of the world's largest fishing tackle manufacturers. "As a businessman," he continued, "I grade the international pharmaceutical industry with an A+ for . . . marketing, and a D for performance of product for major degenerative diseases. . . . If one has a product that is not very effective, it is greatly in your interest to keep everything else out of the market. The problem is, in this case, we are not talking about fishing lines or golf clubs. We are talking about people's health."

Bedell's historic speech drove to a prophetic climax: "Make no mistake, there is a worldwide battle going on. It is whether the international pharmaceutical drug industry is going to be successful in maintaining a monopoly and preventing the use of lower-cost, nontoxic treatments. . . . There is a growing army of angry people who are demanding a greater say in their health care. They have seen the limited effectiveness of conventional treatment for major diseases. In increasing numbers they are demanding the right to be treated by the treatment of their choice."

RECLAIMING OUR FREEDOM OF CHOICE IN HEALTH CARE

The first half of the 1990s saw a series of fierce battles in which the movement for health freedom gained ground. In 1990, despite overwhelming opposition from the Alaska State Medical Association, the state of Alaska enacted the nation's first statutory protection of alternative medicine. In the next four years, the states of Washington, North Carolina, Oklahoma, and New York passed laws designed to protect alternative doctors from prosecution, and to support patients' rights to make unconventional medical choices. And in 1992, the U.S. Congress directed the National Institutes of Health to open the Office of Alternative Medicine.

At the same time, Canada's most populated province, Ontario, was beginning to recognize that many current medical licensing laws are monopolistic. Instead of protecting consumers from fraud and incompetence, as was their original purpose, they more often only protect orthodox medicine from competition. In 1993, Ontario enacted landmark legislation, making consumers in the province now free to seek the health care they desire in the community at large, from whomever they wish, without putting that health care giver at risk of prosecution for "practicing medicine without a license."

As the 1990s rolled along, the movement for health freedom continued to build. In 1995, a bill supporting access to alternative medicine in the state of Oregon passed by a walloping margin of 23–0 in the Senate, and 55–1 in the House. But it still needed the signature of Governor John Kitzhaber. The Oregon Medical Association put tremendous pressure on the governor, himself a physician, to veto the bill, which he did. It appeared that the Oregon Medical Association had defeated the bill. On the last day of the legislative session, only 10 of the 52 bills vetoed by the governor ever reached the floor, and only two were passed. But one was the alternative medical treatment bill, which passed by a staggering 27–2 in the Senate, and 55–4 in the House.

I have noticed a consistent and unusual feature of these legislative efforts — they have almost invariably received bipartisan support. For liberals, the issue is often seen as a matter of civil liberties and consumers' rights. For conservatives, the issue is individual freedom and the creation of a more open medical marketplace with greater competition between health and medical professionals.

In the summer of 1995, Senator Thomas A. Daschle and Congressperson Peter DeFazio introduced the Access to Medical Treatment Act to the U.S. Congress (S 1035/HR 2019). With an identical number of Republicans and Democrats as original cosponsors, this landmark bill sought to give Americans the right to be treated by alternative practitioners if they should so desire. The bill's supporters believed that the choice of medical treatments should be left to the person involved, rather than mandated by the government.

In 1996, former Surgeon General C. Everett Koop, M.D., was developing an alternative medicine center at Dartmouth College in Hanover, New Hampshire.

That same year, the state of Washington began requiring health insurance to cover acupuncture, massage therapy, and other alternative forms of licensed health care. Meanwhile, the King County Council of Washington State established the nation's first government-run natural medicine clinic. Kent Pullen, the chairperson of the council, which governs the most populous county in the Pacific Northwest, spoke proudly of this landmark event for health freedom and alternative medicine: "A program such as this, where natural medicine is integrated with conventional medicine, maximizes treatment options and gives patients more opportunity to prevent illness and achieve high-quality health care."

With each passing month, the campaign for self-determination in health care continues to awaken the conscience of more Americans. The public is sick of living under a medical monopoly, and growing ever less comfortable with the idea of the doctor as dictator. They are calling for a new role—the doctor as collaborator.

There is still an awfully long way to go, but as the value of alternatives is becoming increasingly recognized, the holistic health explosion is coming to represent one of the most powerful grassroots political movements in American history.

Part Four

12
Must We
Kill to Cure?

*The natural healing force within each one of us is the greatest force
in getting well.*

—Hippocrates

EVERY FORM OF MEDICINE IS A LANGUAGE that bespeaks an entire
philosophy of life. Each path to healing holds assumptions about the
nature of the universe, about the meaning and purpose of the human experience, and about how we ought to live. Representing an entire world-
view, each has its own understanding about health and sickness, about the
appropriate role of health professionals, and about how it is best to respond to
illness. The conventional and the alternative approaches to healing tend
to differ from one another, not only in their practices and techniques, but
also in the belief systems that underlie their activities. They presuppose
fundamentally different outlooks on the nature of birth, life, and death.

**The medical paradigm that currently prevails in our society, and
which the AMA stalwartly represents, has become so deeply entrenched
that we often do not realize that it is simply one option among many.
But there are other forms of medicine that represent different ways of
understanding life and of promoting healing, and that, contrary to what
the dominant medical establishment would have us believe, have
demonstrated outstanding records of success.**

Generally speaking, the alternative approaches seek to enhance recuperative power and immunity, decrease drug reliance, and contribute
to an overall sense of greater well-being and ability to resist disease. They
believe that the human body possesses profound abilities to heal itself, and
that the role of the physician is to support and augment these inherent
capacities.

Although the alternative forms of medicine are each unique, they are characteristically respectful of the body's inner self-correcting mechanisms, seeking to assist the body's natural and spontaneous healing intelligence. They typically have in common the belief that health is the natural state of humanity, and involves being in harmony with ourselves and the natural world. In this vision, all living processes are seen as a mosaic of interconnected relationships and conditions, guided by an underlying wisdom, integrity, and coherence. The human body is viewed as an ecosystem within a greater ecosystem, and the art of healing is seen as bringing the body, mind, and spirit into greater balance and wholeness.

The orthodox medical approach that prevails in our society, on the other hand, operates according to a very different set of assumptions, and proceeds according to a very different set of metaphors. Its underlying belief system is perhaps most fully expressed in what has come to be called the "war on cancer."

The orthodox approach to cancer is based on the idea that the human body is a battlefield and its primary images are drawn from the language of warfare. Cancer cells do not simply multiply, they "invade." The tumor is "the enemy," which we must annihilate, whatever the cost. If in so doing we employ techniques that destroy the quality of our lives and wreak havoc on our immune systems, that's considered, by most American medical authorities, to be an unfortunate but acceptable price to pay. War, after all, involves casualties on both sides.

In seeing medicine as a military enterprise, the conventional cancer treatment community is simply writing large the prevailing philosophy of modern Western medicine. A *Time* cover story on the immune system was typical. Words like *enemies, target, invade, assault, warfare, kill,* and *carnage,* were found in virtually every sentence.

In orthodox medical thinking today, the ill human body is rarely described as mobilizing to repair itself, working to restore balance, or seeking to eliminate accumulated toxins. If you are sick, you are not seen as involved in a potentially transformative experience and your body is not understood as an ally or a friend. Instead, you are described as being "attacked" and your body is a victim that is "under siege." Illness is not a challenge to grow nor an opportunity to heal. It's a war.

When diseases are seen as an attacking enemy, the body which spawns them is seen, in its seeming unpredictability, as an environment that must be subdued and controlled. It is not understood as a guide in the healing process, nor a well-spring of healing potential, but as a continuing source of danger. Disease is not a messenger trying to get your attention, or a life process which can activate your body's self-healing resources. Instead, it is an evil force against which your best hope is to enlist the full powers of organized medical technology. The role of medical care, then, is not to champion your body's self-regulating and self-healing mechanisms. It is to intervene with external agents to obliterate the enemy.

The implication of such battlefield thinking is that if you are ill, it hardly matters what this experience might mean to you personally. There is rarely respect given to the role that emotional intelligence or prayer can play in the healing journey. There is little honoring of the intuitive and receptive modes of being, and barely any appreciation for the contribution these states of mind might make to healing. Your experience of yourself and your feelings about what is happening to you are secondary to the "battle" being waged on your behalf by the heroic warriors of Western medicine, whose goal is to extinguish the disease.

THE WAR ON CANCER—RADIATION

Like the costs of military spending, the costs of fighting cancer are astonishing. Treating a typical cancer patient today runs about $100,000. A bone marrow transplant can cost $150,000. In the United States there are now more people making a living off cancer than dying from it.

Of course, we all want people with cancer to be provided the best treatments available. If the enormous amount of money spent on cancer treatment was actually saving lives and sparing human suffering, then most of us would consider the costs worthwhile. But are people really being helped?

Like most of us, I grew up trusting that physicians would only use procedures that had been proven safe and effective. Knowing that radiation was often used in cancer treatment, for example, I assumed that it must be a procedure that provided valuable aid to the healing process.

But while radiation therapy is given today to about half of all American cancer patients, I have discovered that it is extremely controversial. The reason for the controversy is simple: the procedure has actually been proven to be useful in only a small number of cancers—early Hodgkin's disease, lymphosarcoma, inoperable local prostate cancer, and localized tumors of the head, neck, larynx, and cervix. **With these significant and noteworthy exceptions, the vast majority of studies show that radiation cannot cure cancer, and that it does not usually extend life for people with the disease.**

Consider, for example, the use of radiation in the treatment of breast cancer. Radiation is used routinely following lumpectomies, because it decreases the chance of recurrence in the affected breast. But does it significantly increase overall survival time?[1] Studies published in *Lancet* and elsewhere have questioned whether radiation following breast surgery might increase death rates.[2]

Many radiation oncologists are growing weary of watching their patients die, and tired of hearing that progress is just around the corner. Seymour M. Brenner, M.D., who treats cancer patients with radiation at Peninsula Hospital in Far Rockaway, New York, recently traveled to Washington, D.C., to make a major public statement: "I am a radiation oncologist who treats cancer in New York," he said. "I've been doing it for 39 years. I have a rather successful practice, in that I see 100 to 150 patients a day. My great frustration is that, in 39 years of practicing medicine and treating cancer, I have seen no significant progress."[3]

HOW THIS CAME TO BE

How has it come about, then, that radiation is so frequently used in the "war" on cancer? Part of the answer dates from August 1945, when the U.S. military dropped atomic bombs on the Japanese cities of Hiroshima and Nagasaki. From that moment on, the issue of radioactivity became the center of an intense international debate. As the U.S. military pressed forward with the atmospheric testing of its developing nuclear arsenal, it ran into a rising tide of public opposition. In pursuit of its nuclear goals, the military saw tremendous public relations advantage to be gained from the development of "the peaceful atom."

With no evident medical justification, reports began appearing in the media hailing radiation cancer treatments as "one of the most fantastic events in human history" (*Reader's Digest*), and "The Sunny Side of the Atom" (CBS documentary). As early as 1947, the AMA pitched in with the preposterous claim that "medically applied atomic science has already saved more lives than were lost in the explosions at Hiroshima and Nagasaki."[4]

The chairman of the Atomic Energy Commission, Lewis Strauss, was not completely objective on the subject. "The focusing of the powerful beams of deadly radiation on cancerous growths," he enthused, would be an example of the good use of atomic energy, and would help the nuclear cause.[5] He soon became a member of the Board of Trustees at Memorial Sloan-Kettering Cancer Center.

Memorial Sloan-Kettering (now the world's largest private cancer treatment and research center) was already committed to the use of radiation in cancer treatment. The cancer center had accepted tremendous donations from an immensely wealthy businessman named James Douglas in 1913. But, according to Memorial Sloan-Kettering's former official historian, Bob Considine, "Douglas's enormous gifts came with strings attached."[6] Douglas owned vast numbers of radium mines, and stood to profit enormously if the medical use of radiation caught on. He had insisted, as a basic condition of his contributions, that the center routinely use radiation in all of its cancer treatments.

In defense of the medical community, I must point out that at that time little was known about the risks of radiation. And after World War II, while many scientists were seeking to educate the public about the deadly dangers of radioactivity, the Atomic Energy Commission was busy hiding the evidence, not only from the general public, but also from the medical community. What many thought to be an honest debate comparing the dangers of radiation with its possible medical value was actually rigged. Documents uncovered in recent years reveal that the nuclear advocates deliberately covered up what they knew to be the real dangers of medical radiation and atomic fallout in order to sway public opinion in a pro-nuclear direction.

THE DANGERS ARE REAL

The effort bore fruit. Today, although cancer specialists know that very few cancer patients are cured by radiotherapy, they continue to recommend it widely because they consider it to be a relatively harmless procedure.

But is it? In Goiania, Brazil, a man happened upon an abandoned radiotherapy machine, opened it, and was fascinated by the glowing blue granules he found inside. He and his friends put samples of the pretty material into their pockets to take home. After they began to die, the material was identified as Caesium-137. The men had to be buried in 1,400 pound lead-lined coffins.[7]

Are there dangers to patients from radiation? John Laszlo, M.D., senior vice president of the American Cancer Society, acknowledges that indeed there are: "It is impossible to give radiation treatments without injuring normal cells. . . . Depending on the site treated, large doses of radiation can cause nausea and vomiting, loss of appetite and reduction in bone marrow function."[8]

The radioactivity used to kill cancer cells can cause normal cells to mutate, creating new cancer cells of other types. A number of studies have found that people who undergo radiation therapy are actually more likely to have their cancers spread to other sites in their bodies. Early studies at Memorial Sloan-Kettering Cancer Center actually found that patients who received radiotherapy died sooner than those left untreated.[9]

In the 1970s, Dr. Irwin Bross, director of biostatistics at Roswell Park Memorial Institute in Buffalo, New York, led an important project studying the alarming increase in rates of leukemia. The Tri-State Leukemia Survey, as it was called, used the tumor registries in New York, Maryland, and Minnesota to follow 16 million people.[10] One of Dr. Bross's chief researchers was Rosalie Bertell.

"We looked at just about everything you could think of" in the records of people with leukemia, she recalls. "That included family background, cause of death for parents and grandparents, the person's own health history, complete occupational history, residential history, whether they'd been exposed to farm animals or not, whether they had pets, and whether those pets had ever been sick."[11]

After four years of work, it became disturbingly clear to the research team that the main cause of the rising rates of leukemia was medical radiation, in the form of diagnostic medical X-rays.

The use of radiation in cancer treatment employs high-intensity X-rays. Much higher doses are involved in cancer treatment than in diagnostic X-rays, because the purpose is to kill cells, or at least cripple their ability to reproduce. While a typical diagnostic X-ray might deliver one or two rads (radiation absorbed doses) of radiation, a six-week course of radiotherapy delivers about 5,000 rads.

While dead cells don't themselves become cancerous, there is invariably extensive damage to cells in adjacent tissues and organs, which can then become cancerous. "The cancer danger in radiotherapy," says Bertell, "is at the edge of the beam, where you can't control it."[12]

Dr. Irwin Bross, director of the study, is an eminent researcher who has held prestigious positions at major medical centers including Roswell Park and Johns Hopkins. The results of the Tri-State Leukemia Survey were published in the respected *American Journal of Public Health*. Almost immediately, however, under pressure from the pro-nuclear camp, the National Cancer Institute cut off Dr. Bross's funding, and the research team had to find other work. They also lost permission to use even basic data from the tumor registries, which made it impossible for them to do any further investigation. Their effort, in short, was sabotaged.

In 1979, after the near meltdown at the Three-Mile Island nuclear plant in Pennsylvania, the journal *Science* discussed the controversial termination of Dr. Bross's work in a special article titled "Low-Level Radiation: Just How Bad Is It?" The report concluded that it was difficult to accurately assess the hazards posed by the radiation used in X-rays and cancer therapy because of the political nature of the radiation issue. It was hard to get clarity about the dangers, *Science* noted, because the matter fell within "the domain of the atomic energy establishment."[13]

It is perhaps only from within the nuclear establishment itself that the true dangers of medical radiation can ever be told. Fortunately, in recent years, a few of its most preeminent members have been unwilling to allow the veil of obfuscation to remain in place. They have chosen to speak out, often at the risk of their jobs and careers.

John William Gofman, M.D., is professor emeritus of Molecular and Cell Biology at the University of California at Berkeley, and professor at the University of California School of Medicine in San Francisco. He is the codiscoverer of protactinium-232, uranium-232, protactinium-233, and uranium-233, and proved the slow and fast neutron fissionability of uranium-233. Working under the direction of Manhattan Project head J. Robert Oppenheimer, he was responsible for producing the plutonium-239 that was indispensable to the production of the first atomic bombs.[14]

In the early 1960s, working for the Atomic Energy Commission, John Gofman established the Biomedical Research Division at Lawrence Livermore National Laboratory, for the purpose of evaluating the health effects of all types of nuclear activities. There, he came to the distressing conclusion that human exposure to ionizing radiation was far more serious than had been previously recognized.

Dr. Gofman's work led to his 1995 book *Preventing Breast Cancer*, in which he came to a stunning conclusion: "Our estimate is that about three-quarters of the current annual incidence of breast cancer in the

United States is being caused by earlier ionizing radiation, primarily from medical sources." John Gofman does not underestimate the role in cancer causation played by pesticides, hormone pills, fatty diets, and other environmental stressors. He states: "There is no inherent conflict or competition between carcinogens," because they multiply each other's carcinogenic effects. But he finds the medical use of radiation to be so crucial that it bears repeating: "An estimated 75 percent of recent and current breast-cancer cases would not have occurred as they did, in the absence of earlier medical [and other] irradiation."[15]

Although ionizing radiation, the type delivered by X-rays and radiotherapy, is one of the few environmental contaminants known unequivocally to cause many forms of cancer, it is routinely recommended for many cancer patients. This, despite the fact that, with the few exceptions I noted earlier, there is no proven benefit to survival, and the treatment often causes exhaustion, weakness, and nausea. Doctors are desperate that they are losing the "war" against cancer, and want to do everything they can to fight the disease. Knowing little of radiation's dangers, they figure they'll throw everything they've got into the battle against the dreaded enemy. Patients are frightened and yearn for a magic bullet. The idea of technology riding to the rescue can be enormously appealing.

CHEMOTHERAPY

As with radiation, the use of chemotherapy in cancer treatment is intimately interwoven with the world of warfare. In December 1943, the U.S. battleship *John Harvey* was moored in the harbor of Bari, Italy (the main supply point for the Allied armies in Italy). Unbeknownst even to its crew, the *John Harvey* carried 100 tons of poisonous mustard gas. On the afternoon of December 2, British Air Marshall Sir Arthur Coningham demonstrated the truth of the adage that "pride goeth before the fall." He called a press conference to announce proudly that the Allies now had total air supremacy over southern Italy. That evening, however, a fierce attack by the German Luftwaffe produced the worst seaport disaster for the Allies since Pearl Harbor. The mustard gas was released, and many thousands were killed.[16]

In the aftermath, medical officers noted that sailors who survived the explosion and exposure to the chemical warfare agent suffered from severe depression of their bone marrow and depletion of white blood cells. The idea developed in medical circles of deliberately administering varieties of chemical warfare agents to patients with cancer. These agents kill all the cells in patients' bodies that are dividing at the time of use. Since cancer cells divide rapidly, the hope was that they could be totally destroyed and the cancer annihilated while preserving enough of the more slowly dividing cells of the body to keep the patient alive. Unfortunately, patients treated with these cytotoxic [cell-killing] drugs all tended to have reactions similar to those experienced by victims of chemical warfare.

After World War II, Memorial Sloan-Kettering Cancer Center chose Cornelius P. "Dusty" Rhoads, who had been the head of the U.S. Army Chemical Warfare Service, as its new research director. At Sloan-Kettering, he enthusiastically promoted the testing of 1,500 kinds of nitrogen mustard gas as anticancer agents.[17]

On June 27, 1949, Rhoads and the institute were featured on the cover of *Time* magazine. In 1953, he proclaimed, "Inevitably, as I see it, we can look forward to something like a penicillin for cancer, and I hope within the next decade." With characteristic military fervor, he spoke of the "magic bullet" that would destroy cancer once and for all.

Rhoads was consistently adamant that victory was almost at hand; he could see the light at the end of the tunnel. His words left little room for doubt: "It is no longer a question of if cancer will be controlled, but when and how soon."[18] A *Reader's Digest* article on chemotherapy in 1957 echoed the excitement: "There is, for the first time, a scent of ultimate victory in the air."[19]

All that was needed to win the war, said Rhoads, was "a frontal attack with all our forces."[20]

There were, however, some researchers who were not entirely caught up in the excitement. As the former Memorial Sloan-Kettering Cancer Center science writer and noted cancer author Ralph Moss, Ph.D., remembers, "Some scientists recoiled at the horrendous toxicity. . . . Patients were retching, their hair was falling out, and they were dying from drug-related destruction of their bone marrow."[21]

Undisturbed, the director of the M. D. Anderson Hospital and Tumor Institute in Houston told the U.S. Congress in 1969 that "with a billion dollars for ten years we could lick cancer."[22] In 1971, President Nixon responded by declaring the War on Cancer, and pledging the money.

And a war it was. Doctors spoke of "weapons," "strategies," and the "therapeutic arsenal" of cell-killing drugs. A medical text called oncologists "soldiers on the front lines" with "armor forged for them in medical school."[23]

The 1960s, 1970s, and early 1980s were giddy times for the chemotherapy community. Belief in technology was at an all-time high. The U.S. had put a man on the moon, and the power of antibiotics seemed to suggest that any disease could be conquered if only the right drug were found. Hundreds of billions of dollars were poured into chemotherapy research and treatment. Although patients suffered tremendously, extended remissions were achieved for some forms of childhood cancer, most notably acute lymphocytic leukemia, as well as for cancers that primarily struck adolescents, such as Hodgkin's disease. It became possible to cure a number of childhood cancers that had previously been fatal. Further, chemotherapy contributed to the successful treatment of other rare kinds of cancer, such as Burkitt's lymphoma, choriocarcinoma, lymphosarcoma, Wilms' tumor, and Ewing's sarcoma. There were breakthroughs in the use of chemotherapy for testicular cancer, and promising signs of an ability to at least somewhat prolong life in ovarian cancer. There was widespread belief that with enough money spent on the effort, researchers would eventually discover how to conquer the most common cancers, the solid tumors. Surely, these cancers would be the next to fall. One leading chemotherapy advocate called the effort to defeat cancer with cytotoxic drugs "the greatest mobilization of resources . . . ever undertaken to conquer a single disease."[24]

It was a time of grand hope.

UNFORTUNATELY

But as the years passed by, the successes remained isolated to a few comparatively rare forms of cancer. The hoped-for breakthrough in the "war" against cancer was always "just around the corner," and never really materialized. Tens of billions of dollars were spent on research, and hundreds of billions more on treatment, and yet there was little real improvement in survival rates for the vast majority of cancers. The sober truth was that, for most people with cancer, chemotherapy continued to be a disappointment.

The inescapable fact that researchers could never manage to circumvent was that the amount of chemotherapy necessary to kill every

last cancer cell in a human body was almost invariably lethal to the body itself.

As time went along, the bad news began to be announced in the scientific journals. In 1985, a professor of microbiology at the Harvard University School of Public Health, John Cairns, M.D., published a seminal article on the war on cancer in *Scientific American* in which he showed that chemotherapy was able to save the lives of only 2 to 3 percent of cancer patients. Despite the overwhelming investment the medical community had made in chemotherapy, he said, it was not capable of defeating any of the common cancers.[25]

The next year, John C. Bailar III, M.D., Ph.D., published a landmark study in the *New England Journal of Medicine*. Dr. Bailar was held in extremely high regard in medical circles, as he was the former editor of the *Journal of the National Cancer Institute*, and was now with the Department of Biostatistics at the Harvard School of Public Health. Simply looking long and hard at the data, Dr. Bailar said, had compelled him to lose faith in chemotherapy, and indeed in the entire war on cancer: "Some 35 years of intense and growing efforts to improve the treatment of cancer has not had much overall effect on the most fundamental measure of clinical outcome—death. Overall, the effort to control cancer has failed, so far, to attain its objectives."[26]

These critiques of chemotherapy were not arising from professional critics with axes to grind against the cancer establishment, but from members in good standing who simply could no longer ignore the contrast between the great hopes that had once been held for chemotherapy, and the dismal reality that had so far come to pass.

In 1990, another ranking member of the cancer establishment, Dr. Ulrich Abel, biostatistician at the Institute for Epidemiology and Biometry at the University of Heidelberg, Germany, went a step further. While Cairns and Bailar had shown that chemotherapy could do little to cure the vast majority of cancers, many in the cancer treatment community still believed the drugs at least extended life. Abel had for years studied the effectiveness of chemotherapy, and his attitude had been basically sympathetic. But now, in the most comprehensive study ever undertaken of cancer chemotherapy, he stated: "A sober and unprejudiced analysis of the literature has rarely revealed any therapeutic success. . . . There is no evidence for the vast majority of cancers that treatment with these drugs exerts any positive influence on survival or quality of life."[27] This toxic and expensive treatment, he said, was not only rarely a cure, but in the majority of cases actually had little beneficial effect.

Meanwhile, the number of deaths due to cancer was continuing to rise. In 1962, more than 275,000 Americans died of cancer. By 1995, the figure had doubled. The numbers showed a continual and significant increase even after biostatisticians made adjustments for the growth and aging of the population.[28] In 1997, cancer had become the leading cause of death due to disease among U.S. children. By the year 2000, cancer was expected to replace heart disease as the leading killer of Americans.

QUESTIONING CHEMOTHERAPY

Could part of the reason chemotherapy and radiation have had such disappointing results be that they are actually hostile to the natural healing processes of the body? Very often, the effort to "destroy the enemy" at all costs ends up counterproductive because it destroys the body's own immune and defense systems. Despite the imagery of the "war on cancer," the human body is not really a battleground, but a sensitive and complex multilayered system of profound possibility, with inherent capacities for self-regulation and self-healing. In conducting medicine as if it were an activity of war, there is no attempt to assist the body's instinctive wisdom. Rather than activating the body's healing resources and supporting its innate recuperative powers, chemotherapy often damages the body's mechanisms for self-repair and renewal.

It does, however, typically shrink tumors. When people with cancer see their tumor shrink, possibly to the point of disappearance, they are often deeply grateful, and filled with hope. The experience may have been horrendous, but at least, they think, the treatment has gotten results.

If the tumor comes back, however, or cancer appears elsewhere in their body, as it so very often does, they tend to believe that the fault is with themselves. Unfortunately, doctors frequently reinforce this self-judgment, by saying "the patient failed the treatment." Rarely do they say, "the treatment failed the patient."

Patients are told that the cancer has come back in spite of the aggressive medical care they have been fortunate enough to receive. They are rarely told how often this happens.

The problem is that malignant cells have a virtually incorrigible tendency to develop resistance to the assault of cytotoxic drugs. It is extremely common, after an apparently successful treatment, for the cancer to reappear; and when it does, it frequently roars back with a vengeance. Once a relapse occurs, the chances of a second complete remission are remote.[29]

People with cancer always ask, "What are my chances? What are my odds if I take chemotherapy?" In reply, doctors often speak encouragingly of "response rates" approaching 60 or 75 percent. The patient is impressed, willing to undergo the ordeal, and grateful to be in the hands of high-tech modern medicine with its pharmaceutical wonders.

But in his outstanding 1995 book *Questioning Chemotherapy*, Ralph Moss, Ph.D., writes: "The doctor talks 'response rate' but the patient hears 'cure.' These same patients and their family members may be furious when they realize that 'response rates' do not often correlate with increased survival or improved quality of life." Although the assumption that tumor shrinkage leads to increased survival "is almost universally believed, it happens to be wrong. This is well known to some chemotherapists. . . . Response rates simply do not predict survival. . . . [It is] a common linguistic dodge to confuse tumor shrinkages with 'success' in cancer treatment. . . . Tumor shrinking responses are the main yardstick in evaluating chemotherapy drugs. The significance of this is that doctors routinely and regularly seek to bring about such 'responses' and tell patients that this is a most desirable goal in their treatment. The reason for this is their belief that such 'responses' correlate with increased survival. However, this is not true, and constitutes one of the primary illusions in the field of cancer."[30]

Could it actually be that cancer doctors simply assume that tumor shrinkage will lead to prolonged life, and that this supposition is, in fact, unwarranted? I have not wanted to believe this could be true. Yet, in 1988, a leading scientist at the National Cancer Institute published data in the prestigious *Cecil's Textbook of Medicine* that support this alarming possibility. For many forms of cancer, including cancer of the breast (Stages III-IV), stomach, prostate, head and neck, bladder, and other sites, the response rate to chemotherapy was found to be an impressive 75 percent. And yet, for these cancers, outcomes of disease-free survival were almost nonexistent.[31]

Today, chemotherapy remains the dominant mode of cancer treatment in the United States. Its use, often along with surgery and/or radiation, has become almost routine. Approximately one million people with cancer, nearly four out of every five people with the disease, receive some form of chemotherapy every year in this country. And yet enormous and troubling questions persist. Writing in *Lancet* in 1991, oncologist Albert Braverman, M.D., observed that "Chemotherapy should be prescribed only when there is a reasonable prospect either of cure or of benefit in quantity and quality of life." By these standards, he says, the procedure is vastly overused. "Many medical oncologists recommend chemotherapy for virtually any tumor, with a hopefulness undiscouraged by almost invariable failure."[32]

Chemotherapy practitioners do not want to think that the weapons they employ to kill cancer cells are of little or no use to their patients. They want to believe they are helping people, and in their defense they point to the substantial increases in the "five-year-survival" rates for many cancers that have occurred during the years of chemotherapy use. Unfortunately, these improvements have been repeatedly shown to be mainly statistical artifacts. Thanks to new, sophisticated diagnostic techniques (MRIs, CAT scans, biochemical and DNA markers), and more widespread screening for cancer (mammograms, PSA tests for prostate cancer, Pap smears, etc.), many cancers are discovered today much earlier than they used to be. Thus the meter that measures "five-year survival" from time of diagnosis starts running sooner.

The improvement is only on paper. In truth, little time has been added to most patients' lives.

HYPOCRISY?

What do oncologists (cancer specialists) themselves do when they get cancer? Ralph Moss tells of his days at Sloan-Kettering, and of a "celebrated chemotherapist [there] who, when he found out that he had advanced cancer, told his colleagues, 'Do anything you want—but no chemotherapy!'"[33]

This physician was not unique in refusing to undergo a treatment that he prescribed to others. In 1986, McGill Cancer Center scientists surveyed 118 oncologists who specialized in the treatment of lung cancer. The physicians were asked what they would do if they developed the disease. Remarkably, three-quarters said they would not participate in any of the current chemotherapy trials. Their reasons? "The ineffectiveness of chemotherapy and its unacceptable degree of toxicity."[34]

An analysis of the study discovered that the more familiar physicians were with particular forms of chemotherapy, the less willing they were to undergo them.

In 1989, some 150 oncologists at research units around the world were surveyed about the cancer treatment choices they would make for themselves. The researchers noted that "the personal views of many oncologists seem to be in striking contrast to communications intended for the public."[35]

Other polls have come to remarkably similar conclusions. With alarming regularity, oncologists say that they would not allow chemotherapy to be given either to themselves or to their families.[36]

For the most part, these physicians went into their profession at least in part because they wanted to do something about the toll cancer takes on humanity. But, as the saying goes, "If the only tool you have is a hammer, every problem looks like a nail." Unfortunately, writes Dr. Ralph Moss, "The tools oncologists are working with are barely effective, and are in fact inappropriate to most cancers. The whole military philosophy behind their efforts seems misguided."[37]

A SLIGHT PROBLEM WITH TOXICITY

How toxic is chemotherapy? One authority explains that with some agents: "If the intravenous needle through which they are being delivered leaks or slips out of the vein, the resulting scar tissue may cause the patient to lose the use of the arm."[38] Current textbooks tell nurses who administer cytotoxic drugs to wear long-sleeved gowns, face shields or goggles, shoe covers, and extra-thick latex surgical gloves, which are to be changed every half hour. They are told never to eat, drink, smoke, or apply cosmetics in the drug preparation area. They are warned that merely handling the drugs poses "significant risks" to health care workers, including reproductive abnormalities, liver and chromosomal lesions, and hematologic problems.[39]

If these are the risks faced by nurses who simply prepare the injections, what are the dangers to the patients who have these agents injected or infused into their veins, or who put them into their mouths and swallow them?

When chemotherapy agents (and their metabolites) are excreted from patients' bodies in their urine and feces, they eventually wind up in the environment, where, researchers have pointed out, "they may become a source of cancer for future generations."[40]

Chemotherapy agents are among the most poisonous substances ever intentionally introduced into the human body. Oncologists sometimes walk a fine line, trying to give enough to kill the cancer cells, without killing the patient.

The drugs can be so toxic that a miscalculation proves fatal. In 1994, Betsy Lehman, a well-known health columnist for the *Boston Globe*, underwent chemotherapy at the Dana-Farber Cancer Institute, a prestigious hospital affiliated with Harvard Medical School. A three-time winner of the top journalism award from the Massachusetts chapter of the American Cancer Society, she was given "the best" of what modern medicine had to offer.

During chemotherapy, her electrocardiogram showed enormous stresses to her heart, and she began, during treatment, vomiting sheets of tissue. The whole lining of her gut, from one end to the other, was shedding. Yet doctors considered her violent reaction to be normal, and continued with the treatment. Even after she died from the ordeal, they did not suspect anything amiss had occurred. Her reactions, even her death, were considered to be within the range of the normal and expected.[41]

When an autopsy found no visible signs of cancer, doctors stated that "the treatment had worked."[42]

Two months later a clerk happened to realize that Betsy Lehman had been accidentally given four times the specified dose.

It is hard to overstate the toxicity of some forms of chemotherapy. In 1995, a report in the *Journal of Clinical Oncology* discussed the effects of a particular chemotherapeutic regimen that is used in metastatic breast cancer, non-Hodgkin's lymphoma, ovarian, and some other cancers. The regimen is called ICE (ifosfamide + carboplatin + etoposide). The authors concluded, "In summary, ICE is well tolerated, with acceptable . . . side effects and predictable organ toxicity."[43]

What did they mean by "acceptable" side effects, and "predictable" organ toxicity? The study found that "67 percent of the lower-dose patients had mucositis [shedding of the lining of the gut]. . . . In the mid-range-dose patients, [an additional] 50 percent suffered central nervous system and lung complications. And in some of the higher-dose patients, [an additional] 61 percent suffered liver toxicity, 81 percent suffered ear damage, 70 percent suffered kidney toxicity, 92 percent suffered adverse pulmonary events, while 94 percent suffered damage to their hearts [cardiotoxicity]. . . . Eight percent of the group actually died of the effects of the drugs themselves, so-called toxic deaths. Such deaths took place at almost every dose level."[44]

If this is an "acceptable" level of side effects, I'd hate to see what would be considered unacceptable.

The mentality is similar to a state of war in which one side desperately bombs the battlefield with all they've got, knowing that in so doing they will kill some of their own soldiers.

In 1993, researchers from the National Cancer Institute compared the outcomes obtained by women with ovarian cancer who had undertaken different treatments. They found that women who had taken the chemotherapy drug melphalan developed 100 times the incidence of leukemia compared to women who received no chemotherapy.[45]

Chemotherapy agents typically carry warnings about "the possibility of fatal or severe toxic reactions." In many cases, amongst the lengthy list of serious side effects that can be expected, is death.

In 1994, Robert Kotlowitz wrote in the *New York Times Magazine* of watching his wife go through chemotherapy: "I begin to think of the photographs I have seen of the first debilitated casualties of poison gas during World War I. . . . My wife suffers from the same helplessness, the same enfeeblement after chemotherapy, with one major difference: she suffers under medical guidance."[46]

IS THIS A FORM OF MEDICINE?

In defense of chemotherapy, oncologists point to real successes with leukemia. But even here, I'm sorry to report that the benefits from chemotherapy are not as impressive as we would like. Although often thought of as a childhood disease, leukemia actually develops ten times more frequently in adults than in children, and results for chemotherapy aren't nearly as good past childhood. In 1995, 26,000 Americans developed leukemia, and 21,000 died of the disease. For adult leukemia, chemotherapy has few answers.

The type of leukemia in children that can most effectively be controlled by chemotherapy is lymphocytic leukemia. This is the greatest feather in chemotherapy's cap, representing a genuine therapeutic advance, and yet, sadly, here too the treatment has drawbacks. Children undergoing chemotherapy frequently suffer seizures and brain diseases associated with alterations of brain structure. An article in *Pediatrics* acknowledged the high frequency of "acute mental status changes."[47]

Even in those cases where it is effective, chemotherapy can be brutal.

Some oncologists justify chemotherapy on the grounds that it improves the quality of their patients' lives by giving them hope. "I don't ever give up on my patients," a prominent California chemotherapist told me in 1995. "And my patients love me for it. When they die, they die knowing that somebody cared about them, somebody was on their side. They die knowing that medical science didn't abandon them. I give them chemotherapy right up until the end. I don't just stand there with my hands in my pockets and watch them die."

This doctor's attitude is not unusual among aggressive chemotherapists. Like many, he does not allow himself to be restrained by the fact that the treatments he employs are toxic, often ineffective, and enormously expensive. Evidently he believes that his patients are better off with poisonous drugs dripping into their veins, ensconced in a cloud of denial not of their own choosing, than they would be if honestly told the truth about chemotherapy's limits and drawbacks. I pointed this out to him, and asked how he justified what he did in terms of the patients' welfare. "It's terribly hard for patients to be told they have cancer," he said with what appeared to be genuine concern. "I give them hope. I help them to stay optimistic. There's always the possibility of a miracle, you know."

Not wanting to side against hope or the possibility of miracles, I nevertheless ventured to ask whether any of his end-stage patients had ever recovered as a result of the chemotherapy he gave them. "No," he said, shaking his head. "I'm afraid not."[48]

There are certainly times when chemotherapy can improve life for a person with cancer. Shrinking a tumor that is pressing on a nerve, or that is making a vital aspect of life impossible, is a legitimate use of the procedure. But such circumstances are comparatively rare. In many cases, chemotherapy seems instead to diminish the quality of life.

Unless, of course, you happen to like vomiting uncontrollably. Patients sometimes retch incessantly for hour upon hour, even breaking bones or rupturing the esophagus. One called it a form of "medieval torture."

John Laszlo, M.D., of the American Cancer Society commented: "We have seen patients drive into a hospital parking lot and promptly begin to vomit when they smell the alcohol sponge used to clean off the arm prior to chemotherapy, or even vomit when they see the nurse who administers the chemotherapy, even if that person is encountered out of uniform in a supermarket or elsewhere away from the hospital."[49]

There are new drugs that offer better control of vomiting. Yet many of these drugs are extremely expensive, are given by intravenous drip requiring the patient to lie for hours in a hospital bed, and have side effects of their own that typically require additional medication. Furthermore, they sometimes only delay the vomiting rather than actually prevent it. One 1994 study actually found that ondansetron yielded no better results than a placebo.[50]

While not all chemotherapy patients vomit, and some drugs are certainly much easier to take than others, oncologists characteristically downplay the level of suffering involved when they recommend chemotherapy to people with cancer. Only rarely are patients given accurate and complete information in an understandable fashion so that they can make truly informed choices. Far more commonly, chemotherapists think they know what's best for the patient, and only give lip service to the ritual of obtaining consent.

In one study, it was found that "giving chemotherapy to elderly patients with [a particular type of] cancer prolongs their lives by an average of a few months but also causes them severe, intractable, drug-induced vomiting."[51] Most American physicians judged that the few added months justified the chemotherapy, and said they would proceed with the treatment. British doctors, on the other hand, did not feel the trade-off was worth it. And yet none of the physicians seemed to consider the possibility of accurately informing the patients and their families of what was involved, and then letting *them* decide.

RELENTLESS OPTIMISM

It must be difficult for oncologists to face how poorly their patients often fare. Perhaps that is why the conventional cancer treatment community so often speaks in platitudes.

When Senator (and former Vice President) Hubert Humphrey developed cancer of the bladder, he was treated with radiation. In May 1976, his physician, Dr. Dabney Jarman, spoke glowingly of the senator's progress, and said the radiation had been successful. An American Cancer Society vice president cowrote a popular book that called Humphrey "a famous beneficiary of modern radiation therapy."[52]

A few months later, however, the cancer was back, worse than ever. In October, Senator Humphrey was operated on at Memorial Sloan-Kettering's Memorial Hospital. Afterwards, his surgeon, Willard Whitmore, announced at a nationally televised news conference, "As far as we are concerned, the senator is cured."[53]

Less than a year later, after undergoing extensive chemotherapy, Humphrey was dead. All these "successful" treatments had left him emaciated and enfeebled. Before he died, he called chemotherapy "bottled death."[54]

The recent NBC special *Destined to Live* featured famous people speaking of their experiences with cancer. The overall tone of the show was chipper and upbeat. Everyone was feeling fabulous and looking great. "When life kicks you, let it kick you forward," said one woman. "Cancer was the best thing that ever happened to me," said another. "I laughed at it and I beat it," said someone else.

You'd never have suspected anyone had ever died of cancer. People spoke of their fear when they were first diagnosed, and how they got over it. No one was grieving. No one was sad. No one spoke of loss. As Sharon Batt noted, "The sick were not mentioned and the dead were not mourned."[55]

I'm sure that the people who put this show together thought they were doing something for others, providing hope and a positive message to people with cancer. I'm sure they never considered that less noble purposes might be served by the relentless optimism.

But the denial of the fact that orthodox Western medicine has few answers to cancer keeps a dysfunctional system in place. It keeps the public marching obediently and blindly through treatments that often mutilate without providing benefit. It prevents public support for alternative treatment approaches from building to a sufficient level of intensity to create real change. It keeps public outrage from demanding that tobacco advertisements be curtailed, carcinogenic chemicals restricted, and the hazards of radiation made fully public. It allows people to merrily munch on their hot dogs and junk food, naively trusting that when they become ill the medical technocracy will be there to take care of things.

And it keeps money rolling into the organizations that have already spent hundreds of billions of dollars of public funds in pursuit of a victory that has never really materialized.

"REACH TO RECOVERY"

The American Cancer Society is one of the world's wealthiest private charities, with a net worth of nearly half a billion dollars. The organization has done much good, particularly in raising public awareness about the health consequences of tobacco. Some of its programs, however, seem to leave a little bit to be desired.

Recognizing that people with cancer have a great need for social support, the organization has come up with a program called Reach to Recovery. After breast cancer surgery, a woman is visited in her hospital room by a volunteer who has herself recovered from a similar operation. While the concept seems laudable, many patients report that in practice the program does not really serve the women in need.

All volunteers must first be approved by the American Cancer Society. They are told to avoid any discussion of doctors, hospital staff, or treatment options, and are given puffs of lamb's wool to give to patients to stick in their bras.

One woman with breast cancer, the poet Audre Lorde, recalled that after her breast surgery she ached to talk to a woman who would understand what she was experiencing. But after a Reach to Recovery volunteer visited her hospital room, she ended up "feeling even more isolated than before." The volunteer talked about "what man I could capture . . . [and] whether my two children would be embarrassed by me in front of their friends."[56] What was on Lorde's mind, however, was her chances of survival, the changes in values and life direction she was experiencing, whether the cancer could have been prevented, and what she could do to keep it from recurring. She was trying to face the reality of her breast amputation, and integrate the experience into her life. She wanted to come to terms with her pain and loss, and thereby find the inner strength to grow through this time of challenge. The visitor told her to look on the bright side of things, and gave her stuffing to put in her bra.

The feelings of isolation were increased for Lorde when she went to an appointment with her surgeon at his office, and was reprimanded for not wearing a prosthesis. She was told that they really would like her to wear one when she came in for appointments. "Otherwise it's bad for the morale of the office."[57]

Each patient in this office, Lorde thought, either has had a breast removed, or is afraid of the possibility. And each of them "could have used a reminder that having one breast did not mean her life was over, nor that she was less a woman, nor that she was condemned to the use of a prosthesis in order to feel good about herself and the way she looked."[58]

Breast prostheses, she thought, offer the "empty comfort of 'nobody will know the difference.'" But it was that very difference that was now such a big part of these women's lives, and it was that very difference that they needed to come to terms with and affirm.

Lorde felt that she was being asked to deny her bodily reality, that her right to define and to claim her own body was being undermined. It's not that she felt there was necessarily anything wrong with wearing a prosthesis, but if she wore one she wanted it to be her choice. Most of all, she wanted the chance to accept her new body without shame.

She was in touch with one of the most basic truths about facing loss: Only by opening ourselves to the genuine conditions of our lives can we gain the knowledge and experience necessary to become able to respond to life's challenges.

Darlene Betteley, of Waterloo, Ontario, would understand. She had both breasts removed in a double mastectomy. A few years later, she became a Reach to Recovery volunteer, and was told that she would have to wear breast prostheses if she were to visit patients. "We like our volunteers to look normal," the Cancer Society administrator explained cheerfully.[59]

Darlene had been a model, and took pride in her ability to dress becomingly after her surgery. She nearly capitulated, but something about it just didn't feel right, so she went back to the Cancer Society, and said that she didn't see why she should have to wear prostheses. "I am happy with myself. You have to like yourself before you can share your happiness and love with other people."[60]

In that case, came the answer, we can't have you in the program.

Darlene looked up the matter in the Reach to Recovery handbook, and, sure enough, found the directives: "Wear casual clothes. Must be well-fitted over the bustline." And there were other restrictive rules: "Do not be persuaded to show your scar, or look at the scar of the person you are visiting."

In 1988, the American Cancer Society launched a new program, called Look Good, Feel Better. But I'm sorry to say that this program, like Reach to Recovery, seems more devoted to helping women keep up appearances than to providing genuine healing support. Women undergoing cancer treatment are now invited to go to their local hospital and attend a workshop where they receive tips on beauty techniques and applying make-up, plus a package of free cosmetics. The Look Good, Feel Better program is sponsored by cosmetics manufacturers and the beauty industry.

The people involved in the program no doubt mean well, but what price do women pay for so much focus on facade? Isn't part of the pain that women carry, and part of what takes such a toll on their bodies and their health, the pain of having been reduced for centuries to objectified sexual conveniences? What has it done to women to value themselves primarily in terms of appearances, to conceal their suffering and keep it to themselves as a private burden? Does the American Cancer Society really believe that what women with a life-threatening disease need is tips on applying makeup?

When a woman is told to hide her wounds, it becomes difficult for her to find the strength that can only come with facing, and sharing, the truth of her situation. It becomes hard for her to truly connect with other people, because masks and pretense can be isolating.

"When your life is at risk," writes Sharon Batt, "play-acting that you are well exacts an emotional price. It creates barriers of communication between the woman with cancer and those she loves. These tricks to keep surgery and baldness secret make us invisible to each other and to society at large. . . . Wigs, breast prostheses, make-up, and optimism-at-all-costs, keep us isolated in our grief."[61]

As I've seen how much emphasis the American Cancer Society puts on keeping up appearances, I've had to wonder what purpose is being served by so much masquerade. Are these women, whom the system so often fails, being asked to collude in covering that up? The same question occurred to Judy Hoffman in 1996, after she underwent treatment for breast cancer. "The surgery was disfiguring and painful, and the radiation made me feel like death warmed over. My life was in danger, and they start talking to me about which brand of lipstick to use. I don't think anyone could be that superficial and shallow unless they want to hide something. Maybe they don't want us to face how lousy we feel because they're afraid we might stop coming to them. Maybe they want to keep us hooked into the system. Maybe they don't have any answers and don't want us to know it. It's as if they are terrified of the possibility that we will leave the fold and seek alternatives."[62]

Sure enough. The Reach to Recovery handbook specifically instructs volunteers to "always maintain a positive attitude toward conventional treatment methods." Volunteers are told never to "promote unconventional therapies."[63]

13
Alternatives
for Cancer

Never ask a barber whether you need a haircut.

IN 1991, THE TABLOIDS OF AMERICA were riveted on the plight of Michael Landon. The popular actor, whom tens of millions of people had come to feel was almost part of their families through watching him in *Bonanza*, *Little House on the Prairie*, *Highway to Heaven*, and other television shows, had been seriously stricken with pancreatic cancer.

The conventional prognosis for this disease could hardly be more grim. By the time symptoms of this type of pancreatic cancer become apparent, the disease has almost invariably spread. Each year in the United States, there are 24,000 new cases, and an equal number of deaths. Most patients die within a few weeks or months of diagnosis.

Conventional medicine has next to nothing of value to offer for cancer of the pancreas. Less than 10 percent of pancreatic tumors can be removed by surgery. The operation is complex and arduous, and up to 30 percent of patients die on the operating table.

Many people with cancer of the pancreas, however, receive some form of chemotherapy, and Michael Landon was no exception. Remarkably, there is no evidence that the procedure can either cure the disease or extend life for the person who has it. In fact, the opposite seems to be the case. In one study, published in the journal *Cancer*, the median survival for untreated patients after diagnosis was 3.9 months. For those who received chemotherapy, however, the median survival was 3.0 months.[1] Patients who underwent chemotherapy actually died sooner.

Like many people, Michael Landon did not particularly enjoy chemotherapy: "It can have a hideous effect on the body," he said. "First you get sores in the mouth, then peeling skin. Then your hair and eyebrows fall out, then major organs start to break down. You can die of the cure before you die of the disease."[2]

The actor came to reject conventional cancer treatment, and to seek alternatives. And he discovered that there were approaches to his disease with far better track records than orthodox medicine. "Some alternative therapies sometimes work with pancreatic cancer," he said. "I've talked with several survivors of pancreatic cancer who were evidently cured by alternative therapies. I talked with one man right in my living room, a medically certified case of pancreatic cancer who today, ten or eleven years after he was diagnosed, was completely clean. No tumors left, just scar tissue on his pancreas."[3]

Although Michael Landon eventually died of his cancer, his willingness to forsake conventional treatment in favor of alternative approaches stirred something deep in the hearts and minds of millions of people with cancer. Could there be a better way than surgery, radiation, and chemotherapy?

A BETTER WAY

Some of the most remarkable, documented results of an unconventional cancer treatment were those achieved by Dr. William Donald Kelley. Even in the most dire types of cancer, such as cancer of the pancreas, where conventional treatment has nothing to offer, he often achieved stunning results.

Nicholas J. Gonzalez, M.D., met Kelley in 1981, and thought he had to be a charlatan. Expecting to expose him, Gonzalez began to research Kelley's records, thinking it would take only a few weeks to prove the man a quack. But Gonzalez ended up spending the next six years analyzing the results Kelley obtained in treating cancer patients, and studying his methods.

Nick Gonzalez was not a man to be fooled. He had studied medicine at Columbia University and Cornell University Medical College, and he undertook his investigation of Kelley's work under the sponsorship of Dr. Robert A. Good, then president of Memorial Sloan-Kettering Cancer Center. Medical historians say the analysis is "widely regarded as the finest case review ever conducted concerning an alternative cancer therapy."[4]

The deeper Gonzalez probed, the more impressed he became. To his amazement, he found that Kelley actually seemed to be "curing the incurable" utilizing individualized diet, intensive nutritional support, pancreatic enzymes, and detoxification.

During the years covered by the study, Gonzalez found that 22 patients who were diagnosed by medical authorities as suffering from terminal pancreatic cancer came to see Kelley. All patients were evaluated by independent medical specialists at a number of stages, so there could be no doubt about the accuracy of their diagnosis and outcome.[5]

For one reason or another, 12 of the patients never started the program, and their median survival was about what would be expected, eight weeks. Five of the patients undertook Kelley's program, but only partially followed the treatment protocol, and their median survival was eight months.

There were five other patients, however, who followed through with Kelley's complete treatment regimen. Sickened with a disease that orthodox Western medicine considers utterly hopeless, for which the expected survival time is typically measured in weeks, four of the five were still alive, at last report, more than 15 years after starting the program. And the patient who had died had lived for many years after treatment by Kelly. He died of Alzheimer's disease, with no sign of cancer in his body.[6]

Kelley's success rate for those pancreatic cancer patients who stayed with the program was 100 percent. Conventional medicine's success rate for this disease, remember, is zero.

Gonzalez thoroughly studied the records of 455 Kelley patients who suffered from a variety of cancers, and found that it was not only with cancer of the pancreas that Kelley achieved spectacular successes. After the late Dr. Harold Ladas, a biologist and former professor at Hunter College, reviewed Gonzalez's study, he wrote: "Gonzalez has given us convincing evidence that diet and nutrition produce long-term remission in cancer patients almost all of whom were beyond conventional help. Because the cases represent a wide variety of cancers . . . the paradigm has wide applicability to cancer treatment. . . . The evidence is in, and it is stunning."[7]

Did the American Cancer Society or the National Cancer Institute immediately follow up these encouraging findings with a major study on Kelley's work? Not exactly. They completely ignored it. You see, back in 1971 the American Cancer Society had put Kelley's therapy on its Unproven Methods list, where it has remained ever since, stigmatized and discredited. To this day, no American Cancer Society or National Cancer Institute representative has ever attempted an impartial evaluation of

Kelley's methods and results. And to this day, the American Cancer Society warns cancer patients against involving themselves with the treatment.

Although the cancer establishment continues to shun Kelley's approach, Nicholas J. Gonzalez, M.D., was so impressed with the results Kelley achieved in treating "terminal" cancer patients that after completing the study in 1987, he returned to New York and began treating cancer patients with the Kelley method. Though he had set out to discredit Kelley as a quack, he was so impressed that today, with Kelley retired, he now provides patients a variation of Kelley's approach to cancer.

What kind of results is Gonzalez getting? With the American Cancer Society and National Cancer Institute steadfastly refusing to objectively evaluate his work, we have only the testimonials of cancer patients who tell their individual stories. Many say that Gonzalez's approach has healed them when conventional medicine could not.

In 1991, Robert Maver, vice president and research director of Mutual Benefit Life, added credence to the many personal testimonials. Writing in a leading insurance industry journal, he announced: "The Research Division has been evaluating Dr. Gonzalez's results over the last four months, including numerous site visits. The results are indeed extraordinary."[8]

THE AMERICAN CANCER SOCIETY
JUDGES ALTERNATIVE TREATMENTS

Many of the proponents of unconventional cancer treatment methods are sincere and well-intentioned people, but that doesn't mean that the procedures they advocate are sound. Just because they are impassioned is no guarantee that their treatments are valid.

Further, the world of health care is not immune from deceit. With conventional medicine having so little to offer people with cancer, many are left desperately grasping at straws. Is it surprising, then, that in the cancer world we do not seem to have a shortage of people selling straws? In the midst of the many unconventional cancer treatments, some no doubt are pushed by people who are self-deluded, and others who would take advantage of the ignorant, the gullible, and the vulnerable.

How, then, is a person with cancer to evaluate the competing claims of various alternatives? How can someone who is relatively medically illiterate separate the charlatans who are only peddling dreams from the practitioners whose methods represent legitimate therapeutic advances with real healing potential? How do we know which of the unorthodox cancer treatments truly have something to offer, and which are mere fantasies?

There is a profound need for impartial and open-minded analysis of the many innovative and unconventional approaches to cancer treatment. We need clear, objective, accurate, and unbiased information. Just because a treatment is alternative certainly doesn't mean it is effective. If a given treatment is ineffectual, we need to know that. If an approach works only rarely and in special cases, that information can be crucial and provide the basis for further discovery. If a method cannot work when the immune system has been incapacitated by chemotherapy, but shows promise or has use when the immune system is intact, then this knowledge can save lives. We need to know which treatments work best with which types of cancers, how they complement one another, and what percentage of the time they accomplish what kinds of results.

For years, the American Cancer Society has presented itself as a reliable and established guide to the world of cancer, and has published a directory of unorthodox procedures called *Unproven Methods of Cancer Management*. The American Cancer Society gives the unmistakable impression that the unconventional methods listed in *Unproven Methods of Cancer Management* have been subjected to a disinterested and unbiased appraisal, and found wanting.

And yet when Ralph Moss studied the American Cancer Society data on the methods included in *Unproven Methods of Cancer Management*, he found: "Seventy-two percent of the methods on the unproven methods list have never been shown to be ineffective by any sort of rational scientific procedure. . . . For less than 20 percent does the American Cancer Society offer any documented evidence of failure. . . . Many of these methods have been tested and condemned in a one-sided manner. In *no* case, for example, was a clinical double-blind study carried out on any of these procedures before it was condemned."[9]

I'm sure there are many ineffective methods among the unconventional treatments listed in *Unproven Methods of Cancer Management*, and probably some downright frauds. But others of these new ideas might seem bizarre at first glance, without necessarily being invalid. The only way to know is to study them with an open mind, and see if they work. This, the American Cancer Society has not done.

Much of the medical profession, as well as legislators, judges, juries, and the lay public, have taken the opinion of the American Cancer Society on alternative practitioners as representing objective analysis. Doctors listened when the *New England Journal of Medicine* editorialized in 1992: "Unbiased information about alternative medicine is hard to acquire, but the American Medical Association and . . . the American Cancer Society . . . are useful sources."[10]

But in effect, the American Cancer Society's *Unproven Methods of Cancer Management* functions as a blacklist, not entirely unlike the list of "subversive" organizations that was maintained by the House Un-American Activities Committee during the McCarthy era. Researchers whose names appear on the list have been branded as quacks, their funding and insurance reimbursements cut off, and their work stigmatized. In some cases, their medical licenses have been taken away, their clinics closed, and they have had to flee the country in order to continue to offer treatments that thousands of people with documented cases of cancer say have given them life.

There are countless physicians in the United States who would like nothing better than to integrate the best of alternative health care with the best of orthodox medicine. And yet every time a physician's license has been revoked because he or she offered patients an unapproved therapy, a signal has been sent to physicians throughout the country who are curious and would like to explore unconventional approaches. The message is brutally simple: If you dare step outside the confines of what has been approved, you risk your career, your reputation, and your livelihood.

Today, as a result of the suppression of alternative cancer treatments, Americans with cancer who want to try these treatments often have to break the law, or else leave their country and go to Europe, the Bahamas, or Mexico.

Why is it that so many people are willing to take such risks? Partly because there are indications that some of the blacklisted approaches are more effective than orthodox treatments. And also because these therapies often provide significant "healing" even when they cannot provide permanent "cure."

"CURE" AND "HEALING"

There is a critical difference between "cure" and "healing." "Cure" is basically a physical reality; it means that your body is rid of its symptoms and you are returned to a familiar state of functioning. "Healing," on the other hand, takes place in many dimensions of life. You can heal emotionally, psychologically, and spiritually, whether or not your body is cured. But very often, while conventional cancer treatments are failing to cure, their toxicity is undermining healing.

Healing has to do with your experience of yourself and your experience of life. Even if you do not recover physically, it is possible to find renewed meaning in your unique journey, to move into greater wholeness and fulfillment. Whether or not your health is restored, it is possible to develop greater appreciation for the value of what is emerging in your life adventure, and to gain greater clarity about what is important to you.

Illness, even terminal illness, can be an opportunity for healing.

Everyone has the capacity for healing, though it means different things to different people at different times. For some, it involves increasing self-acceptance, and an awareness that, given the limitations of their lives, they still have a contribution to make. For others, healing means taking more responsibility for their lives, giving up self-destructive habits, and making more life-affirming choices. For others, it may include coming to terms with a sense of loss or frustration, and allowing new life to awaken in its time.

Cancer can bring a serious confrontation with mortality. Faced with the possibility of their own demise, some people with the disease feel a profound urge to reassess what is truly valuable and worthwhile, and to reexamine how they want to live the remainder of their lives. For some people with cancer, healing involves finding a creative balance between the will to live and the awareness of death. For others, it includes forgiving life for its injustices, forgiving themselves and others for various assorted failings, and allowing love to flow again where it has been missed.

Quality of life is a difficult thing to measure. You can't put it in a test tube, or calibrate it on a scale. Perhaps for this reason, it has not been fully considered in the criteria by which medical science assesses its treatments. Hard data, like the number of days of survival after a particular procedure, are more amenable to scientific determinations. And yet, for many people, the opportunity to live out their last years in an atmosphere of dignity and self-determination is of supreme importance.

Many of the novel and innovative approaches to cancer may turn out in the end to be no more successful than orthodox treatments at actually curing cancer, but that doesn't mean they can't have enormous value to people with cancer. Methods that can mobilize patients' inner resources, add to their feelings of well-being and comfort, support their healing process, and also sometimes prolong their lives are no small achievement.

Even for people who are near death, activities that enhance health can provide wonderful benefits. Many of the holistic and nontoxic treatment alternatives can assist people with end-stage cancer in accomplishing critically important kinds of healing. By alleviating physical pain and other symptoms, reducing anxiety, and providing a feeling of control, they can supply a basis of support in the quest for self-understanding and spiritual insight. By providing the strength to fulfill needed tasks, to recognize and complete any remaining "unfinished business," these treatments can help dying people's precious remaining days be ones of accomplishment, peace, and satisfaction.

Many of the orthodox cancer regimens, on the other hand, are notoriously debilitating and exhausting to patients, who come to experience themselves as losing control over their lives. Large, complex medical bureaucracies seem to have a knack for depleting patients' sense of responsibility and incentive. Caught up in the machinery of orthodox medicine, many people with cancer do not feel that they can participate in their own healing process. Too frequently, at what could be a time of profound spiritual significance, they become apathetic, despondent, and cynical.

CANCER CARE—AMERICAN STYLE

On April 25, 1992, the *New York Times* published a tale that illustrates the devastating loss of control that cancer patients sometimes experience in hospitals. Entitled "Making a Living off the Dying," the piece was written by Norman Paradis, M.D., director of emergency medicine at New York University's Bellevue Hospital.

The story began when the writer's father, who was also a physician, and who had been in perfect health all his life, was diagnosed at the age of 75 with terminal pancreatic cancer. "Norman," implored his father, "I have been a surgeon for almost 50 years. In that time, I have seen physicians torture dying patients in vain attempts to prolong life. I have taken care of you most of your life. Now I must ask for your help. Don't let them abuse me. No surgery, no chemotherapy."

Paradis assured his father that he would make sure nothing like that would happen to him. He spoke to the attending physicians and the hospital staff, and made it clear that his dying father only wanted, and was only to receive, medication to keep him comfortable.

Soon thereafter, however, Paradis discovered that his father was being subjected to a barrage of surgical and radiological procedures. He repeatedly pointed out to the attending doctors that what was being done was futile, painful, debilitating, and was not wanted by his father or by anyone else in the family.

The doctors agreed to stop the procedures. But once again, Paradis found that the procedures were continuing.

"I quickly realized what was going on," he wrote. "Our health care system is structured to meet reimbursement rather than patient's needs. . . . Consulting surgeons get paid thousands of dollars an hour when they 'decide' to operate. So that was what they were deciding to do. It's an old story of inflated fees charged by sub-specialists with procedure-based practices. When I finally got my father's physicians on the phone, I insisted that he be cared for only by internists who had no incentive to do anything but make him comfortable. They assured me they understood my concerns and would keep in close contact. I never heard from them again."

Despite Paradis's persistent efforts, the series of procedures continued unabated. At this point, he was joined by his brother, an attorney, and together they mounted a full-scale campaign to get the hospital to stop performing fruitless and invasive procedures on their father without consent. Each time, they were told that things would be corrected, and yet each time they returned to the hospital to find that the insanity continued. Once, they found their father in a hallway where he had been left alone after yet another "test." The dying man pleaded, "They are treating me like an animal. Please get me out of here."

The brothers again contacted the doctors in charge, and were once again assured things would improve. "I can't describe the anger I felt," Paradis wrote, "when my mother called to say that they had continued the endless procedures as soon as we left. My father had been in the hospital for two weeks. He had spent most of that time receiving unnecessary, 'billable,' high-tech therapy that could not possibly cure him or relieve his pain. Many things had been done to correct problems caused by earlier 'therapies.' When my mother put him on the phone, he was incoherent."

At this point, the brothers, one a physician and the other an attorney, called an emergency meeting with the hospital administrators and chief of staff. After being told the surgeons were "too busy" to attend, the brothers became adamant. "Despite our clear instructions," they bristled, "you have continued to perform invasive procedures on our father. He is now incompetent, so we are invoking our power of attorney and explicitly forbidding you from doing anything that is not directed at relieving his suffering."

That night, however, their father was subjected to yet another surgery. Infuriated and desperate, the brothers tried to transfer their father to another hospital or to a hospice, but each time they arranged for him to be moved, "a test or procedure would be performed, making him temporarily too unstable to be transported." After finding their father sitting alone in yet another hallway after yet another procedure, skeletal and barely alive, the brothers were finally able to move him to a New York hospice. He died the following morning.

If this were an isolated case, it would be tragic enough. But unfortunately, it represents a pattern in cancer care that is repeated far too frequently in American medicine. If a physician and an attorney could not break the chain by which their father was so violated and disempowered, a father who was himself a physician, what chance would the average American have?

Medicare paid the hospital bill totaling more than $150,000, even though, according to Paradis, his father "needed only a bed and some morphine." When he went to file a complaint against the hospital, Paradis was told by the Medicare inspector general's office that billing for unauthorized procedures was a violation, but there were so many pending cases of fraud representing more than a million dollars that a case involving a mere $150,000 could not possibly be investigated.[11]

CANCER CARE IN OTHER COUNTRIES

The atmosphere that often makes cancer patients feel powerless is so common in American medicine that we may accept it as the inevitable price we pay for advanced technological medical care. But it is not shared to nearly the same degree by the other advanced scientific societies, whose treatment results are at least the equal of our own.

As an American, I am conditioned to believe that we have the best of everything, and so it has come as something of a surprise for me to learn that American medicine in general, and American cancer treatment in particular, while uniquely aggressive, are often no more effective than the treatment approaches of many other nations, where patients often play a more active and involved role in their healing process, and alternatives treatments are more recognized and available.

In European nations today, there is far more access to alternative cancer treatment methods that allow for greater patient participation, which is one of the reasons these countries have far less expensive health-care systems than the United States, and longer life expectancies.

Germany has been called "one of the great innovators in the field of alternative approaches to cancer."[12] Strong traditions of naturopathic, herbal, homeopathic, and spiritual approaches to medical care exist side by side, and work in tandem with conventional methods. By American standards, German cancer patients have an extraordinarily wide choice of cancer therapies.

"Nowhere, perhaps, is the beauty of German cancer medicine more visible than in its anthroposophical hospitals," writes Michael Lerner in his lengthy study of alternative cancer treatment options.[13] These hospitals are based upon the anthroposophical principles first articulated by Rudolph Steiner, which are perhaps best known to Americans through the "Waldorf schools" for children.

"The hospitals are aesthetically beautiful," Lerner continues. "There is a strong emphasis on treatments that will enable the patient to make the best possible use of his life; and nursing and medical care are strikingly humane by American standards."[14]

At the world-famous Lukas Klinik, an anthroposophical hospital in Arlesheim, Switzerland, self-expression is a component of all cancer treatments. Art, music, and movement are part of the daily activities, along with herbs and a vegetarian diet based on organic fresh fruits, vegetables, and whole grains. The underlying belief is that when patients express their passions, talents, and gifts, they activate their innate forces of self-healing. "Artistic activities like painting, clay modeling, creative speech, and color therapy lift the patients out of fixed habits and help them unblock their creative faculties," said one observer.[15] Movement exercises are designed to help both the body and the soul to breathe freely again. At the Lukas Klinik, cancer is seen, not as a punishment, but as an impetus for a change in lifestyle that can allow new life impulses and possibilities to be realized. It is seen as a process of self-discovery, and an opportunity to undergo inner spiritual change and find new direction.

When I first learned of these hospitals, I thought they sounded lovely, but I wondered if they were actually helpful to people with advanced disease. "The Anthroposophical hospitals," Lerner concludes, "are widely known and admired in Germany, and are frequently used by Germans with life-threatening cancer diagnoses."[16]

In July 1994, the chairman of the German Commission on Anthroposophical Medicine, Jurgen Schurhold, M.D., told the U.S. Congress that alternative therapies "have repeatedly been shown to be safer, more efficacious, and cost-effective" in German medical practice. "In Germany," he said, "there is a long history and tradition associated with the use of natural therapies. In 1978, Germany passed the Medication Law of 1978, to provide a regulatory framework for legalizing alternative medicines. At the time the bill was being debated in our Congress, critics made all kinds of insupportable claims that the public would suffer harm or fail to use 'effective' conventional therapies. After more than 15 years of experience, these criticisms have proven to be wrong."[17]

Legislation has existed in Germany since 1978 legalizing, and paying for, all forms of alternative medicine. All German medical students are taught natural therapies, and must become knowledgeable about them to pass their medical board exams. More than 60 percent of all German orthodox physicians practice homeopathy, or prescribe other alternatives. They also have a great respect for the healing power of nature, with widespread use of spas, herbs, mud baths, and other natural methods.

It's not only Germany. In England, physicians are much more sensitive than are Americans to the side effects of treatments that may damage a patient's quality of life. To their eyes, the uncritical acceptance of chemotherapy in America is unconscionable.

The English medical system has much more respect for the patient's experience, and doesn't strive to keep people alive at any cost. Far more emphasis is put on helping people to die comfortably with dignity. It is no accident that hospices for the dying originated in England, where there is far greater understanding of the importance of kindness in medicine.

English acceptance of vegetarian and vegan diets, naturopathy, homeopathy, acupuncture, spiritual healing, and many other alternative forms of health care is remarkable by American standards. Cancer patients have a wide range of options in treatment, and can blend unconventional and conventional approaches in a variety of ways.

Homeopathy is widely practiced, fully recognized, and paid for by health insurance plans in England, as it is in Germany, France, the

Netherlands, Italy, and many other countries worldwide. The Queen of England has her own personal homeopathic physician, and the entire Royal Family has been looked after by homeopaths for 150 years.

In Israel, too, alternatives are far more widely available than in the United States. All major university hospitals have homeopathic departments run by licensed physicians. At Assaf HaRofe Hospital, the Department of Integrated Medicine offers patients 11 types of alternative therapies.[18]

In France, physicians have a deep concern for what they call the "terrain"—the vitality of the inner field of the body. They do not see cancer as an alien invader, but as a product of the living system of the body-mind itself. Accordingly, they tend to favor cancer treatments that build up the "terrain," rather than those that merely try to annihilate the disease. Lynn Payer, former medical correspondent for the *International Herald Tribune,* writes: "The French are leaders in fields that concentrate on shoring up the 'terrain,' such as immunotherapy for cancer. . . . If the 'terrain' is more important than the disease, it becomes less important to fight the disease aggressively and more important to shore up the 'terrain.' While American [cancer] doctors love to use the word 'aggressive,' the French much prefer 'les medecines douces,' or 'gentle therapies' . . . with patients doing equally well in both countries."[19]

While the French are still keen on both nuclear power and the medical use of radiation, the limitations of orthodox treatments are being increasingly acknowledged. In 1995, a prominent Paris oncologist, Laurent H. Schwartz, M.D., called conventional cancer treatment "the most important failure of modern medicine."[20]

In France, gentler alternatives are rapidly gaining in favor. The bestselling prescription drug in the country is actually an herbal extract, gingko biloba. So many French doctors prescribe homeopathic medicines (more than 40 percent) that the nation's 23,000 pharmacies are required by law to stock homeopathic remedies.[21]

In Japan, hospitals have an entirely different atmosphere than in the United States. Local people typically enjoy their hospital stays, and develop lasting friendships with the staff. Hospitalized patients always wear their own nightclothes. In fact, one prominent Japanese physician said that requiring hospital nightclothes would cause legal suits, and would be considered a human rights violation. "It would be in all the newspapers."[22] Family members help with the patient's care, mingle with the hospital's staff, and frequently cook the meals. One Japanese doctor explained, with refreshing candor: "We certainly cannot expect a sick person to eat the hospital food, which is not edible even for a healthy person."[23]

Although Japanese physicians still often make all the decisions for patients, who are not expected to ask too many questions, they have a great respect for traditional forms of health care, including herbs and acupuncture, and also deep regard for the spiritual significance of the disease process. In Japanese cancer centers and hospitals, acupuncturists and herbalists practice right alongside physicians trained in Western approaches, and they generally work quite happily together to help patients.

All this stands in marked contrast to the United States, where orthodox medicine has unrelentingly opposed the practice of alternatives, resulting in flagrant antagonism between conventional and unconventional methods. In other countries the alternative and orthodox approaches may occasionally compete, but they typically proceed in a spirit of cooperation, not conflict. There is mutual respect, and a willingness to work together in order to help patients.

VITAMIN C AND THE CANCER ESTABLISHMENT

Not too long ago, I believed that if advocates of unconventional cancer treatments found themselves outside the scientific mainstream, it must be because something was amiss with their work. I pictured them as eccentrics, possibly incompetent, and maybe even unethical. They must be pseudoscientists, I thought, or perhaps even frauds. Surely, anyone who played by the rules of valid research would be given a fair hearing by serious scientists.

The American Cancer Society has certainly nurtured this way of thinking. In 1995, the organization stated: "Proponents of questionable cancer treatment or prevention methods . . . tend to be isolated from established scientific facilities and association. Their clinical and scientific records are weak and sometimes nonexistent. They may have . . . unusual degrees from obscure institutions of higher learning or even correspondence schools."[24]

It's hard to see how that description would fit Dr. Linus Pauling.

A brilliant scientist who won the Nobel Prize for Chemistry in 1954, Pauling worked tirelessly for human health and world peace. While the Atomic Energy Commission was propagandizing for the open-air testing of nuclear weapons and the medical use of radiation with reassuring press releases that claimed "generations of fruit flies raised in radioactive containers showed more vigor, hardiness, resistance to disease, and better reproductive capacity," Pauling translated the physics of nuclear explosions into language people could understand.[25] Using the Atomic Energy Commission's own figures, he showed that then-scheduled weapons tests would cause 55,000 children to be born with gross physical and mental defects, result in more than 500,000 miscarriages, stillbirths, and newborn deaths, and cause a tremendous increase in cancer rates. In 1958, Pauling presented a petition calling for an end to nuclear weapons testing, signed by 11,000 leading scientists, to Dag Hammarskjöld, secretary-general of the United Nations. When he was invited to dinner with other Nobel laureates by President Kennedy, he spent the afternoon picketing outside the White House for an end to nuclear testing.

Spurred by the international citizen movement to which Dr. Pauling gave so much support, the superpowers eventually signed a treaty to suspend above-ground nuclear testing. Poignantly, it went into effect on the very day that Dr. Pauling was awarded the 1962 Nobel Peace Prize.

The only man in world history to win two unshared Nobel prizes, Linus Pauling received honorary doctorates from 48 universities, including Oxford, Cambridge, Yale, and Princeton. Unfortunately, however, the way the American cancer establishment treated this extraordinary man exemplifies its attitude toward alternative treatments.

In 1973, Pauling went to the National Cancer Institute to show a dozen top specialists the case histories of the first 40 patients with advanced cancer who had been treated with 10 grams of vitamin C a day by Dr. Ewan Cameron, a physician at a hospital in Scotland. "My objective," he said, "was to ask these specialists to carry out a controlled trial of vitamin C."[26] The response was not favorable. One witness said she had "never before seen a group of medical researchers with less interest in new ideas."[27]

Though the specialists at the National Cancer Institute refused to study the matter, they did suggest to Pauling that he might apply to the institute for funding to undertake the study himself. This he did, but he was turned down, as he was each subsequent time he applied, seven in all.

Meanwhile, Dr. Cameron continued, with Pauling's support, to administer vitamin C to people with advanced cancer and monitor the results. In 1976, Pauling and Cameron presented a groundbreaking report in the *Proceedings of the National Academy of Sciences*. One hundred "terminal" cancer patients had been given large doses of vitamin C, and their outcomes compared with a control group of 1,000 "terminal" patients cared for by the same physicians, in the same hospital. Neither group received chemotherapy. The only difference was the supplemental vitamin. The controls were matched as to sex, age, tumor type, and clinical status. Outside experts were brought in to critique the procedure, to insure that no bias would interfere with impartiality.[28]

The results, said Pauling, "were surprising, even to us."[29] The patients receiving vitamin C had lived, on average, almost a year longer than the controls, and some of those who were still alive gave every impression of having been completely cured. At the time of the report, all 1,000 of the controls had died (as would be expected with terminal patients), whereas 18 of the 100 patients receiving the vitamin C were still alive. In addition, the vitamin C recipients had shown dramatic improvements in quality of life. Many who had been receiving large doses of morphine had been able to entirely stop taking the narcotic drug.

In comparison, bear in mind that chemotherapy can only extend life in less than 20 percent of advanced cases of cancer, and these extensions often last only a few months and even then are purchased at enormous human cost. While chemotherapy agents can entail a host of devastating side effects, vitamin C is completely nontoxic.

Pauling never claimed that vitamin C "cured cancer," though he described cases that seem to deserve this label.[30] He said, rather, that it "significantly prolongs the life of the cancer patient . . . [and] improves the condition of the patient to such an extent that his life during his remaining months or years is comfortable, contented, useful, productive and satisfying."[31]

Instead of funding Pauling's work, the National Cancer Institute sponsored a study at the Mayo Clinic the next year that seemed to refute the value of vitamin C for people with cancer.[32] The Institute claimed the study was closely modeled on the Pauling/Cameron work, but Pauling pointed out there was a crucial difference. In the Pauling/Cameron studies, very few of the patients who received vitamin C had previously undergone chemotherapy or radiation. But most of the patients in the Mayo Clinic study who received vitamin C had already received heavy doses of radiation and chemotherapy—treatments known to damage the immune system and interfere with the action of the vitamin.

Pauling had specifically warned the National Cancer Institute about this very issue the year before, telling them: "The cytotoxic drugs damage the body's protective mechanisms, and vitamin C probably functions largely by potentiating these mechanisms. . . . You should be careful to use only patients who have not received chemotherapy."[33]

The Mayo Clinic researchers responded that the administration of chemotherapy was routine treatment for cancer patients in the U.S., and if high-dose vitamin C was incompatible with such treatment, it was therefore useless. It was "not conscionable," they said, to withhold "accredited" treatments in order to substitute the "scientifically unproven" vitamin C.[34] Chemotherapy was so entrenched in their treatment repertoire that to "deprive" patients of this toxic treatment seemed "unethical."

LINUS PAULING KEEPS TRYING

As the years went by, Pauling and Cameron undertook further studies, which continued to find dramatic improvements in quality of life and significant life extension for people with cancer taking large doses of vitamin C. And they kept finding a small percentage of seemingly permanent cures, even in cases that had been considered "hopelessly terminal."[35]

At about the same time, an independent Japanese study found that "terminal" cancer patients given high doses of vitamin C (more than five grams a day) lived substantially longer, needed less pain-controlling medication, had better appetites, and showed increased mental alertness, compared to those who received lower amounts of the vitamin.[36]

And when Abram Hoffer, M.D., analyzed the cancer patient outcomes from his 40 years of medical practice, he was electrified. Those cancer patients who did not take vitamin C (and other nutrients) in high doses survived an average of six *months*. But those who did take large doses of vitamin C (about 12 grams a day) and other nutrients, lived an average of more than six *years*. The results for women with cancer of the breast, ovary, uterus or Fallopian tube were even more spectacular. Those who took high daily doses of the vitamins lived an average of *21 times longer*. At the time of the analysis, all of the 22 such patients who didn't take vitamin C were dead, while half of the 40 women who took the vitamin were alive.[37]

Faced with mounting public pressure, the National Cancer Institute decided to fund a second Mayo Clinic study, which it said would duplicate the Pauling/Cameron work, in order to settle things once and for all.

In the Pauling/Cameron studies, as well as Hoffer's work and the Japanese study, the patients who received vitamin C took it every day for as long as they lived, which was in some cases decades. But in the second Mayo Clinic study, headed by Dr. Charles G. Moertel, the vitamin C patients received the supplement *for an average of only ten weeks.* Moertel claimed the "duration of treatment made no difference whatsoever."[38] He simply tested vitamin C as he would any cytotoxic drug which is administered for short periods of time, and whose therapeutic impact is measured primarily in terms of tumor shrinkage.[39]

None of the vitamin C patients died while taking the vitamin. But, tested as a chemotherapeutic drug, vitamin C did not measure up in the short run. It didn't kill cancer cells the way cytotoxic drugs do. A spokesperson for the National Cancer Institute announced that the Moertel study showed "finally and definitely that vitamin C has no value against advanced cancer." Moertel himself went on national television to denounce vitamin C as "absolutely worthless."[40] In something other than a spirit of open-minded scientific inquiry, the National Cancer Institute concluded that no more studies of vitamin C should be undertaken.

This study did not justify these conclusions, since patients only died after being deprived of vitamin C. If anything, the study showed that people with cancer should continue taking vitamin C. Pauling and others made repeated requests to see the raw data from which the negative conclusions about vitamin C were drawn, but the National Cancer Institute refused to make them public, or share them with him.

Pauling never claimed that the vitamin killed cancer cells. In fact, he repeatedly repudiated the entire militaristic ideology behind the "war" on cancer, much as, in his work for world peace, he continually rejected the concept of a "winnable nuclear war." He consistently said that vitamin C was not a cytotoxic weapon, but an agent of healing that could restrain cancer cells, stimulate the immune system, and improve the general health and well-being of people with cancer. And he continually said that vitamin C had to be taken daily on an ongoing basis to achieve the desired results. But somehow, Charles Moertel and the National Cancer Institute didn't quite grasp the concept.

As I've immersed myself in this controversy, I've wondered how science, which at its best can be so elegant, could ever become so twisted. I once believed that doctors and researchers would never want to suppress good medicine. But in this case, I've had to wonder: Is it possible that vested interests were intruding on what should have been an impartial evaluation of vitamin C?

After Moertel took the patients in his study off vitamin C, he put most of them on a powerful chemotherapeutic drug that he had acknowledged in scientific publications to be unable to "produce benefit or extension of survival" in such circumstances.[41] I couldn't understand why Moertel would give patients toxic drugs he knew would not help them, until I saw a remarkable paper he published in the *New England Journal of Medicine* on the use of chemotherapy in gastrointestinal cancer, which explained his thinking to me.

Moertel began the article by noting that, in these situations, chemotherapeutic agents can produce a "response in only about 15 to 20 percent of treated patients, [and adding that] these responses are usually only partial and very transient."[42] He then said that in order to achieve "this minor gain for a small minority of patients" all patients would have to be subjected to the toxicity, cost, and inconvenience. And even in those few cases where a response (tumor shrinkage) is achieved, he said, there is no evidence that this results in life extension.

You or I might not think chemotherapy was appropriate under these circumstances, but Charles Moertel saw things differently. He continued: "By no means, however, should this conclusion imply that these efforts should be abandoned. Patients with advanced gastrointestinal cancer and their families have a compelling need for a basis of hope. If such hope is not offered, they will quickly seek it from the hands of quacks and charlatans."[43]

Evidently, to Charles Moertel, anyone who offered a treatment that was not approved by the cancer establishment was so to be feared that it would be better to subject people with cancer to highly toxic chemotherapy, even while knowing it would not do them any good, than to risk losing them into the hands of such people.

Such people as Linus Pauling.

THE CANCER INDUSTRY

It has been anything but pleasant for me to consider the possibility that the cancer establishment not only often blacklists alternative treatments that it has not tested, but is also apparently quite capable of unfairly testing those it does. I have not wanted to believe that the scientific study of medicine could be so sullied. But it is difficult to avoid such an impression when seeing a man of Charles Moertel's stature (professor of oncology, Mayo Medical School; chairman, Department of Oncology, Mayo Clinic; member, Council on Cancer, AMA; past president, American Society for Clinical Oncology) testing a nontoxic, inexpensive, health-supporting agent like vitamin C as if it were simply another agent of chemotherapy, and then finding it of no value because it does not kill cancer cells the way cytotoxic drugs do. Vitamin C, of course, works on an entirely different principle than chemotherapy. It builds up the patient's natural resistance to the disease. **Testing vitamin C as if it were a chemotherapy drug is like measuring the value to national security of peace ambassadors and international diplomats by how many "enemy" troops they can kill.**

The leading members of the cancer establishment have a vested interest in the war on cancer and the practice of chemotherapy. They have risen to prominence in their profession by virtue of their advocacy of this approach. It can be nearly impossible for them to admit that there might be a better way, when so many people have suffered and died as a result of the direction they have taken. Unfortunately, the consequence is that even more people continue to needlessly suffer and die.

Another reason that chemotherapy is so difficult to dislodge is that enormous profits are involved. In 1995, worldwide revenues from the sale of chemotherapy drugs totaled $8.6 billion.[44]

The leaders of the cancer war often have financial interests that are intimately connected to the drug manufacturers. Many own stock in the drug companies, and are highly paid as consultants for them.

In 1995, when Samuel Broder, M.D., resigned as the director of the National Cancer Institute, he entered into a new position, at twice the salary, as a director of Ivax, Inc., a Miami chemotherapy company. To find a replacement for Broder at the National Cancer Institute, a search committee was created, headed by Paul Marks, M.D. Would Marks look for someone less attached to the chemotherapy approach? Marks, the president of Memorial Sloan-Kettering Cancer Center in New York (where his salary in one year alone was $2.2 million), was also a director of Pfizer, Inc., a prominent manufacturer of chemotherapy drugs.[45]

In the world of chemotherapy, the big players are companies like Pfizer, Merck, Roche, and Upjohn, but the dominant player is Bristol-Meyers Squibb. This one company, which by itself accounts for nearly half of the chemotherapy sales in the world, does not suffer from under-representation in the upper echelons of the cancer establishment. In 1995:

• Richard L. Gelb, chairman of the board of Bristol-Meyers Squibb, was also the vice chairman of the Memorial Sloan-Kettering Cancer Center Board of Managers.

• James D. Robinson III, director of Bristol-Meyers Squibb, was also the chairman of the Memorial Sloan-Kettering Cancer Center Board of Overseers and Managers.

• Richard M. Furlaud, president of Bristol-Meyers Squibb until 1994, and a former director of the Pharmaceutical Manufacturers Association, was also a director of Memorial Sloan-Kettering Cancer Center.

In addition, many drug company officials serve on National Cancer Institute advisory committees.[46] In at least one instance, the American Cancer Society has actually coowned the patent for a key chemotherapy drug along with a drug company, thus sharing in the profits from the use of the drug, and having a direct stake in its use.[47]

In warning the public to avoid the use of "unproven methods," the American Cancer Society positions itself as fighting the unethical and unscrupulous charlatans who would take financial advantage of people in their time of pain and need. Frankly, it has been difficult for me to avoid the impression that the cancer establishment sometimes accuses others of its own vices.

While the costs of the various unconventional approaches vary a great deal, none of them to my knowledge approaches the costs of surgery, radiation, and chemotherapy.

In fact, some of them are extremely inexpensive.

ESSIAC

Essiac, a nontoxic herbal preparation, was developed by Canadian nurse Rene Caisse (Essiac is her last name spelled backwards), from a formula used by an Ontario Indian medicine man. She successfully treated many thousands of cancer patients with Essiac until her death in 1978, at the age of 90.

As Richard Walters writes in his comprehensive and optimistic review of alternative cancer treatments, *Options*, "Refusing payment for her services, instead accepting only voluntary contributions, the Brace-bridge, Ontario nurse brought remissions to hundreds of documented cases, many abandoned as 'hopeless' or 'terminal' by orthodox medicine. She aided countless more in prolonging life and relieving pain. Caisse obtained remarkable results against a wide variety of cancers, treating persons by administering Essiac through hypodermic injection or oral ingestion."[48]

In a notarized statement made on April 6, 1990, Dr. Charles Brusch, cofounder of the prestigious Brusch Medical Center in Cambridge, Massachusetts, and former personal physician to President Kennedy, declared: "I endorse this therapy today for I have in fact cured my own cancer, the original site of which was the lower bowels, through Essiac alone."[49]

Today, Essiac is not approved for the treatment of cancer in either the United States or Canada, even though it has never been disproven through scientific clinical trials. The pattern of disinterest (if not downright hostility) to Essiac by the cancer establishment has been long-standing. Way back in 1926, when Rene Caisse was first beginning to demonstrate the efficacy of the compound, nine Canadian doctors petitioned the Canadian federal health department to test the remedy on a large scale. In their signed petition, they testified that Essiac reduced tumor size, extended life, and showed "remarkable beneficial results," even when "everything else had been tried without effect."[50]

The response from the authorities was not precisely what the doctors had in mind. In one of those moments that seem as if they never should have happened, Ottawa's Department of Health and Welfare sent two investigating doctors to arrest Nurse Caisse for practicing medicine without a license. When the two physicians discovered, however, that she was treating only "terminal" cases, and accepting only voluntary contributions, they refused to arrest her. In fact, one of them, Dr. W. C. Arnold, became so intrigued that he stayed to study her results, and became one of her advocates.

Word of the impressive outcomes Caisse was obtaining with a wide variety of cancers spread quickly. In 1937, John Wolfer, M.D., director of the tumor clinic at Northwestern University Medical School, arranged for her to treat 30 "terminal" cancer patients at his clinic. After supervising more than a year of Essiac therapy, a panel of five doctors at

Northwestern declared that Essiac "prolonged life, shrank tumors, and relieved pain."[51]

At about the same time, a Los Angeles physician, Emma Carson, M.D., took it upon herself to investigate the Bracebridge, Ontario, clinic. Originally quite skeptical, she ended up staying nearly a month, scrutinizing clinical records and examining more than 400 patients. She wrote:

"The Rene M. Caisse 'Essiac Treatment' for cancer is the most humane, satisfactory, and frequently successful remedy for the annihilation of cancer that can be found at this time. . . . As I examined each patient regarding intervening progress during the preceding week and recorded notes of indisputable improvements . . . I could scarcely believe my brain and eyes were not deceiving me. . . . The vast majority of Miss Caisse's patients are brought to her for treatment after surgery, radium, X-rays, etc., have failed to be helpful, and the patients are pronounced incurable. . . . The actual results from Essiac treatments and the rapidity of repair are absolutely marvelous."[52]

But Nurse Caisse provided her treatment under the constant threat of being arrested for practicing without a license, and the strain on her was growing. Finally, more than 55,000 people, many of them patients, their families, and doctors, signed a petition calling for Caisse to be allowed to legally practice without the threat of being arrested. A special Ontario parliament bill that would have accomplished this failed by just three votes. Justifiably fearing imprisonment, Caisse closed her clinic, and thereafter practiced only from her home, shunning all publicity.

In 1959, she was invited to the Brusch Medical Center in Massachusetts, where she spent three months working under the supervision of a panel of 18 doctors. In the end, the physicians stated: "Clinically, on patients suffering from pathologically proven cancer, it [Essiac] reduces pain and causes a recession in [tumor] growth. Patients have gained weight and shown an improvement in their general health. . . . Remarkably beneficial results were obtained even on those cases at the 'end of the road' where it proved to prolong life and the quality of that life."[53]

Can Essiac cure cancer? Both research and clinical experience indicate that Essiac often helps people suffering from cancer, but how often, and in which cases, there is no way now to say. We have no evidence from controlled studies large enough to make clear-cut judgments. Certainly, many of Nurse Caisse's patients died of cancer, despite her efforts. But many others, evidently, were cured, and a great many of those who were not cured nevertheless achieved substantial improvement in quality of life, freedom from pain, and life extension. Why, then, have those organizations entrusted by the public with the financial resources that are required to open-mindedly evaluate cancer therapies been unwilling to study Essiac?

Essiac is an herbal preparation, and so it cannot be patented. The principal ingredients include burdock root, sheep sorrel, turkey rhubarb root, and slippery elm bark. (For a recipe to make it yourself, see Sheila Snow's book *The Essence of Essiac*. Made from purchased herbs, a two-year supply costs about $25—less than four cents a day.) A commercially available product, Flor-Essence, marketed as a cleansing tea, is modeled after and virtually identical to Essiac.

Defenders of the cancer establishment's disinterest in Essiac point out that Nurse Caisse's work was done many years ago, as if this makes it irrelevant to today. If modern medical science had since developed medications that worked well for cancer, Essiac might be of merely historical interest. But Western medicine's ability to cure most forms of cancer has hardly improved in the last 50 years.

Perhaps the closest thing we have to a final word on Essiac can be found in a letter dated August 3, 1991, from Charles Brusch, M.D. This eminent physician, who had worked closely with Rene Caisse while one of his personal patients was the President of the United States, declared: "I have been taking Essiac myself since 1984 when I had several cancer operations, and I have every faith in it. Of course, each person's case is different as well as each person's own individual health history. . . . Someone may respond in a week; someone else may take longer. Whether or not someone is cured of cancer, Essiac has been found to at least prolong life by simply strengthening the body."[54]

If I had cancer, would I take Essiac? I would seriously consider including it in a complete therapeutic program.

THE QUACK WHO CURED CANCER

At first glance, Harry Hoxsey might appear to be the "premier quack." He claimed to have inherited herbal cancer remedies from his grandfather, who had devised them after seeing a cancerous horse cure itself by grazing on medicinal herbs. The AMA has given absolutely no credence to his work, and has attacked it viciously. But a deeper look reveals a most intriguing story.[55]

In the 1950s, Hoxsey operated clinics in 17 different states. His center in Dallas was the world's largest privately owned cancer center. His formula, which interestingly enough contained some of the same herbs found in Essiac, was attested to by thousands of cancer patients who said it had cured them.

In fact, Hoxsey's cancer treatments might have been accepted into the mainstream of Western medicine were it not for the activities of one man, the long-time editor of the AMA *Journal* by the name of Morris Fishbein. This was the same Morris Fishbein who supplemented his AMA salary by acting as a highly paid consultant for a number of tobacco companies.

Fishbein was actually quite impressed by the Hoxsey formula, and apparently tried, in secret, to buy it. Hoxsey said later that he had been all set to sell the formula to Fishbein and the AMA, but had pulled back when they would not promise, as part of the contract, to provide the treatment free of charge to those who could not pay. Hoxsey had promised his father on his deathbed that he would never turn away any cancer patient who could not afford to pay, and he held that promise as sacred.

Fishbein retaliated by waging what has been aptly called "a battle of historic proportions" against Hoxsey. Never one to find himself trapped in patterns of saccharine speech, he called Hoxsey "a ghoul feasting on the bodies of the dead and the dying." As a result of Fishbein's efforts, Hoxsey was arrested more times than anyone in medical history, usually for practicing medicine without a license. And yet no cancer patient ever lodged a complaint or testified against him. In fact, each of the many times Hoxsey was put in jail, hundreds of former patients would surround the jail, praying and singing until he was set free.

Dallas Assistant District Attorney Al Templeton had personally arrested Hoxsey more than 100 times when his younger brother, Mike Templeton, developed colon cancer. Mike had a colostomy, but the cancer continued to spread. After his doctors told him there was nothing more they could do for him, he secretly went to Hoxsey, whose treatments cured him. Al Templeton was so moved that though once a hostile prosecutor, he now became Hoxsey's lawyer.

This kind of story was repeated again and again. *Esquire* magazine sent reporter James Burke to Dallas to do a story exposing Hoxsey as a "worthless, dangerous quack," but after staying six weeks, Burke was so impressed by what he learned that he became an ardent supporter, and titled his story "The Quack Who Cures Cancer." He was particularly impressed by the fact that Harry Hoxsey, true to the pledge he had made to his father, never turned away a patient who had trouble paying. An exceedingly generous man, he treated nearly a third of his patients for free, and often paid for the food, lodging, and travel expenses of his poor patients.

Mildred Nelson, the woman who was eventually to become Harry Hoxsey's chief nurse, and who is today the most prominent practitioner of the Hoxsey method, was another doubter when she was first introduced to the Hoxsey approach in 1946. Her mother, Della Mae Nelson, had decided to go to Hoxsey for her cancer, even though Mildred, a conventionally trained nurse, was sure Harry Hoxsey was a quack, and was vehemently opposed. But Della Mae Nelson went ahead with the treatment, was cured, and at last report was alive and well nearly 50 years later, having outlived all her doctors. Mildred has since selflessly devoted her life to helping people with cancer through the Hoxsey treatments.

Hoxsey repeatedly pleaded with the AMA and the National Cancer Institute to conduct a scientific investigation of his formulas, even offering to pay for the studies himself. But they refused, and Fishbein continued his relentless attack. One of his articles, none-too-tenderly titled "Blood Money," called Hoxsey the worst quack of the century, and said that Hoxsey's most enthusiastic supporter was the undertaker. This diatribe was published in the Hearst papers' Sunday supplement, reaching 20 million people.

Finally, Hoxsey could take it no more. He sued Fishbein and the AMA for slander and libel. In a contemporary enactment of David against Goliath, Hoxsey became the first individual ever to win a judgment against Morris Fishbein and the AMA. In the process, two different federal courts found that the Hoxsey cancer formulas had therapeutic value. In one epic court scene, Fishbein himself admitted under oath that the treatment had in fact cured melanoma and other skin cancers.

In 1953, Benedict F. Fitzgerald, Jr., special counsel to the U.S. Senate Commerce Committee, conducted an in-depth investigation to determine whether a conspiracy existed to suppress Hoxsey and other innovative cancer treatments. The Fitzgerald Report, released on August 3, 1953, declared that a conspiracy had indeed been undertaken by the AMA, the National Cancer Institute, and the FDA to suppress a fair investigation of Hoxsey's methods.[56]

Shaken by the Fitzgerald report, an independent team of ten physicians decided that if the cancer establishment wouldn't fairly investigate Hoxsey, they would look into it for themselves. After examining hundreds of case histories and interviewing patients and ex-patients, the physicians released a signed report:

"[The Hoxsey Clinic] is successfully treating pathologically proven cases of cancer, both internal and external, without the use of surgery, radium or X-ray. Accepting the standard yardsticks . . . established by medical authorities, we have seen sufficient cases to warrant such a conclusion. Some cases we have seen have been free of symptoms as long as 24 years, and the physical evidence indicates that they are all enjoying exceptional health at this time. We as a Committee feel that the Hoxsey treatment is superior to conventional methods. . . . We are willing to assist this Clinic in any way possible in bringing this treatment to the American public."[57]

By now the Hoxsey clinic in Dallas had 12,000 patients in its care. Harry Hoxsey kept repeating his pleas for an impartial investigation of his results. He even considered running for governor of Texas in order to instigate an unbiased investigation into his therapy. There was talk of surrounding the White House with a circle of 25,000 recovered Hoxsey patients. But the medical establishment steadfastly refused to evaluate Hoxsey's formulas.

Recently, Oliver Field, former director of the AMA Department of Investigations, explained why the medical establishment still refuses to investigate the Hoxsey method. "He's like all the rest of them. They all say they're treated unfairly; that medicine won't pay attention to them. And it's true, medicine doesn't, because we know that their products are worthless."[58]

What about people who say they've been cured? These people suffer, says this AMA official, from an "unwillingness to face reality."[59]

The medical establishment won't investigate the Hoxsey and other unconventional treatments because they "already know" they aren't effective. How do they know? Because they have spent hundreds of billions of dollars looking for answers, and haven't come up with any. Therefore, these "quacks" couldn't possibly have found anything useful.

William Grigg, Public Information Officer of the FDA, put the reasoning rather colorfully: "The idea that the American Indians, or this person or that person . . . would accidentally stumble upon some herb that would cure [cancer] is rather far-fetched. It's like the idea that if you put three billion monkeys in a room, one of them might write a Shakespearean sonnet."[60]

Based on this reasoning, the FDA in 1960 closed the Hoxsey clinics in all 17 states where they were flourishing. Treating Hoxsey like some sort of notorious public enemy, the FDA posted prominent public warnings against his treatment in all 46,000 post offices nationwide.[61]

Hoxsey's chief nurse, Mildred Nelson, went to Mexico, where she has since operated the Bio-Medical Center, and where Americans with cancer must go today if they want to receive the Hoxsey treatment. Harry Hoxsey himself died in 1974, but Mildred has carried on, even though it has meant living and working in Tijuana. Her faith in the treatment is strong, based on years of seeing its results.

A superb documentary film on the entire Hoxsey controversy, and the swirling medical politics that surround alternative cancer care, is available from Realidad Productions, P.O. Box 1644, Santa Fe, NM 87504 (505-986-0366). Titled *Hoxsey: How Healing Becomes a Crime*, it was produced and directed by Ken Ausebel, and I recommend it highly.

Does the Hoxsey treatment cure cancer? Thanks to medicine's obstinate refusal to fairly evaluate the treatment, we don't have any hard data to go on. Mildred Nelson says that approximately 80 percent of the patients seen at the Bio-Medical Center benefit substantially from the treatment, but what this precisely entails is hard to know. It's a nontoxic treatment that often adds to the quality of life even for those cancer patients to whom it cannot bring cure.

When Ken Ausebel first visited the Hoxsey clinic, he was stunned by the atmosphere. "My only direct experience with cancer had been the horror of my father's death. Visiting him in Memorial Sloan-Kettering Cancer Center in New York had branded my psyche with the indelible imprint of a medical concentration camp. Hopeless patients in blue smocks hovered like ghosts, their emaciated bodies ravaged by radiation and chemotherapy. Bald-headed children surrounded a color TV spewing out violent cartoons and commercials for sugar-coated cereal. It smelled of death and despair. The doctors, aloof and cold, seemed to have hardened themselves against the incredible pain and their own helplessness. . . . At the Hoxsey Clinic, the mood definitely was not what we expected. People laughed, joked, and circulated freely. As time wore on, we came to recognize the new patients. They were the ones looking anxious and depressed. As time passed, they shared the same experience we did, listening to countless older Hoxsey patients cheerfully tell of how Mildred had healed them three, five, and twenty years ago. And healed their mothers, their neighbors, and their best friends. The stories were miraculous, and they were legion. They involved almost every type of cancer, including the most deadly forms such as pancreatic, lung, and melanoma. In addition we heard several accounts of relatives who had died not long after trying Hoxsey, but who had experienced a pronounced relief of pain, enough to stop taking painkillers."[62]

In the late 1980s, Dr. Steve Austin of Portland, Oregon, conducted a preliminary survey of results obtained at the Hoxsey clinic. He began, as so many have, dubious: "I was a skeptic about the Hoxsey program. Initially it felt pretty hokey to me. But Mildred Nelson told me, 'Everything is open here. Go out there and talk to any of the patients. They all know somebody who has been cured by the treatment.' When I mingled with the patients and spoke to them, Mildred's statement turned out to be true."[63]

Austin and his colleagues stayed in touch with 16 of the patients for five years thereafter (or until they died). After five years, ten had died, while six were not only still alive but evidently totally free of cancer.

Although Austin's survey is only rudimentary, it does suggest considerable healing power in the Hoxsey treatment. It's important to note that all six of the cancer-free survivors had been previously diagnosed in the U.S. by medical doctors, and that patients commonly only go to clinics in Mexico when their doctors have pronounced them "terminal." At least two of the six survivors were confirmed to have been given fatal prognoses before undertaking the Hoxsey treatment. "Finding between two and six miracles in a group of 16 cancer patients impressed us," Austin wrote in 1994.[64]

If I had cancer, would I take the Hoxsey treatment? I would have to consider it seriously, even though it is not legally available in the United States.

One thing is sure. I wouldn't be deterred because the American Cancer Society includes the Hoxsey therapy on its list of Unproven Methods. No representative of the American Cancer Society has ever visited the Hoxsey Bio-Medical Center, or scientifically tested any of the Hoxsey remedies.

14
Heretics
and Healing

Great spirits have always encountered violent opposition from mediocre minds.

—Albert Einstein

MANY OF THE ALTERNATIVE CANCER METHODS that seek to build up the body's ability to overcome disease call for a vegetarian or vegan (no animal products at all) diet. For some of the approaches, such a diet is of central importance.

Max Gerson, M.D., could be called the father of these nutritional approaches. His cancer therapy involves a raw vegetarian diet, with many glasses a day of freshly prepared vegetable and fruit juice, coupled with a vigorous detoxification program. Gerson was also one of the first advocates of organic farming, and would refer to the soil, which nourishes the food we eat, as our "external metabolism." Fifty years ago, long before the environmental crisis had become a matter of public awareness, this prophetic man said that the earth's well-being was intimately interwoven with our own.

German by birth, he fled to the United States as Hitler was coming to power, and soon was achieving superlative results for people with cancer. Yet, according to medical historians, this "scholar's scholar . . . presented his remarkable cases modestly, concluding that he did not yet have enough evidence to say whether diet could . . . alter the course of an established tumor. He claimed only that the diet, which he described in considerable detail, could favorably affect the patient's general condition, staving off the consequences of malignancy."[1]

The editor of the AMA *Journal*, Morris Fishbein, was not pleased. The AMA had staked out a position on the subject of diet and cancer, and Gerson was being uncooperative. "There is no scientific evidence whatsoever," stated the AMA doctrine, "to indicate that modification in the dietary intake of food or other nutritional essentials are of any specific value in the control of cancer."[2] To Fishbein, anyone who claimed changing your diet could have any effect on cancer was a "quack."

Fishbein had another reason to dislike Gerson. Max Gerson spoke strongly about the hazards of tobacco. Philip Morris was then the AMA *Journal's* chief source of advertising, and one of Fishbein's main sources of income.[3]

But what really angered Fishbein and the AMA was that Gerson had warned Congress that the government's cancer efforts should not be controlled by the AMA or any other group seeking a monopoly over American medicine. Furious, the AMA sought to discredit Gerson, but he presented the U.S. Senate with a string of cancer patients who had not responded to conventional therapies and been pronounced "terminal," only to succeed on his program. The medical director of Gotham Hospital in New York was among the witnesses who called Gerson's successes "miracles."[4] An independent physician who carefully reviewed Gerson's records for Congress stated: "Relief of severe pain was achieved in about 90 percent of cases."[5]

Gerson, ever the gentleman and scholar, was more modest in his claims, and said only that his treatment warranted a fair trial. But Fishbein and the AMA would not hear of it. Shortly after the Senate hearing where Gerson made his presentations, he was attacked in the AMA *Journal*, remembers one scholar, for "treating cancer patients with diet and warning against cigarettes."[6]

The soft-spoken, kindly Gerson was no match for the AMA's campaign of smear tactics and dirty tricks. He was expelled from the New York Medical Society, and deprived of his hospital affiliations and malpractice insurance. His manuscripts were stolen, and his work was literally driven out of the country.

Can the Gerson treatment cure cancer? No one knows how often, nor which types of cancer it treats best. Patients often do well while at the Gerson clinic which is now based in Tijuana, Mexico, and run by Max Gerson's daughter, Charlotte. But the program is arduous, and I have to wonder how many are able to stay on it fully when they return home. There is no doubt in my mind, however, that Gerson patients frequently experience healing on many levels.

No controlled trial of Gerson's methods has ever been done. In 1989, however, a British insurance company sent a research team headed by Karol Sikora, M.D., professor of clinical oncology at the Royal Postgraduate Medical School, University of London, to visit the Gerson Clinic in Mexico. The researchers found a "very marked enhancement of quality of life and of pain control without the need for opiates, even in advanced cancer."[7]

Writing in *Lancet*, they reported: "A striking feature was the high degree of control the patients felt they had over their health and . . . the high ratings for mood and confidence. Particularly intriguing were the low pain scores and analgesic requirements for all the patients, despite the presence of extensive metastatic disease."

For some types of cancer, the treatment does seem to generate markedly enhanced survival rates. **In 1995, Gar Hildenbrand, an advisor to the Office of Technology Assessment (OTA) in its attempt to assess the status of unconventional cancer therapies in the United States, coauthored a thorough retrospective analysis of five-year survival rates of melanoma patients treated with the Gerson therapy. The results were extremely impressive. Some 82 percent of Gerson patients with Stage IIIA melanoma were alive five years after commencing treatment, compared to 39 percent with conventional treatment. For Stage IVA melanoma, the results were even more exceptional: 39 percent were alive at five years, compared to 6 percent.**[8]

In a time when organized medicine insisted there was no connection between diet and cancer, Dr. Max Gerson dared to say otherwise. Though he has not been widely recognized as the pioneer he was, many of his insights have come to be accepted, and the flame he carried in the darkness for so long has become a light to millions.

The American Cancer Society, with its customary level of open-mindedness to unorthodox methods, has never sent a representative to the Gerson Clinic or tested his work. To this day, however, the organization tells people with cancer that the Gerson treatment is worthless.[9]

Humanitarian, physician, and Nobel Peace Prize winner Albert Schweitzer wouldn't agree. He knew Max Gerson's work well, and hailed him as "one of the most eminent geniuses in medical history."[10]

MACROBIOTICS AND CANCER

Macrobiotics is probably the best known of the current dietary approaches to cancer. Its leading exponent in the United States is Michio Kushi. Born in Japan, he was deeply affected by the bombing of Hiroshima and Nagasaki, and decided to devote his life to peace. His philosophy and approach to cancer stem from his belief that by returning to a traditional diet of whole, natural foods, humanity can regain its physical and mental balance, become more peaceful, and achieve optimum health.

Kushi does not claim that a macrobiotic diet cures cancer, but rather that it is part of a way of life that can prevent much disease, including many cases of cancer. And yet there have been repeated reports from both physicians and patients of cures that have occurred when people with cancer have switched from the typical American diet to a macrobiotic diet.

One of the most credible of these reports came from Anthony Sattilaro, M.D., chief executive of Methodist Hospital in Philadelphia, and formerly chairman of the anesthesiology department. This doctor suffered from severe metastatic prostate cancer, and received the "best" of conventional therapies, but to no avail. He was told he had at best only a short time to live. In desperation, he turned to a macrobiotic whole-foods diet, and experienced a complete physical recovery. Ten years later, still adhering to the diet, he was youthful and vigorous, and his cancer seemed to be totally gone. In his later years, however, he deviated from the diet, adding chicken and fish, at which point the cancer returned and proved fatal.[11]

Another fully credible source regarding macrobiotic successes with cancer is Vivien Newbold, M.D., a specialist in emergency medicine in Philadelphia. "Five patients with advanced, medically incurable cancer," she wrote in the *Townsend Letter for Doctors*, "achieved complete remission for five years or more after beginning a macrobiotic diet. These remissions cannot be explained by any medical treatment the patients received. One additional patient obtained remission after trying macrobiotics, failed to continue the diet, and died when the cancer recurred."[12] Newbold had all of these cases reviewed independently, and had their diagnoses confirmed by pathologists and radiologists.

After carefully documenting each of these instances, she sent her findings to the AMA *Journal* and other leading establishment publications. None chose to publish it, saying their readership would have "insufficient interest."[13]

What do I think of macrobiotics for cancer? I wouldn't expect a great number of cancer cases to be cured by the diet alone, but I recognize that some people with cancer have experienced enormous improvement. It is indisputable that many people with cancer have enhanced their quality of life, and gained significant life extension on the diet. James Carter, M.D., chairman of the Department of Nutrition at Tulane University, conducted a controlled study of the macrobiotic diet in prostate cancer. He found that men who made the shift to macrobiotics lived, on average, three years longer than those who did not. Even more remarkably, a 1994 study published in the *Journal of the American College of Nutrition* found that the median survival time for men with prostate cancer who received aggressive treatment was six years; the median survival time for men with prostate cancer who went on a macrobiotic diet was 19 years.[14]

If I had cancer, would I eat a Gerson or Macrobiotic type of diet? I already do. I've eaten a low-fat, whole-foods, completely vegetarian diet for almost all of the last 30 years. But if I hadn't, and I were to develop cancer, one of the first things I'd do would be to eliminate meat, eggs, dairy products, sugar, and junk food, and start eating natural foods.

In 1988, Dr. Harold Foster of the University of Victoria, British Columbia, reviewed 200 cases of spontaneous regression from cancer, and found that nearly 90 percent of these people had made major dietary changes before their dramatic improvement "spontaneously" occurred. Usually, their changes involved switching to a strictly vegetarian diet, and dispensing with white flour, sugar, and overly processed foods. Many of them also used vitamin and mineral supplements, and drank herbal teas.[15]

In 1995, the American Cancer Society commented simultaneously on vitamin C, the Hoxsey herbal therapy, the Gerson diet, the macrobiotic diet, and several similar dietary methods. "None of these approaches is supported by adequate clinical data," the organization began, neglecting to mention that a major reason for this is its own refusal to conduct or support any sort of testing that would provide adequate clinical data.

"Some involve a diet that is nutritionally inadequate," the report continued. "Some involve potentially toxic doses of vitamins and/or other substances."[16]

I see. This leading advocate of chemotherapy seeks to fulfill its public trust by warning the public that vitamin C, herbs, carrot juice, and brown rice are potentially toxic.

THE MOST CONTROVERSIAL OF THEM ALL

Based in Houston, Texas, Stanislaw Burzynski, M.D., is probably the most controversial figure in the world of cancer today. The American Cancer

Society considers his treatment of "highest concern," and wants him stopped at almost any cost. Yet there are many, even within the establishment, who feel his discoveries are the most important ever attained in the struggle with cancer. Even some of his most zealous opponents admit that if his theories are correct, the man deserves a Nobel prize.

Born in Poland in 1943, Burzynski was a child prodigy, graduating first in his class from medical school, and becoming one of the youngest men in Europe ever to receive doctoral degrees in both medicine and biochemistry. In 1970, rather than join the Communist Party, this independent-minded physician left his homeland and emigrated to the United States, becoming a research professor at Baylor University, where he quickly became recognized as a truly outstanding scientist with an extraordinary genius for original research.[17]

Burzynski discovered that people with cancer have a dramatic shortage of certain substances that occur naturally in the human body. These substances, a group of peptides and amino-acid derivatives, inhibit the growth of cancer cells.

Burzynski named these substances antineoplastons because they inhibit "neoplastic" (cancerous) growth. He discovered that they play an indispensable role in the biochemical defense system, upon which the body depends to correct defective cells.

Based on his original research, Burzynski eventually developed an entire approach to treating cancer. In 1993, health writer Richard Walters reported, "By reintroducing the peptides into the patient's bloodstream, either orally or intravenously, he brings about tumor shrinkage or complete remission. In many cases, just weeks after the start of treatment, tumors have shrunk in size or disappeared. Most types of cancer respond to the therapy, which is safe and nontoxic. The natural substances used are well tolerated by the body, even in high doses, without any of the disastrous side effects routinely associated with toxic chemotherapy and radiation. Since the Burzynski Research Institute opened in 1977, Dr. Burzynski has treated some 2,000 cancer patients, most of them in advanced stages. He has saved or prolonged hundreds of lives with his innovative approach. A significant number of persons treated have been in complete remission for five years or more, even though they were pronounced 'terminal' or 'incurable' by their conventional doctors."[18]

But early on, Burzynski ran into a roadblock. **Antineoplastons are largely species-specific. This means that although they might be mar-**

velously effective in human beings, they would not generally be effective in other animals. The problem was that the FDA was (and is) entrenched in requiring success in animal experiments before allowing human trials.

Burzynski was faced with a formidable obstacle. He knew that the medicines would not pass the FDA's animal-test requirements. At the same time, he believed deeply that they were an answer for many people with cancer. Faced with this impasse, he made a decision to go ahead and begin treating patients, even without FDA approval.

How could Burzynski have known what this might trigger? "Coming from Poland," he said later, "where everybody has a saintly opinion of the United States, I was convinced that this would be the country where democracy is everywhere."[19] He believed that once he showed that the treatment could save many lives, the bureaucratic obstacles would somehow be removed.

Unfortunately, this was not what happened. Ever since the fateful moment that Burzynski decided to place saving people's lives ahead of following rules that would not allow his medicine a fair chance, he has experienced "the full-scale legal and regulatory terror of county, state, and national authorities."[20] On one occasion, for example, agents of the FDA entered Burzynski's clinic and seized 200,000 medical documents and business records. Ten years later, no charges had been filed, and yet the documents had never been returned.[21]

The ongoing attacks upon Burzynski's work have hardly created the ideal conditions for scientific inquiry and compassionate healing to take place. And yet somehow this remarkable man has persevered, treating cancer patients with sometimes stunning success, and conducting original research that is extraordinarily promising. Additionally, he has always made his therapy available for independent assessment.

No patient has ever testified against Burzynski. And in all the actions against him, no one has ever suggested that Burzynski has harmed a single patient.

When the American Cancer Society put Burzynski's antineoplaston therapy on its list of *Unproven Methods of Cancer Management*, the organization's report cited one particular study as part of its proof that his treatment didn't work. How they reached this conclusion I have no idea, because the study had involved treating people with advanced cancer (of the breast, bladder, colon, leukemia, and other sites) with antineoplastons, and 86 percent of them had shown clinical improvement. Some 19 percent of the patients had complete remissions.[22] Yet somehow the American Cancer Society managed to conclude from this that his treatment was worthless.

The thousands of patients who have gone to Burzynski for treatment don't seem to agree. Every time the government or medical authorities try to stop Burzynski from practicing, they are deluged with letters from patients and their families. One such 1992 letter, to Texas District Attorney Dan Morales, read:

"I understand that you are currently engaged in efforts to prevent Dr. Burzynski in Houston from practicing medicine. I understand and appreciate your desire to protect the public from fraud and I am certain you would be interested in hearing any valid information about him.

"I investigated Dr. Burzynski for my father, who is suffering from glioblastoma multiforme, a viciously aggressive brain tumor that rarely responds to radiation or chemotherapy, and then only briefly. It is basically a death sentence. . . .

"I spoke to Dr. Patronas, a National Cancer Institute neuroradiologist with 20 years experience, whose knowledge of Dr. Burzynski came not from rumors but from a site visit during which he audited a number of cases. He told me that he believes in Burzynski's results, that he found the evidence 'extremely impressive,' and that 'in 20 years in this business I haven't seen anything that looks so promising.'

"But the most impressive evidence is my father. A recent scan shows that the tumors have stopped growing and there is some necrosis [cancer cell death] within the tumors. . . . I would be happy to send the radiology reports at your request. I know that many in the medical establishment are hostile to Dr. Burzynski. We should keep in mind how often the medical establishment has been proven wrong. . . . Mr. Morales, I am sure that you have only the public's interest at heart. I urge you to consider the possibility that Dr. Burzynski's treatment is in fact saving lives. I urge you to keep in mind the very real possibility that had your effort to prevent him from treating patients succeeded, my father might be dead. . . ."[23]

Some of the most touching letters come from children, who in their simple way speak eloquently of basic human realities: "I am 13 years old and I have a 7 year old brother. We love our father very much. Thanks to Dr. Burzynski's treatment, my father's tumor has stopped growing. All of the doctors in my home state of Missouri said there was no cure for my father's disease. Dr. Burzynski gave him a chance for life again. Please don't take that away from us."[24]

If you were looking for someone to speak ill of Dr. Stanislaw Burzynski, you'd have a particularly rough time with Sharon Hermann, of Marlboro, New Jersey. Testifying before Congress in 1993, she described what happened to her son Ryan, who was ten years old when he was diagnosed in 1989 with an advanced and highly malignant brain tumor. Orthodox doctors told the boy's parents that he had only months to live, and the disease was incurable.

The boy underwent radiation that proved ineffective. It did, however, burn out most of his pituitary gland, stunt his growth, and disturb his mental functioning. After it was over, Ryan's mother felt betrayed: "We were never told about radiation's possible long-term effects."[25]

The doctors wanted next to proceed with a highly toxic experimental chemotherapy treatment, which, they said, could at best extend his life 12 to 18 months, although in a progressively debilitated condition. But Ryan's parents were fed up, and took him to Burzynski in Houston. His mother recalls: "The doctors really beat us up over not doing chemo. We were discouraged at every turn from pursuing a safe, nontoxic therapy. They also told us Burzynski was a quack. The American Cancer Society said they have an arrangement with the Hilton to keep rooms available for cancer patients' families, but when we mentioned Dr. Burzynski's name, they said to 'forget it.' The Corporate Angel Network, which boasts in TV ads how it flies young cancer patients around the country for free, refused to fly our son because the National Cancer Institute won't let them fly Burzynski's patients."[26]

Young Ryan began treatment with Burzynski in April 1990. His mother could hardly believe what happened. "It felt as if a miracle had occurred," she said. After four weeks, an MRI scan of the brain found only barely visible tumor remnants. By November, Ryan was in complete remission. Since then, brain scans have repeatedly found him to be completely free of cancer.

When the boy's mother called the radiologists back home to tell them the good news, their reaction was utter disbelief. They were sure she was calling to tell them the boy had passed away. When they later examined Ryan and his brain scans, they said they had never in their lives seen anything like it.

Another woman no force on earth could get to testify against Burzynski is the mother of Jimmy Kilanowski. In May 1989, doctors at Memorial Sloan-Kettering told her that her ten-year-old son had brain cancer and would live less than three months without treatment. If he received both radiation and chemotherapy, they gave him a year. When a make-a-wish foundation offered him his dream, Jimmy said he'd like to meet President Bush. It was arranged, and he did. The president was told he was shaking hands with a dying boy.

But little Jimmy crossed up all the prophets of his doom when his parents took him to Dr. Burzynski. When the boy arrived in Houston, he had five brain tumors visible in his CT scan, and the prognosis could hardly have been worse. By May 1991, however, all traces of his tumors were gone, and orthodox doctors at North Shore University Hospital stated he was in complete remission.[27]

Burzynski does not claim to have a cure for all cancers. Although his treatment often gets outstanding results with prostate cancer and many brain cancers, and also often achieves excellent outcomes with non-Hodgkin's lymphomas and pancreatic cancers, the results with breast cancers are not as consistent, thus far, nor are those for certain types of lung and colon cancers. It speaks well of Burzynski that he is the first to acknowledge when antineoplastons aren't likely to be useful, and will only accept patients that he thinks he can help.

THE PERSECUTION OF A GENIUS

Despite the remarkable results Burzynski has obtained, and his outstanding level of personal integrity, the Texas Medical Board has been trying since the early 1980s to prohibit him from using his non-FDA approved medicines within the state. In 1993, Administrative Law Judge Earl Corbitt ruled that it was legal for him to use his non-FDA approved medicines in the state of Texas. Unfazed, the state Medical Board simply voted to overturn the judge's decision, and in 1994 declared it illegal for Burzynski to use antineoplastons in Texas. **The state Medical Board came to this conclusion despite acknowledging that there was no evidence that the treatment was harmful, and despite accepting the undisputed evidence presented by a National Cancer Institute investigator that antineoplastons were effective and necessary for the survival of many of Burzynski's patients.**[28]

In ordering Burzynski to cease providing his medicines, the Medical Board was in effect condemning hundreds of patients (who were in the process of recovering thanks to his treatment) to death. Astonishingly, the board ruled that the "mere survival of patients did not qualify as an immediate need under the law."[29] The board also suspended his medical license for ten years, then stayed the suspension providing he complied with its orders to cease providing his medications, and placed him on probation.

Burzynski's attorneys immediately appealed, and on February 3, 1995, District Judge Paul Davis rendered a verdict that reversed and vacated the Medical Board's order. In a stinging rebuke to the Medical Board, he declared that the board's attack on Burzynski was "in excess of the agency's statutory authority, not reasonably supported by substantial evidence, capricious and arbitrary, and characterized by abuse of discretion."[30]

By this time, both Administrative Law Judge Corbitt and District Court Judge Davis had rendered decisions in favor of Burzynski, but the Medical Board simply undertook yet another appeal.[31]

Meanwhile, for the fifth time in ten years, a federal grand jury was convening to investigate Dr. Burzynski. Like the previous grand jury investigations, the focus of attention was the alleged illegal shipment of non-FDA approved medicines across state lines. All four previous grand juries had investigated these claims, and all four had refused to press charges against him, noting that he had FDA approval to ship his medicine around the country to various sites for clinical trials, as well as to patients who have received a compassionate use permit. (Burzynski does not ship the medicines out-of-state without the explicit permission of the FDA. There is in fact a long-standing policy at Burzynski's Institute that any employee who does so will immediately be terminated.)[32]

Texas Congressperson Joe Barton called the investigation "an extraordinary abuse of the legal system. . . . It is extraordinarily rare for a grand jury to fail to indict at the request of the U.S. Attorney. To fail to indict some four times successively may be unprecedented. It would appear that the FDA and the Justice Department have no case and are abusing the grand jury process to harass and punish Dr. Burzynski."[33]

As the grand jury convened, Burzynski's attorney, Richard Jaffe, commented: "Unfortunately, there is no statute of limitation limiting the number of times the U.S. Attorney's Office and the FDA can present the same tired allegations to a grand jury, and I doubt that this grand jury knows much about its four predecessors."[34]

It didn't. And as a result, in 1995 the grand jury indicted Stanislaw

Burzynski, M.D., placing this extraordinary physician in jeopardy of spending the rest of his life in jail.

Meanwhile, Burzynski's impressive success in treating people with cancer was getting national exposure. In March 1995, Burzynski appeared on the "Eye on America" segment of the CBS-TV/*Evening News*. The response to the show was so tremendous that the network asked him and several of his patients to appear the following week on CBS-TV's *This Morning* show. On both national shows, Burzynski spoke clearly and accurately about the biochemical defense system in the human body, antineoplastons, and his results with cancer.

The patients who appeared with him presented compelling stories. Two had suffered from non-Hodgkin's lymphoma, and one from brain cancer. All three had been told they were medically incurable, and yet all were now in complete remission due to Burzynski's treatment. Their statements were profoundly moving, and after the nationally televised programs Burzynski's Institute was flooded with thousands of calls from people with cancer.

And yet on the very day of Burzynski's second CBS appearance, while he was in New York doing the show, the FDA raided his Institute. Seven agents herded his employees into a conference room, and proceeded to seize medical records, message books, and patient lists. When office manager Barbara Tomaszewski asked the agents to please wait while she contacted Burzynski's attorney, they told her not only would they not wait, but they would conduct the search by force if necessary. The raid went on for more than six hours.[35]

What did the FDA want with a list of Dr. Burzynski's cancer patients? The FDA threatened some with grand jury subpoenas for nothing more than receiving and taking antineoplastons for their own use. In New York, FDA agents actually turned up at a cancer patient's home, demanding that his wife turn over his medicines.

Ironically, the National Cancer Institute and the FDA were at that very moment conducting controlled clinical trials of Burzynski's medicines at Memorial Sloan-Kettering Cancer Center, the Mayo Clinic, and several other sites. But after the raid, without consulting Burzynski, they arbitrarily changed the terms under which antineoplastons would be tested. In a maneuver eerily reminiscent of the vitamin C tests, patients would now be included who had previously received massive chemotherapy and radiation.[36]

Impartial scientists were horrified, saying the change seemed designed to produce a negative result. In May 1995, the independent *Cancer Chronicles* reported: "A patient who has already failed to respond to surgery, radiation, and/or chemotherapy, who has numerous large tumors, metastases in the liver and lungs, and a declining performance score can now be enrolled to 'test' this gentle nontoxic treatment, whose protocol was designed to treat patients in earlier stages. It is known to all that these antineoplastons, at the dosages given, will almost certainly not work in this situation. Patients will die."[37]

Asking why the tests would be skewed like this, the *Cancer Chronicles* noted that Burzynski's successful nontoxic treatment of many cases of cancer threatened the very basis of the "War on Cancer," and represented a profound threat to the vested interests of the cancer establishment. The report concluded: "The failure will be loudly announced to the public, most probably on national television, and will deal a heavy blow to this treatment and to alternative medicine in general."[38]

In 1995, the American Cancer Society warned that they would "strongly urge individuals afflicted with cancer not to participate in treatment with antineoplastons."[39]

As if they had a better answer.

DECIDING WHAT TO DO

Not that long ago, whenever I heard someone claim he was persecuted by the medical establishment for holding controversial beliefs, I'd check my crackpot meter. The idea of there being a conspiracy to suppress cancer cures seemed paranoid. Sure, I thought, the system isn't particularly open to new ideas that come from outside its domains, but certainly, once a treatment is shown to be valuable, doors will open, scientific studies will be carried out, and if sober analysis finds a method effective, it will be accepted and put to use.

The American Cancer Society supports this view, stating that you can identify "the proponents of questionable or totally worthless remedies [by the] claim that established medical and scientific organizations have conspired against them."[40]

But the more I've learned, the more I've come to realize that when it comes to American medical politics, those in power have a vested interest in the belief systems and methods by which they have attained their position. It is a sad and unfortunate fact that they often dismiss alternative approaches as false or even fraudulent without being willing to evaluate them impartially.

If the advocates of alternative methods can sometimes seem a little paranoid, perhaps they have reason. Some of them have worked tirelessly their whole lives to develop alternative approaches that show great ability to relieve suffering, only to find themselves and their ideas ridiculed and criminalized.

Of course, some unconventional practitioners exaggerate their results out of wishful thinking, and others stretch the truth in order to generate business. And even those practitioners who are scrupulously honest may not be able to provide reliable statistical data, for they often lack the resources necessary to compile comprehensive statistics or do thorough follow-up. Establishment organizations like the American Cancer Society have the resources to objectively evaluate unorthodox treatments, but they don't seem overly eager to do so. The result is that people living with cancer who are interested in trying an alternative approach are often left bewildered and overwhelmed, and in a quandary over how to choose wisely.

In this book I can only mention a few of the many alternative treatments that are available and worthy of serious consideration. If I had cancer, I would certainly take advantage of at least one of the expert personalized services available to help people make informed decisions on the most promising therapeutic options for their type of cancer. Such services include Ralph Moss's *Healing Choices* (718-636-4433), and Patrick McGrady's *Can-Help* (206-437-2291). A list of other organizations and additional resources can be found in the resource guide at the back of the book.

People living with cancer are faced with many difficult choices, and I believe passionately that they deserve the best of all available worlds. If an aspect of conventional medical treatment can be of use, I'm all for it. If surgery can help them (and it often can), then they should have that option. If chemotherapy or radiation, provided at just the right time with ample nutritional and emotional support, can truly help them, then wonderful. And yet, by the same token, if blends of herbs, or dietary changes, or other alternative methods can be useful, as they often can, then these options, too, should be made available. What we don't need is an inquisition-like atmosphere, where any practice or belief that does not conform to the dominant paradigm is considered heresy.

Today, some of the most outstanding and inspiring results are being obtained by health-care practitioners who bridge the two worlds, combining the best of both conventional and alternative methods for the benefit of their patients.

INTEGRATING THE BEST OF ALTERNATIVE AND ORTHODOX MEDICINE

Most people with cancer who are cured by conventional medical treatment are cured by surgery. And yet, the procedure is often severely traumatic. Alternatives can play a role in making operations not only more humane, but also more effective.

One example of integrating the best of both worlds is the use of acupuncture for anesthesia in cancer surgery. David Eisenberg, M.D., of Harvard Medical School, and an advisor to the National Institutes of Health Office of Alternative Medicine, was the first U.S. medical exchange student to study in the People's Republic of China. Eisenberg, who speaks Chinese, describes watching major brain surgery being done on a patient with pituitary cancer. The patient, named Lu, was a 58-year-old professor at Beijing University.

The anesthesiologist was a woman with ten years of Western anesthesiology training, who preferred acupuncture because of its far fewer side effects. She placed needles in six key points—two in the eyebrow area, two near the right temple, and two near the left ankle—and then connected them to a low-voltage electronic stimulating machine that sent current through the needles at regular intervals. Twenty minutes later, writes Eisenberg:

"The anesthesiologist gave the go-ahead to begin, and the surgeons took up their scalpels. They made an incision along three sides of the rectangle outlined by the marking pen, and proceeded to lift a three-sided flap of full-thickness skin from Lu's skull. At the moment of incision, Lu failed to wince, grimace or give any hint of pain. He remarked he was aware of the surgeons applying pressure to his skin but that he experienced no discomfort. His pulse and blood pressure remained at preoperative levels. . . .

"Throughout the entire procedure, which continued for more than four hours, Lu remained conscious, and his vital signs remained stable. We conversed the whole time he was on the operating table.

"After the completion of the surgery, Lu sat up from the operating table, shook the hand of the surgeon, thanked him profusely, shook hands with the anesthesiologist and me, then walked out of the operating room unassisted."[41]

Another example of the wise integration of alternative methods in cancer surgery is found in the work of cancer surgeon (and noted author) Bernie Siegel, M.D. As a surgeon, he offers his technical skill and training in orthodox medicine, but he also seeks to enlist the assistance of the patient's innate healing abilities. Here he describes how he blends the two approaches in a surgical setting:

"After my patients are relaxed, I instruct them to divert the blood away from the operative site so that they won't bleed; I tell them that when they awaken they will feel comfortable, thirsty, and hungry and will have no difficulty voiding; and I give them whatever other messages might be appropriate to their particular situation. When the anesthesiologist says, 'You'll be going out,' I may talk about going out on a date, so that the image becomes something positive. I stand by, holding my patients' hands and gently guiding them into the anesthesia with soothing words and healing music. Afterward, some of my patients have even asked if I operated with one hand, because they had the impression I continued to hold their hands after they fell asleep.

"I keep talking to patients throughout the operation, telling them how things are progressing and enlisting their cooperation if I need it. For example, I may suggest that they stop bleeding, or lower their blood pressure or pulse. People who have worked with me in the operating room know how effective these suggestions can be. One day, as I was preparing to leave after finishing an operation, the anesthesiologist tore off a foot or two of electrocardiogram and said to me, 'Here, you fix it.' I looked and saw that the patient, who was still under anesthesia, was having an arrhythmia, so I whispered in his ear, 'You are on a swing. It's going up and back, in a nice and steady, even rhythm. Up and back, slow and steady.' And his cardiogram reverted to a normal rhythm.

"Often when a patient's pulse rate is too high during an operation I'll simply say, 'We'd like your pulse to be 86.' I always pick a specific number because I want everyone to see the pulse go down to that exact number. Something in the body hears these messages and knows how to respond to them."

Siegel mentions the damage done to patients when a surgical team does not acknowledge that patients hear and process information while unconscious. Not only do they fail to give healing messages during the operation, "they may do the opposite, wisecracking and even making abusive remarks about the patient who lies unconscious on the operating table, or offering their opinions about the patient's dismal prognosis." Afterwards, patients rarely consciously remember such destructive remarks, but callousness can take a toll nevertheless, expressed in postoperative pain, slow healing, prolonged depression, and worse. Patients who are unconscious are in a particularly suggestible state, and the way they are spoken to and treated can make a tremendous difference in their outcomes.[42]

SUPPORT GROUPS THAT HEAL

In 1989, David Spiegel, M.D., of Stanford Medical School announced the results of a remarkable ten-year study. His report on the life-extending potential of breast cancer support groups, published in *Lancet*, is another outstanding example of how much is to be gained when conventional medicine expands to include alternative approaches instead of blocking them.

Spiegel's randomized controlled study compared the outcomes for women with "terminal" breast cancer who received standard medical treatment, to the results obtained by women with the same diagnosis who received the same treatment, but who also met weekly in a support group and received lessons in self-hypnosis. "I undertook the study," he confessed later, "expecting to refute the often overstated notions about the power of mind over disease."[43]

But that's not what happened. Instead, Spiegel and his colleagues found that, while the women who received orthodox medical care alone lived an average of 19 months, those who in addition met once a week to talk about and express their feelings lived an average of 37 months.

Why would participation in support groups extend the lives of people with cancer? Repressing strong feelings causes emotional strain and tension that all too often turns into physical problems. When feelings are stifled, they are pushed underground where they fester, sometimes producing a situation conducive to the development and growth of diseases, including cancer. This was Woody Allen's point when he said in one of his movies, "I can't express anger. I internalize it and grow a tumor instead."

The women who participated in these groups had the opportunity to unburden themselves and to gain one another's support in dealing with their pain. As a result, they felt less isolated, less like they had to bear their ordeal alone. They could discuss their fears and challenges with others who understood. Some felt that the resulting gains in the quality of their lives were even more important than the added life extension. The experience of opening their hearts to others not only added years to their lives, but also life to their years.

VITAMINS, TOO

Most doctors would scoff at the idea that high doses of vitamins could have an appreciable influence on the course of cancer. But in 1994, the *Journal of Urology* reported a remarkable randomized, double-blind, placebo-controlled trial that assessed the effect of megadoses of vitamins on the recurrence rate of cancer of the bladder. Half the patients were put on a multivitamin and mineral supplement that provided the RDA of these and many other nutrients. The other half received a megavitamin supplement that included 40,000 IU of vitamin A, 100 mg of vitamin B6, 2000 mg of vitamin C, 400 IU of vitamin E, and 90 mg of zinc. After five years, the results were more than impressive. Those people with cancer who received the RDA level of vitamins and minerals had a tumor recurrence rate of 91 percent. Those who took the megadose vitamins, in contrast, had a recurrence rate of only 41 percent.[44]

MARIJUANA AS MEDICINE

I continue to be amazed by the benefits that can occur when natural methods are used to complement orthodox medical procedures. While nausea and vomiting are not the only toxic and dangerous side effects from chemotherapy, they can be profoundly debilitating. Remarkably, the marijuana plant has been repeatedly shown to be far more effective for these problems than any drug currently available in the pharmaceutical repertoire. In 1988, the *New York State Journal of Medicine* published a study of 56 chemotherapy patients who got no relief from standard antiemetic (antivomiting) agents. Nearly 80 percent actually became symptom free when they smoked the leaves of this plant.[45]

Why, then, is this plant not commonly used to reduce the nausea and vomiting from chemotherapy? Because it is illegal, even for medical purposes.

Keith Nutt, of Beaverton, Michigan, developed testicular cancer at the age of 22, and was given chemotherapy. His mother explains: "He would vomit violently for eight to ten hours, and afterward was so profoundly nauseated that he could not bear to look at or smell food. Antiemetic drugs provided no noticeable relief. In less than two months, our son lost at least 30 pounds. He began to vomit bile. When there was nothing to vomit, he would simply retch and convulse. It was horrible for us to watch our son suffer such anguish from the disease and the treatment. . . .

"One evening I read a newspaper article that said marijuana could reduce the severe nausea and vomiting caused by many anticancer therapies. The idea that marijuana had medical uses was new to my husband and me. As a parent I was strongly opposed to marijuana and other illegal drugs. My husband and I made sure our sons had no illusions about our stern opposition to drug use. . . .

"[But] shortly after my husband and I read these materials, Keith had another round of chemotherapy, and, as always, it made him dreadfully sick. We could not stand by and watch him suffer, but, as an older couple, we did not have the slightest idea where to find marijuana. In desperation, we asked a close friend for help, an ordained Presbyterian minister who worked with local youth groups. Several days later he appeared at our door with some marijuana. It was the first time we had ever seen any.

"The next day we took the marijuana to Keith in the hospital. After he smoked it, his vomiting abruptly stopped. The sudden change was amazing to see. Marijuana also put an end to his nausea. He actually began to put on weight. His mental outlook underwent a startling improvement. . . . Marijuana was the safest, most benign drug he received in the course of his battle against cancer."[46]

Keith's parents came to resent that marijuana was illegal for medical purposes. Honest, simple people, they felt like criminals, having to sneak around to obtain some in order to help their son. As their original supply ran out, they hated having to ask their friend, the minister, and their other son to risk arrest in order to obtain for Keith the medicine he desperately needed. Knowing that there were many other cancer patients who could benefit greatly from marijuana, they decided to go public with their experience and to testify before the Michigan State Judiciary Committee.

Shortly after a newspaper article told their story, an Episcopal priest knocked on their door. He brought some marijuana, and said simply that he thought they would know who might benefit from it. Another woman in the community gave them a cigar box filled with marijuana. She said that her husband had smoked it to control his terminal cancer pain. Now that he was deceased, she had no use for it, and hoped that it would help their son.

At the hearings, the family met another family, the Negens, of Grand Rapids, whose 21-year-old daughter, Deborah, was receiving chemotherapy for leukemia. The Negen family also testified to the tremendous benefits their daughter had received from marijuana. The Reverend Negen was pastor of a very conservative Dutch Christian Reform Church in Grand Rapids, and was vehemently opposed to illegal drugs. But his daughter was suffering so badly from her chemotherapy that he could not just stand by and allow this to continue when marijuana could be of so much help. He prayed for guidance, and eventually decided that if using marijuana to help his daughter was not acceptable to his congregation, then he would have to leave the church.[47]

Marijuana can be of extraordinary value in reducing the nausea and vomiting that often accompany chemotherapy, and can contribute enormously to the quality of life of a person undergoing the treatment. Such comfort is certainly rationale enough for its medical use.

But there is also substantial evidence that, in those cases where chemotherapy can sometimes produce a cure, marijuana can greatly improve the odds. The reason is simple: long periods of uncontrollable and intense nausea destroy people's spirits and will to live, and can make it impossible for them to eat. Dispirited and wasting away, they become prone to all kinds of diseases and complications, some of which can be fatal.

The world-famous Harvard geologist Stephen Jay Gould says that marijuana helped to save his life when he came down with a rare kind of cancer, abdominal mesothelioma. "When I started intravenous chemotherapy, absolutely nothing in the available arsenal of antiemetics worked at all. I was miserable, and came to dread the frequent treatments with an almost perverse intensity. I had heard that marijuana often worked well against nausea. I was reluctant to try it, because I have never smoked any substance habitually (and didn't even know how to inhale). Moreover, I had tried marijuana twice (in the usual context of growing up in the sixties) and had hated it. I am something of a Puritan on the subject of substances that, in any way, dull or alter mental states, for I value my rational mind with an academician's overweening arrogance."[48]

But realizing that the nausea was so intense he might not be able to complete a chemotherapy treatment that had a realistic possibility of producing a cure, Gould tried marijuana.

"The rest of the story is short and sweet. Marijuana worked like a charm. I disliked the side effect of mental blurring, but the sheer bliss of not experiencing nausea, and then not having to fear it for all the days between treatments, was the greatest boost I received in all my year of treatment, and surely had a most important effect upon my eventual cure."[49]

Oncologists are legally permitted to prescribe Marinol, a synthetic drug that contains one of marijuana's active ingredients (THC). But there are problems with Marinol. For one thing, it is extremely expensive. And for another, it is taken orally rather than smoked, with the result that the THC is only slowly and erratically absorbed into the bloodstream. When the actual herb is smoked, the THC is absorbed much quicker and more reliably, so patients can learn to adjust their dosage effectively, controlling the amount that reaches the blood and the brain.

Most patients strongly prefer smoked marijuana to oral Marinol, which they say makes them anxious and uncomfortable. There are substances in marijuana smoke, such as cannabidiol, that are not contained in Marinol, and that reduce the anxiety that can be produced by THC alone.

Furthermore, patients who are severely nauseated often cannot keep capsules of Marinol down, vomiting up the drug as they do anything else they swallow.

Due to the medicinal value of marijuana, not only for chemotherapy, but also for other conditions (most notably to reduce interocular pressure in glaucoma patients, but also for multiple sclerosis, paraplegia and quadriplegia, epilepsy, AIDS wasting syndrome, chronic pain, migraines, pruritis, and menstrual cramps), there have been repeated attempts in many states to legalize its use for medical purposes.[50] Time and again, individuals, families, and oncologists have bravely placed themselves at risk in order to testify to the value this plant can provide in cancer treatment, and plead for its humanitarian use. Unfortunately, the established cancer organizations have so far remained firmly seated on the sidelines, preferring to invest public funds in the search for pharmaceutical answers.

In 1995, the AMA *Journal* carried a commentary coauthored by Lester Grinspoon, associate professor of psychiatry at Harvard Medical School, titled "Marijuana as Medicine: A Plea for Reconsideration."[51] Drug Enforcement Administration (DEA) administrator Thomas Constantine immediately reacted to the piece, saying the DEA would continue to strongly oppose any attempt to use or even test marijuana for medical purposes. The reason? "The American Cancer Society," he said, "has rejected marijuana as medicine."[52]

The opponents of medical marijuana believe that the advocates of medical use of the plant are only using the issue as a wedge to open the way for recreational use. Because it would be impossible for anyone to accuse the American Cancer Society of being a front for a recreational drug use agenda, it is likely that if this organization were to actively engage in the effort to legalize medical marijuana, countless patients would be spared untold suffering, and lives would be saved.

STUNNING RESULTS WITH BREAST CANCER

In the waiting room of the Heather M. Bligh Cancer Research Laboratories at the Finch University/Chicago Medical School there hangs a painting of a statement made by the philosopher Pierre Teilhard de Chardin: "The day will come when, after harnessing the ether, the winds, the tides, and gravitation, we shall harness for God the energies of love. And on that day, for the second time in the history of the world, man will have discovered fire."

Georg Springer, M.D., commissioned the painting of those inspiring words. His desk is covered with research papers, test results, and scientific literature. In the windowsill are flowering potted plants, like the ones he sends to his cancer patients each year to honor their continued survival, and to let them know he is thinking of them and holding them in his heart.

A physician who combines love with science, Springer has published numerous articles in the scientific literature explaining his approach to breast cancer. When he isolated antigens, substances that develop on the surface of cancer cells and elicit an immune response, he began to be able to listen for the very first signals within the body that cancer is developing. Since then, he has developed a harmless and inexpensive skin test using the body's own antigens that can detect the presence of cancer cells up to six years before they would show up on a mammogram (and without exposure to harmful X-rays), 90 percent of the time.[53] As of 1994, 1,200 people had taken the test, and there had been no false positives, no times that the test said cancer was present when it actually wasn't. Mammograms, on the other hand, are notorious for high rates of false positives, leading to a tremendous amount of anxiety and unnecessary medical intervention.

When Springer's beloved wife Heather was pronounced "terminal" with breast cancer, he developed a treatment program for her that enabled her to live six additional years. A key component of the Springer program, which he now provides for women with breast cancer, involves injections of antigens to stimulate the immune system. His goal is to fortify the body's natural abilities for self-repair, to harness the power of the immune system to fight malignant disease. His methods, like those of many other alternative practitioners, work to strengthen the immune system rather than destroy it as chemotherapy often does. One of his patients remarked, "I don't get colds anymore. When everybody is moaning and groaning, I'm fine and dandy."[54]

"All human cancer cells differ from their parental healthy cells in the fine architecture of their cell surfaces," says Springer.[55] The body's defense system, sensing the abnormal structure of cancer cells, perceives them as foreign and seeks to eliminate them, just as it does viruses and disease-causing bacteria. Springer's antigen-based injections support the effort, enabling the body's defense system to accomplish its purpose.

He has most of his patients on high doses of vitamin C (4 grams daily) and vitamin E (800 units daily), plus beta carotene and a multiple vitamin. Though his treatment is not covered by most insurance companies, he is able, thanks to a small inheritance he received, to spend his personal funds to support the center. He does not turn people away who cannot afford to pay.

Of course, the real question, with any method, be it conventional or unconventional, is does it work? Does it help people with cancer?

According to the National Cancer Institute, the five-year survival rate for women with breast cancer using the conventional treatments is 41 percent for Stage III patients (large tumors with involvement of the lymph nodes), and 10 percent for Stage IV patients (distant metastases, e.g., to bone, liver, or lung).[56] In comparison, Springer's results are nothing short of spectacular. An astounding 100 percent of the Stage III and Stage IV women in his first study group were alive after five years.[57] Furthermore, they were not only alive, they were in most cases thriving. The vast majority of them appeared to be totally cured, with no detectable sign of cancer present in their bodies. Although the size of this study group was relatively small, subsequent results have been consistent with this sensational beginning.

With conventional treatment, only 20 percent of Stage III women and less than 5 percent of Stage IV women are alive after ten years. In Springer's group after ten years, however, 75 percent of the Stage

III women were alive, and a truly phenomenal 60 percent of Stage IV women.[58]

Linda McCormick of Joplin, Missouri, was 40 when she had a double mastectomy. After the operation, her doctors told her they had found a large tumor at the base of her spine. Authorities at the Mayo Clinic told her she had, at best, another year to live. "All anyone could say was, 'I'm sorry,'" she remembers.

Then she went to Georg Springer, M.D., to see if he could help. Six years later, in 1994, she was well, and looking forward to a long, full life. "But even if I should die now," she said reflectively, "I feel a whole lot better than I did six years ago."[59]

In 1994, *Life* magazine commented in a special article on breast cancer: "Historically, breast cancer has been treated with the triumvirate of surgery, radiation, and chemotherapy. Although these traditional methods have never worked well, maverick researchers like Springer [have been] ostracized by the establishment." *Life* called Springer's results "startling."[60]

If a woman close to me developed breast cancer, would I encourage her to seek treatment from Georg Springer, M.D.? Yes.

BRIDGING THE TWO WORLDS FOR THE BENEFIT OF PEOPLE WITH CANCER

You might not expect the vice president of a Chicago chapter of the American Cancer Society, and the medical director of the cancer care treatment program at Edgewater Hospital, an affiliate of the University of Illinois Medical School, to be particularly open to the use of complementary approaches. But Keith Block, M.D., has treated many thousands of people with cancer, and has not fallen prey to the belief that conventional medicine has nothing to learn from alternatives.

"Chemotherapy, radiation, and surgery can be extremely harsh on the body," he says, "not only wreaking havoc on the immune system, but also leaving the body overly toxic and malnourished."[61] He always begins with the least invasive and least toxic therapies. If they fail and conventional treatments appear to be helpful, he uses them—but only in small "fractionated" dosages and with strong nutritional support.

"With the right support," Keith Block says, "cancer patients can tolerate and respond far better to chemotherapy and radiation. Supplements and food can make a colossal difference in this area of cancer care."[62]

His goal, he says, is to "produce a heightened sense of well-being, vitality, and emotional resilience," and to involve patients fully in the healing process. He believes that "giving the patient personal responsibility and a sense of personal power regarding his [or her] care is as important as prescribing the right medication."[63]

How did he develop such an uncharacteristic attitude for an orthodox physician? While in medical school, Block developed an illness that conventional medicine could not help, but he found relief by switching to a Macrobiotic diet. Today, a low-fat, high-fiber vegetarian diet is a critical ingredient in his cancer treatment. He strongly encourages this form of diet because he has seen that what people eat makes a significant difference in their body's ability to resist disease and maintain health. He says that patients who follow the diet need fewer medical interventions, and get better results with the ones that are required. They suffer from fewer side effects, heal faster, experience less pain, and have more remissions.

Speaking before a large audience of doctors and researchers at a cancer symposium in Tampa, Florida, in late 1995, Dr. Block reported the results of a recent study conducted with ten of his patients. All had cancers that had metastasized, and most had been told they had less than a year to live. While following his program, however, "these ten individuals had continued to thrive an average of more than eight years beyond their previous doctors' grim predictions."[64]

He presented case after case demonstrating the value of his approach. A man diagnosed in 1979 with prostate cancer that had spread to the bone; a woman diagnosed in 1981 with breast cancer that had spread to her lungs; a man diagnosed in 1981 with kidney cancer that had entered his bones; patients with metastasized cancers of the ovary, colon, pancreas, and liver. All were still alive, and all were now cancer-free.

In 1996, Dr. Block told me that he had undertaken a follow-up study to determine how long his cancer patients survive compared to national averages. Though he is using very conservative data regarding survival times for his patients (basing these on their last visit to his office rather than actual survival times which will be much longer), the preliminary data are fascinating. On conventional treatment, only 20 percent of pancreatic cancer patients survive for a year; yet on the Block program, 41 percent survive for a year. On conventional treatment, only 7 percent survive for two years. On the Block program, though, 25 percent survive for two years.[65] When the study is complete, and Dr. Block is able to use actual survival times rather than merely the last visit to his office, the benefits of his methods will loom even larger.

I'm inspired by the fact that Keith Block's humane, patient-centered, and successful approach is taking place in the very haven of orthodox cancer treatment. If more officials in the American Cancer Society and the National Cancer Institute were like Keith Block, the war against alternatives would be over. The importance of a vegetarian diet would be recognized. And the benefit to millions of people with cancer would be incalculable.

"A GENTLE, HUMBLE, AND TREMENDOUS MAN"

Perhaps the most spectacular example of the ability to bring patients the best of both the orthodox and innovative approaches is found in the work of Glenn Warner, M.D., a board-certified oncologist, and one of the most highly qualified cancer specialists in the Seattle area.

Not that long ago, he was a leading figure in the cancer hierarchy. For more than 20 years, he ran the Tumor Institute at one of Seattle's largest hospitals. But as time went along, he began to realize that conventional treatments weren't helping very many people. "It became apparent," he says, "that we were not seeing people lasting very long. We were not prolonging survival. Surgery, X-ray therapy, and chemotherapy are all strongly immunosuppressive, destroying the body's response to disease."[66]

Seeing that the conventional tools were often ineffective, Warner began using them less and less, and began developing a treatment program to help people with cancer take charge of their illness. The program was designed to strengthen the body's inherent capacities for self-healing. It included stress reduction, a healthful diet, a positive mental attitude, exercise, and often (like Burzynski and Springer) supporting the immune system with immune-therapy drugs.

Warner's results were becoming outstanding, particularly when compared to those obtained by his colleagues who stuck exclusively with the conventional methods. In time, he left the Tumor Institute, and formed the Northwest Oncology Clinic. Here, he expanded his treatment program to include weekly support group meetings where patients could tell the stories of their illnesses and treatments, and help one another heal their lives. One patient told me: "The support groups are wonderful. The people who've gotten well come to help the people who are just starting out. These aren't passive cancer patients. They're taking charge of their lives."[67] Warner has attended every one of these meetings for more than six years.

A sense of community has developed among his patients that many find deeply nourishing and meaningful.

I asked Warner about the diet he recommends. "We steer people toward a vegan diet," he answered, "sometimes with a little fish." Does he still use chemotherapy, radiation, and surgery? "A little, but very judiciously, and only when we know it will help."[68]

He has become increasingly outspoken about the damage being done by overreliance on conventional approaches. "We have a multi-billion dollar industry that is killing people, right and left, just for financial gain. Their idea of research is to see whether two doses of this poison is better than three doses of that poison."[69]

By 1995, Warner had treated several thousand cancer patients at the Northwest Oncology Clinic, and attained a phenomenal level of success. His immunotherapy approach had produced a record of achievement with cancer patients that is quite possibly superior to that attained by any other oncologist in the United States.

But there was trouble brewing. Big trouble. In daring to speak out about the damage done by conventional approaches, and in treating cancer patients with "unproven" methods, Warner had drawn the wrath of the cancer establishment. A complaint had first been filed against Warner in 1985 by a physician who was apparently envious of the results Warner was achieving. Although the charges were dismissed, the pattern of harassment continued. For more than a decade, the Washington state Medical Board conducted an ongoing effort to find fault with Warner, and some excuse to take away his license. For more than ten years, he had to defend his right to practice the highly effective techniques he uses to treat a variety of cancers against the state's conventional doctors and their supporting bureaucracies. And yet there has never been any evidence of breach of conduct, nor a single patient complaint. There is only one logical explanation for the vendetta against this outstanding physician—he left the fold. He has not conformed.

Warner's patients are extraordinarily grateful. They have voluntarily donated more than $300,000 to help cover his legal fees. And among the thousands of cancer patients he has treated, the Medical Board has not been able to find a single one who has had anything negative to say about him. In fact, his patients set up a phone tree to spread the word as to when hearings were to take place, so they could attend and speak on his behalf. In an attempt to thwart this unprecedented demonstration of patient support, the Medical Board repeatedly changed the date or location of hearings at the last minute.

In January 1994, hearings were held in Tacoma, Washington. Most of Warner's patients live in the Seattle area, but despite the inconvenient location the hearing room was full every day for 13 days. Patient after patient took the witness stand to testify that they had been told they were terminally ill by other doctors, but then had gone to Warner and, thanks to his treatments, recovered their full health and lived many happy years.

Administrative Judge James Stanford received an outpouring of no fewer than 380 individual letters from patients supporting Warner, each telling someone's story of a personal struggle with cancer that had been successful due to his help. Lois Berry of Mercer Island, Washington, explained: "In 1969, I had a radical mastectomy for breast cancer. I was pronounced cured by my doctor. Four years later, in 1973, my cancer had metastasized to the bone and my surgeon sent me to Dr. Warner. I was treated (by him) with immunotherapy (BCG). I had no chemotherapy, and was never sick a day from my treatment, and have been cancer-free ever since. There are many more patients like me who have led long and productive lives because of the care and therapy recommended by this doctor."[70]

The Medical Board, however, refused to accept Judge Stanford's decision to dismiss most of the charges. They also showed something less than respect for Dr. Warner's patients, declining to read any of the many hundreds of letters patients had written, on the grounds that "the letters might prejudice the members in Dr. Warner's favor."

In July 1995, agents of the Medical Board marched into Glenn Warner's office and took away his license. Hundreds of patients who had come to Seattle from all parts of the country for his innovative treatments were thrown into a panic. Stranded, with no place to turn, many feared for their lives. The *Seattle Post-Intelligencer* spoke of "state officials on a witch-hunt for doctors who stray outside mainstream medicine."[71]

The charges against Warner revolved around the testimony of a few oncologists that the only acceptable standard of care in the treatment of cancer is surgery, radiation, and chemotherapy. Dr. Warner's innovative approaches, they said, were deviant and therefore unacceptable.

And yet, more than half of the thousands of cancer patients Warner had treated had undergone the conventional approaches before coming to see him, and had not been helped. Hundreds had been told they were "terminal," only to have their lives saved and their health restored by the very treatments for which Warner was now being condemned.

When news reached J. T. Quigg, of Lacey, Washington, that the Medical Board had taken away Glenn Warner's license, he flew into action. A former state legislator, Quigg was now president of Panorama City, the largest continuing care retirement community in the western United States. A year before, on August 10, 1994, he had been diagnosed with inoperable Stage IV non-small cell lung cancer. There was no surgery, no radiation, and no chemotherapy, he was told, that could possibly save his life. His oncologist told him that he should buy his Christmas presents immediately, for there was no possible way he could live until December. He was given a few weeks, at best a few months, to live.

Quigg began chemotherapy treatments which he was told might relieve some of his pain, but the side effects hit him hard, including complete numbness in his hands and feet. When a woman he chanced to meet told him she had been diagnosed with terminal cancer ten years previously, and here she was, thriving thanks to Dr. Glenn Warner, he knew what his next step had to be.

When Quigg, who stands six feet six inches and weighs 240 pounds, reached Warner's office, he was virtually beside himself. "Glenn Warner spoke with me and my wife for about 20 minutes, asking me about my children and what I had to look forward to in my life. Then he began quietly pondering the charts and records I had brought with me. Finally, he looked up, put his hand on my shoulder, and said, 'Calm down, big fella. I've seen people a lot sicker than you get well. And I've seen people a lot healthier than you die. What makes the difference is what you have to live for, and your immune system. I can help you with your immune system.'"

Warner gave Quigg a shot to help him deal with the side effects of the chemotherapy. "Bingo," Quigg says, his voice ringing with amazement, "the feeling in my fingers and hands came totally back, and much of the feeling returned to my feet."

Quigg had been under Warner's care for a year, and was feeling terrific, when the Medical Board made its move. Livid, he immediately called all his friends in the state legislature. Warner would not be put out of practice, not if he could help it. "Glenn Warner," he told me, "is an absolutely outstanding physician. He's got the whole range of treatments. There's nothing fringe about him. When the Medical Board first heard the charges against him, they brought in a nationally famous oncologist to assess his records. His report was that Glenn Warner's outcomes were exemplary; his efficacy was outstanding.

"When I first told my oncologist about what I was doing in seeing Warner, he was skeptical. But he's watched me thrive since then, and he's come to have enormous respect for Warner.

"These oncologists who testified against Warner are jealous. They tell people to go home to die, and then two years later bump into them at the country club. They're embarrassed. Warner has repeatedly taken people they've given up on and brought them back to health. They can't take this, particularly from someone who was one of their own.

"The six charges against him are based on patients he treated more than ten years ago, and four of them are still alive! The only thing he did wrong was heal people using innovative methods. He stepped outside the lines. He didn't adhere to the old methods because they weren't helping people.

"Glenn Warner's sin was turning. He was part of the brotherhood. Now they want to hang his carcass high, to remind any other potential heretics of the price of heresy.

"I'm alive for something, and this is it. I'm going to bring in these guys who condemn Warner as a heretic, and in full public view let's look at their records with cancer patients and match them up against Warner's.

"Glenn Warner is a gentle, humble, and tremendous man. He is an example of agape love in the finest sense."[72]

The fact that Warner's immune enhancement programs have enabled hundreds of people to recover from "terminal" cancer is immensely important. And the nearly 400 letters written on his behalf by his patients tell another, equally marvelous part of this man's remarkable saga. These letters are filled, not only with gratitude, but also with an overwhelming sense of respect for him as a human being.

I've had the opportunity to speak with a number of Warner's patients, and they have each independently told me that this wise, caring man is as fine a person as they've ever been privileged to know. They say things like, "He is truly the caring, compassionate doctor that every patient dreams of having on his or her side." "The first time I met him, I just knew I was going to get better." "He's incredibly inspiring." "He's a saint."

I don't know if Glenn Warner is a saint, but I do know that, for decades, this 74-year-old doctor's schedule has been demanding. He has arisen at 5 A.M., read medical literature for an hour, and arrived at his office at 7 A.M. He has seen patients all day, made hospital rounds until 8 or 9 o'clock at night, then gone home to another hour or two of reading. That leaves only five hours a night for sleep, but he says, "I seem to thrive on it."[73]

Will he be allowed to continue? His lawyers have filed for an injunction against the Medical Board, and are optimistic.

I have seen plenty in the world of cancer that gives me reason to despair, but Dr. Glenn Warner gives me hope. He is one of those truly rare human beings who hold the flame steady in the times of darkness when it is most needed. He meets people in their times of greatest challenge, and brings them conviction, compassion, and courage.

He was part of the system not that long ago, as one of its leading figures. And now here he is, having found a better way to help people in need. He was, as one of the many people whose lives he has saved puts it, part of the "brotherhood" of the medical hierarchy. But now he's found a larger brotherhood, and sisterhood, to serve—one to which we all belong.

Glenn Warner reminds me of people like Semmelweis and Pasteur, physicians who saw a light their contemporaries did not, who suffered the scorn and condemnation of their colleagues, and who yet persevered to give something to humanity of immense and sustaining significance. He reminds me, as well, of Linus Pauling, who like Warner was both an eminent scientist and a distinguished humanitarian. And he brings to mind people like Mildred Nelson and Nurse Caisse, humble people who have asked nothing for themselves but the opportunity to be of service to their fellow human beings.

Once, when I was a child, a shiver went through me when I heard a man say that doctors were God's hands on earth.

He must have been thinking of doctors like Glenn Warner.

UPDATE REGARDING DR. BURZYNSKI AND DR. WARNER FOR THE PAPERBACK EDITION

In the section on Dr. Stanislaw Burzynski, I mentioned that this outstanding cancer specialist had been indicted in 1995 by a grand jury. When the case came to trial in 1997, Judge Sim Lake (who was presiding) received a remarkable document addressed to him from Robert E. Burdick, M.D.

Dr. Burdick is on the faculty of the University of Washington Medical School, and has been a cancer researcher and practicing medical oncologist for the last 27 years. He had been asked, as an independent reviewer, to critically examine the case records of 17 patients who were receiving Dr. Burzynski's antineoplaston cancer therapy in 1996 for brain tumors. His task was to assess the patients' outcomes and to compare them with those obtained through current standard treatments.

In his letter to Judge Lake, Dr. Burdick wrote:

"It is very rare, currently, to ever get a complete remission or cure in a patient who has a malignant brain tumor using our standard modalities of surgery, radiation, and chemotherapy. By the time the tumor is large enough to be clinically detected, it has involved such critical structures that to remove it surgically would result in a patient who is left in a vegetative state or was markedly more disabled than he was prior to the surgery. As a rough estimate, neurosurgeons do well to cure 1 in every 1,000 brain cancer patients they operate on. Radiation therapy gains perhaps one month of life, and again may result in a cure in only 1 in every 500–1,000 patients. Similarly, chemotherapy research, despite 30 years of clinical trials, has not resulted in the development of a single drug or drug combination that elicits more than an occasional transient response in primary brain tumors. In fact, to this time, our chances of curing somebody with a brain tumor with chemotherapy are worse than the surgeons' or radiation therapists' and are probably on the order of 1 in 5,000. . . .

"I have carefully reviewed Dr. Burzynski's patients' clinical records to make sure that the responses seen could not be attributed to prior surgery, radiation or chemotherapy, even though the chances of any of those modalities having a lasting long-term effect on tumor regression would be unlikely. . . . The following is a summary of the 17 cases that I reviewed. Of the 17 patients, there were 7 complete remissions. . . . There were 9 partial remissions. . . . "

Dr. Burdick then proceeded in his letter to Judge Lake to carefully analyze each of the 17 cases. He concluded: "To summarize . . . this review, I would have to say that I am very impressed. . . . The responses here are far in excess of any prior series of patients published in the medical literature. . . . The response rate here is astounding. . . . Such remission rates are far in excess of anything that I or anyone else has seen since research on brain tumors began. It is very clear that the responses here are due to antineoplaston therapy, and are not due to surgery, radiation, or chemotherapy."

Dr. Burdick's testimony, along with that of many former patients who credited Dr. Burzynski with saving their lives, presented a formidable obstacle to prosecutors. Aware of the overwhelming scientific evidence that antineoplaston therapy is safe and in many cases effective against cancer, prosecutors fought to have any mention of its efficacy barred from the trial.

In a remarkable pretrial motion, the prosecuting attorneys wrote: "Permitting [scientific evidence as to the therapy's efficacy] will certainly infect the jury's consideration . . . with irrelevant, emotional, prejudicial and misleading concerns regarding whether antineoplaston works. . . . "

When defense attorneys presented a request for the jury to visit Dr. Burzynski's clinic, so that they might see for themselves what was going on, prosecutors were adamantly opposed. Asked to explain his opposition, lead prosecuting attorney Michael Clark made a truly stunning remark: "The jury visit request is a thinly veiled effort to expose the jury to the specter of Dr. Burzynski in his act of saving lives."

Heaven forbid!

Even though evidence for the efficacy of Dr. Burzynski's therapy was ruled inadmissible, the eventual verdict in the case represented a major step forward for medical freedom in the U.S. All the charges against him were eventually dismissed—except one, on which he was found not guilty.

After the trial, jury foreman John Coan remarked on the fact that although the government team had more than four years to prepare for the trial, and virtually unlimited financial resources at their disposal, they could not produce even one disgruntled patient, former employee, business associate, or colleague who would speak ill of Dr. Burzynski. Another juror, Darlene Phillips, was so outraged by the trial that she sent a letter to U.S. Attorney General Janet Reno and various members of Congress, calling the prosecution's case "ridiculous," and adding, "they didn't come close to proving their case."

Juror Sharon Wray summed things up tellingly: "This was a government witch-hunt."

Apparently, America will continue to be exposed for some time to "the specter of Dr. Burzynski in his act of saving lives."

I, for one, am grateful.

In the section on Dr. Glenn Warner, I mentioned that the Medical Board (formally known as the Washington State Medical Quality Assurance Commission) had been attempting, for more than fifteen years, to take away this board-certified oncologist's license, on the grounds that he sometimes deviated from the prescribed standard of care protocols. He was one of the first high profile oncologists to break away from medical dogmas and not rely solely on surgery, radiation, and chemotherapy.

The Medical Board would surely have succeeded long previously, were it not for the dedicated efforts of his many grateful patients, who raised hundreds of thousands of dollars and a huge outcry in his defense. The Medical Board, however, refused to read the more than 400 letters written to them by his former patients, arguing that to read the patients' letters "would prejudice [them] in Dr. Warner's favor."

In June 1996, when the case came before the Court of Appeals, the Medical Board's attorney, Beverly Goetz, addressed the issue of Dr. Warner's many former patients who were speaking out in his behalf. Her remarks, however, did not exactly exude respect for patient empowerment. She argued that cancer patients are "incapable" and "unqualified" to know whether they're getting appropriate care.

One observer remarked that, despite Goetz's protests, cancer patients are eminently qualified to know whether they are alive or dead, whether they are in pain or not, and how long ago it was that their conventional oncologist told them they had only a short time to live.

But speaking for the Medical Board, attorney Beverly Goetz insisted that only a body of experts such as the Medical Board are qualified to assess whether patients are receiving appropriate cancer treatment. She did not mention that not a single one of the members of the Washington State Medical Quality Assurance Commission was a cancer doctor or oncology expert. Nor that no other cancer doctor in the Northwestern United States could claim to match Dr. Warner's more than 1,000 surviving cancer patients.

It may have been a victory for a medical bureaucracy, but it was surely a tragedy for humanity when the court allowed the Medical Board to revoke Dr. Warner's medical license. Judge Robert Lasnik stated that he could not legally overrule the Medical Board, even though he considered their decisions to be wrong.

For many of his patients, this was the final straw. Deprived of his care, a number of them, including J. T. Quigg (whose eloquent defense of Dr. Warner I quoted at length), died.

Unable any longer to legally practice medicine, Dr. Warner sought to find an oncologist who would take over his practice and treat patients as he had done. Yet the state's oncologists were afraid to get involved. If this esteemed and beloved physician, who had been the head of oncology at Seattle's largest hospital for many years, and who had the active and unwavering support of many hundreds of current and former patients, could have his license taken away for using alternative methods, what chance would they stand?

Some months later, I received a remarkable letter from a reader of *Reclaiming Our Health* that helps explain what happened next. Carol Ann Stockton of Poulsbo, Washington, wrote:

"The story I have to tell is nothing short of miraculous, and I couldn't be telling it if you hadn't written *Reclaiming Our Health*. I am inexpressibly grateful to you.

"My brother Chuck was diagnosed with non-Hodgkins lymphoma. He followed his doctor's advice, and took the well-worn path of surgery, chemotherapy, hair loss, chronic sore throat, nausea, fatigue, and remission.

"Predictably (and tragically), however, the path through the medical maze twisted within six months into relapse—with a vengeance! Because Chuck's immune system had been severely suppressed by the chemo, the cancer could now spread through his body unchecked.

"His oncologist, Dr. Frank Senecal of St. Joseph Hospital in Tacoma, brought out the heavy artillery—higher doses of chemo. There went Chuck's hair, humor and hope, and Dr. Senecal explained his last-ditch, no-holds-barred campaign to destroy the cancer: 'Around Thanksgiving we'll check you into the hospital where you will stay through Christmas and into the New Year. The doses of chemo will be so strong that you might die. If you survive, we will perform a stem cell transplant. You will remain in total isolation in the hospital for at least one month, hideously ill with all of your organs and mucus membranes inflamed and infected. You won't be able to eat or drink anything. Then we'll do the stem cell transplant. If you survive (and the odds are not good), then you will be very ill for 6 to 12 months. This is all we have to offer.'

"Hearing this, Chuck was understandably depressed, and began to have reservations about following this path. With no time to waste, I sent him your newly released book *Reclaiming Our Health*.

"Chuck immediately and voraciously read the chapters on cancer. It gave him the hope he needed (the most powerful medicine), and then he began to explore other paths through the maze. Empowered by the clear and compassionate way you presented the strengths and weakness of our current medical system, Chuck told Dr. Senecal that he wanted to explore other options (It's always a good sign when a person stops being a 'good patient' and assumes the leadership role in his own health care!).

"Chuck contacted Dr. Glenn Warner, and within just a few days had a two-hour appointment (cost $100). Dr. Warner reviewed Chuck's medical records and discussed many aspects of the situation with him, including his diet. He recommended a number of things, including that Chuck cut out all the refined sugar and saturated fat, coffee, and alcohol from his diet, that he take megadoses of certain vitamins as outlined in Dr. Quillan's book *Beating Cancer With Nutrition*, and STOP any further chemo. Dr. Warner's approach is to enhance the body's immune system's own ability to destroy cancer cells, in a nontoxic way.

"Chuck then had a meeting with Dr. Senecal, and told him he was choosing to forego the stem cell transplant (and accompanying horrors) and work on enhancing his immune system—reclaiming his health. He asked for and received Dr. Senecal's support.

"Soon Chuck was looking and feeling great! He lost 15 pounds, and his normally gray, straight hair (he's 55) grew back brown and curly. As the months went on and he continued to consult with Dr. Warner, he continued to improve. He saw Dr. Senecal bimonthly for various tests to monitor the condition of the cancer (Dr. Warner couldn't perform this function because his license had been taken away). Six months after his first meeting with Dr. Warner, Chuck's ultrasound results were clear. There was no trace of any cancer activity in his body.

"As you know, at this time there were no oncologists who were willing to take over Dr. Warner's practice, even if they understood his way of treating, because the Medical Board had been so vicious to him. But Dr. Senecal was so taken by Chuck's success during this period while he was following Dr. Warner's advice that he has now taken over Dr. Warner's practice and is practicing in Dr. Warner's old office!

"This isn't some far-fetched testimonial that I heard about seventh hand! This is my very own brother! And none of this would have happened if we didn't have the great good fortune of reading *Reclaiming Our Health*. Whatever happens to Chuck in the future, he has had the best year of his life, when conventional medicine could offer him nothing but agony. Thank you from the bottom of our hearts."

Although divested of his medical license, Dr. Glenn Warner currently has a consulting and counseling practice. He says, "I want people to know there are many possibilities in treatment, not just the few which mainline doctors insist on—surgery, radiation, and chemotherapy. As always, I emphasize the importance of mind-body-spirit. Stress reduction and a tranquil lifestyle are vital components in cancer treatment, and I think there is a gradual awakening in the profession to this. It is my hope that I can expedite the spread of this philosophy."

Part Five

15
Toward Partnership: Integrating the Best of Alternative and Orthodox Medicine

Why do governments tremble when the inflation rate rises, yet no elections are lost over the infant mortality rate or violent deaths among adolescents? Why doesn't national shame over the homeless or deaths from tobacco lead to demands for change in political leadership?

—Jonathan Mann, M.D.

IN HER EPOCHAL WORK *The Chalice and the Blade,* Riane Eisler describes two basic models of society that underlie the great surface diversity of human culture.[1] The first, which she calls the *dominator* model, is commonly known as patriarchy or matriarchy, and is characterized by the ranking of one section of humanity over the other. The second, in which social relations are primarily based on the principle of linking rather than ranking, she calls the *partnership* model. In a dominator society, issues of inferiority and superiority color all social relations, particularly those between males and females. In a partnership society, on the other hand, the relationships between males and females are marked by cooperation, respect, and mutual support.

The significance of this distinction between dominator and partnership types of societies is profound, because Eisler and many others have found distinct correlations between the attitude toward women that prevails in various cultures, and the level of peace and health enjoyed by the people as a whole. Where women are respected as equals, societies tend to be more harmonious and concerned with human welfare, and the health of the people typically flourishes. On the other hand, where women are treated as inferior, societies tend to be far more warlike and indifferent to social justice, and their activities are often damaging to the environment. In such situations, human health deteriorates. Women are relegated to an underling status, and "feminine" values such as caring, nurturing, and non-violence are likewise subordinated.

In dominator societies, life is typically understood as a hierarchy ruled from the very top by a male God, with men, women, children, and finally the rest of nature in a descending order of lesser and lesser importance. Commonly, male leaders speak proudly of their ability to "master" nature, "subdue" the elements, and "conquer" space.

In such a culture, the heroes are violent. Children are taught to obey authority. Power is defined as the ability to control nature, one another, and even ourselves. Success means being better than others.

In partnership societies, on the other hand, giving birth and nurturing are valued more than killing and exploiting. These cultures speak of living in "harmony" with nature. They value cooperation more than competition, and learning more than winning. Daily life is full of artistry, ceremony, and celebration. The role of logical and linear thinking is balanced by an appreciation of intuition and inspiration. Dreaming is treasured as a carrier of wisdom and insight, bringing greater sanity, humor, and meaning into human existence.

In partnership societies, power is experienced as the ability to respond to and nurture life. Children are raised to develop their capacities for empathy, intuition, and imagination. Parenting is based on caretaking rather than coercion. Creativity and caring are valued more than obedience. Happiness and well-being are more important than conquest and victory.

The direct relationship between male dominance, authoritarianism, and warfare can be seen in violent and repressive regimes such as Hitler's Germany, Franco's Spain, Stalin's Soviet Union, Mussolini's Italy, and more recent examples such as Saddam Hussein in Iraq, Zia-ul-Haq in Pakistan, and Ceausescu in Romania.

The Ayatollah Khomeini is another example. He was originally expelled from Iran for leading a riot in protest against the more equal treatment of women. In 1983, after he had returned and taken power, ten Baha'i women, including Iran's first woman physicist, a concert pianist, a nurse, and three teenage college students, were publicly executed for the crime of believing in a faith that encourages equality between women and men.

Perhaps the most extreme recent example of the dominator mentality run amuck is Uganda under Idi Amin. In 1971, the Ugandan military overthrew the elected government, and this semi-literate man became the head of a nation of 18 million people. At that time, Uganda was blessed with a richly productive agriculture, and a well-established infrastructure of schools, hospitals, roads, and trade.

Amin's tactics were a little excessive. When he decided that parts of Kenya, Sudan, and Tanzania belonged to Uganda, he notified the world by publicly executing a group of Kenyan students who were studying at universities in Uganda.[2] By the time the dictator had been in power for six years, he had committed so many atrocities that both the United States and the Soviet Union had broken off diplomatic and trade relations. His human rights practices were said by British sources to include the "wholesale rape of women nationwide, as well as summary executions of tens of thousands of citizens of all ages." When the British condemned these actions, Amin personally executed an Anglican archbishop in front of hundreds of witnesses and television cameras.[3]

A characteristic of dominator societies is that the basic human needs of people often go unmet, subsumed in priority to military campaigns. The result—neglected people and an ecology ravaged by war—creates ideal conditions for pathogenic microbes to thrive.

During Idi Amin's reign, Uganda's entire health infrastructure was shattered, and the country was swept by devastating epidemics of malaria, leprosy, tuberculosis, cholera, and virtually every infectious disease known in Africa.[4] So great was the country's chaos that most cases of these diseases went untreated, and no attempt was made even to keep track of the numbers of dead. By the end of the 1970s, the nation of Uganda was completely out of clean water, sterilizers, antibiotics, aspirin, cotton wool, bed linens, soap, light bulbs, suturing equipment, surgical gowns, and toilet paper.[5] There were numerous outbreaks of strange new diseases, but of these our knowledge is scant, because there were no public health officials to investigate.

Examples of partnership-oriented societies are not as well known to most of us, for their activities rarely make headlines. But the indigenous peoples of Bali, and other contemporary ancient tribes like the African pygmy BaMbuti and the bushmen !Kung are sharing peoples who live in partnership with one another. The Tiduray people (sometimes referred to as the Tiruray), living on the large island of Mindanao in the southern Philippines, are perhaps the most vivid recent example of a fully partnership society.

University of California anthropologist Stu Schlegel, who lived with the Tiduray for two years during the 1960s, remembers them as extraordinarily brave, healthy, and kind. In his book *The Gracious Vision: Spiritual Wisdom From a Rainforest People*, he recalls a way of life that was characterized by a complete equality between the sexes: "All human beings— whether men or women—were of equal worth and equal standing in society. . . . Neither gender was thought superior in any way. Men and women related with empathy and an ethos of interdependence, with a mutual sharing of life, its problems and its delights. There was no sign of anything like a 'battle of the sexes.' Rather there was an abiding spirit of harmony between the sexes as joyful and equal participants in the great dance of life. . . .

"Just about all the positive values, such as caring and nonviolence, warmth and nurturing, sharing and empathy—which were considered 'feminine' in the world I grew up in—were held to be quite general and proper for both genders in Tiduray society. They were neither 'masculine' nor 'feminine' but were simply 'human' values, positively regarded as the right way for both men and women to be. And it was the same with many of what we in the West consider to be positive male characteristics. Bravery and assertiveness, intellectual calm and rationality, sexual and conversational boldness—these were not male qualities but equally valued and fostered in everyone, in women every bit as much as in men. On the other hand, a great many of the values which we see as masculine glories—such as toughness, conquest, and domination—were roundly condemned in Tiduray society for everyone. They were simply not appropriate for either men or women."[6]

The way of life of the Tiduray people, Stu Schlegel remembers, was marked by a "palpable graciousness." He adds that they were "marvelously healthy, living to old ages at least the equal of our own." Though eating fewer calories than Western authorities say are necessary, they were "always robust and vigorous, with no signs of mental illness of any kind."[7]

WHERE ARE WE ON THE CONTINUUM?

In *The Chalice and the Blade*, Riane Eisler documents the mounting evidence from archaeological excavations that our many legends about an earlier, more harmonious and peaceful age are not merely wishful fantasies.

On the contrary, our ancient past included long periods of peace and prosperity during which societies were neither violent nor hierarchic, and the status of women was fully equal to men. Over the course of these great ages, the wear on the environment due to human activities was minimal, and social and cultural evolution moved steadily forward. By all accounts, these were times of great spiritual beauty, and great healing.

Contemporary American society, to my perception, adheres more closely to the dominator model than the partnership model, but we are surely somewhere in the middle. We are certainly not a dominator society in the sense that Iran or Iraq are today, but neither are we exactly a garden of Eden where women and men live in caring, conscious connection with one another and with the natural world. The awe-inspiring opportunity of our situation—and its awful terror—is that our position along this continuum, far from being set in stone, is to some degree still ours to create. At this point in history, we are still capable of moving in either direction. According to *World Military and Social Expenditures*, the cost of developing a U.S. intercontinental ballistic missile is enough to feed 50 million children, build 160,000 schools, and open 340,000 health-care centers.[8] The cost of a single U.S. nuclear submarine is equal to the annual education budget of 23 developing nations.[9] Although there are certain forces that have already been set in motion and will have to play themselves out, the future is still yet to be fully written. We can channel trillions of dollars into technologies of destruction, or we can shift our resources toward pursuits that sustain and enhance life.

The choices we make will help influence the world's direction. **The World Health Organization tells us that an allocation of $20 billion a year would be enough to see to it that no human being on earth goes without access to primary education, health care, family planning services, safe drinking water, and adequate nutrition. Though $20 billion may seem like a tremendous amount of money, it represents only 2 percent of the world's annual military expenditures. The U.S. annual share of such an effort, according to the WHO, would be about $2 billion— less than we spend monthly on beer.**[10]

DOMINATOR MEDICINE

Our current medical system does not exist in isolation from the society out of which it has grown. Like our wider society, medicine today has aspects of both the dominator and the partnership orientations.

When patients are expected to be subservient and compliant, this is dominator medicine. When obstetricians are trained to intervene in normal births with pitocin and fetal monitors rather than patiently supporting women's natural rhythms, this is dominator medicine. When children are pharmaceutically subjugated and healthy alternatives ignored, this is dominator medicine. When normal life events are medicalized, and drugs prescribed to mask problems that have been shown to respond readily to lifestyle approaches, this is dominator medicine.

When obstetrics and gynecology are controlled by males, and when the primary images and practices in cancer treatment are drawn from warfare, this is dominator medicine. When healing becomes an imperial profession where experts reign as royalty, and when doctors speak of treatment success even though their patients die, the dominator principle has indeed become sovereign.

When the American College of Obstetricians and Gynecologists condemns birthing centers and persecutes midwives while running up an outrageous cesarean rate, when the AMA tries to destroy chiropractic and denounces all unconventional approaches as quackery, when the American Cancer Society seeks to banish innovative cancer treatments without bothering to investigate them, this is dominator medicine.

The alternative approaches represent the feminine principle in medicine—they seek to nurture the innate healing forces and potentials of the body and being. When these methods of health care are banished from recognition and practice, people are not only deprived of the health benefits these ways can bring, but of the values and the relationship to life that they represent.

In every society and epoch, there has been a relationship between those who would take their culture in a dominator direction, and those who would move more toward partnership. In one form or another, these two poles of thinking have interacted with each other wherever human beings have lived, suffered illness, and sought help. Most commonly, the nature of their relationship has mirrored the relationship between the sexes. When the sexes have respected and enjoyed each other, there has usually been harmony, not only in the household, but in the wider society including the healing arts. When the female has been considered inferior to the male, then the nurturing and preventive approach to healing has been neglected.

In ancient Greece, doctors worked under the patronage of Asklepios, the male god of medicine, while healers served Asklepios' daughter, the radiant Hygeia, goddess of health. Physicians today may not realize what they are doing when they take the Hippocratic oath, but they are swearing allegiance to both of these archetypes. The oath begins: "I swear by Apollo the Healer and by Asklepios, by Hygeia and Panacea and by all the gods and goddesses, making them my witnesses, that I will fulfill according to my power and judgment this oath and covenant."

The eminent physician Rene Dubos clarifies the meaning of these words: "The myths of Hygeia and Asklepios symbolize the never-ending oscillation between two different points of view in medicine. For the worshippers of Hygeia, health is the natural order of things, a positive attribute to which people are entitled if they govern their lives wisely. According to them, the most important function of medicine is to discover and teach the natural laws which will ensure a person a healthy mind in a healthy body. . . . [On the other hand], the followers of Asklepios believe that the chief role of the physician is to treat disease, to restore health by correcting any imperfections caused by the accidents of birth or life."[11]

In our medical system today, the followers of the Asklepian way utterly dominate those of the Hygeian. And yet, we may soon find ourselves needing the Hygeian tradition more than ever, for it is from this lineage that we can learn how to create health, and how to reown the powers of naturally healing ourselves. Alternative medicine is where most of the followers of the Hygeian tradition can be found today, teaching us the use of natural and inexpensive things such as herbs, hot and cold water, and how to prepare natural and wholesome food. They are reminding us of the power of our attitudes. They are helping us to take responsibility for our lives and to take charge of our health. They are telling us to exercise, to play as well as to work, to be intuitive and artistic as well as rational and logical. They are the health advocates, not only for those who can afford modern technological medicine, but also on behalf of the increasing numbers of people who cannot afford expensive medical interventions. Perhaps most importantly, the Hygeians are today the primary advocates for education, and for public health measures designed to create healthy environments for all people.

It is a great loss that the Hygeian perspective is not given much public recognition today, because it is saying something our culture needs desperately to hear—that health comes from learning to live in harmony with ourselves, with our communities, and with the natural

world. With the dominance of the Asklepian voice, the idea that health is dependent on and derives from medical treatment has come to eclipse the ancient understanding: Health can only be achieved and preserved by an appropriate way of life.

HYGEIA RETURNS

Like all eclipses, this one too shall pass. There are already emerging many physicians who seek to honor Hygeia, who strive to restore people's faith in their bodies and in the activities that generate and protect health. A leader among such physicians is Andrew Weil, M.D. In his book *Spontaneous Healing*, he writes:

"Political debates about how to cover the costs of medical care mostly take place among followers of Asklepios. There has been no argument about the nature of medicine or people's expectations of it, only about who is going to pay for its services, which have become inordinately expensive because of doctors' reliance on technology. I am a dedicated follower of Hygeia and want to interject that viewpoint into any discussions of the future of medicine.

"In the West, a major focus of scientific medicine has been the identification of external agents of disease and the development of weapons against them. An outstanding success in the middle of this century was the discovery of antibiotics. . . . This success was a major factor in winning hearts and minds over to the Asklepian side, convincing most people that medical intervention with the products of technology was worth it, no matter the cost. . . .

"[But] weapons are dangerous. They may backfire, causing injury to the user, and they may also stimulate greater aggression on the part of the enemy. In fact, infectious-disease specialists throughout the world are now wringing their hands over the possibility of untreatable plagues of resistant organisms. . . .

"In the East, especially in China, medicine has had quite a different focus. It has explored ways of increasing internal resistance to disease so that, no matter what harmful influences you are exposed to, you can remain healthy—a Hygeian strategy. In their explorations Chinese doctors have discovered many natural substances that have tonic effects on the body.

"Resistance does not develop to the tonics of Chinese medicine, because they are not acting against germs (and therefore do not influence their evolution) but rather are acting with the body's defenses. They increase the activity and efficiency of cells of the immune system, helping patients resist all kinds of infections, not just those caused by bacteria. Antibiotics are only effective against bacteria; they are of no use in diseases caused by viruses. Western medicine's powerlessness against viral infections is clearly visible in its ineffectiveness against AIDS. Chinese herbal therapy for people infected with HIV looks much more promising. It is nontoxic, in great contrast to the Western antiviral drugs in current use, and may enable many of those with HIV infection to have relatively long, symptom-free lives, even though the virus remains in their bodies.

"The Eastern concept of strengthening internal defenses is Hygeian, because it assumes that the body has a natural ability to resist and deal with agents of disease. If that assumption were more prominent in Western medicine, we would not now have the economic crisis in health care, because methods that take advantage of the body's natural healing abilities are far cheaper than the intensive interventions of technological medicine, as well as safer and more effective over time."[12]

WHO IS RESPONSIBLE FOR OUR ADVANCES IN HEALTH?

As a child of our culture, I grew up believing that the great improvements in human health and longevity that have occurred in modern industrialized societies have been the products of advances such as antibiotics and other Asklepian innovations in high technology medical treatment. But Alfred Sommer, dean of the Johns Hopkins School of Public Health, has a different point of view. He says that public health education and prevention have actually been far more important to the advances in health our society has enjoyed. "Historically," he says, "community-based, societally driven activities and changes in individual behavior have accounted for the vast majority of health gains."[13]

Could this be so? Could it be that the more feminine, Hygeian approach of preventing disease by nurturing the health of the environment and the community has actually accomplished much of what has been gained, though not given the credit? The preeminent work on the role of medicine and the history of human disease was done by a team of researchers led by Thomas McKeown, M.D., emeritus professor of social medicine at the University of Birmingham in England. In his books, *The Role of Medicine* and *The Origins of Human Disease*, McKeown analyzes the many factors that have served to improve human health, and appraises the contributions made by each.[14] His conclusion is that better nutrition and a healthier environment made people more resistant to infectious disease, and reduced the exposure to virulent pathogens. Nutritional, environmental, and behavioral changes, he says, have been (and will continue to be) far more important than medical interventions. They have done (and will continue to do) far more than clinical treatments to promote human health.

The most important reasons for the decline of infectious disease, McKeown says, have not been antibiotics or vaccines, but rather improvements in food production, transportation, and storage, and in hygiene. **It has been the purification of water, the efficient disposal of sewage, the creation of sanitary living conditions, and the safety and sufficiency of the food supply that have been the real medical miracles.** The most important advances in human health have not been attained through the interventions and treatments of clinical Asklepian medicine, but rather through public health measures leading to improved nutrition and sanitation—the arts of Hygeia.

You might think that Christiaan Barnard, M.D., the first surgeon to perform a successful human heart transplant, would take issue with this line of thinking. After all, the surgical advances he pioneered are considered among the proudest achievements of high-tech modern medicine.

Yet this physician, a virtual high priest of Asklepios, says emphatically that the Hygeian approach has been far more productive to humankind. "Today's doctors," he says, "have been blinded to reality by technological gimmicks. Medicine's real function has been obscured under its fixation on the space-age technology of the 20th century."[15]

The actual benefactors of humankind, he says, have been people like Thomas Crapper.

Crapper, according to Barnard, was responsible for "what was probably the largest stride in terms of preventive health measures in the last century." It was Crapper who developed the flush toilet. Knighted by Queen Victoria for his gift to humankind, his name has come to be uniquely commemorated in the English language.

Noting that Crapper was not a doctor, but a plumber, Barnard goes on to mention another person he considers to have also been a great benefactor to human health—an English iron worker who noticed the power in steam and used it to create a pump. "The pump operated the piped water systems of the great cities of Europe," Barnard says, "and did much to wipe out the mass diseases so common in medieval times." Barnard also commends the "builder who first used plastic sheeting to damp-proof the foundations of modern mass housing."[16]

What we have here is the veritable symbol of heroic medical intervention, one of the most highly regarded figures in the history of surgical science, saying in 1996 that: "A plumber, an iron-worker, and a brick-layer did more for the human race than all the surgeons put together. . . . It wasn't the doctor who wiped out typhoid, it was the plumber. It wasn't the drug researcher who halted the advance of tuberculosis, it was the social planner who attacked poverty and overcrowding. Nor was it the pediatrician who cut the infant mortality rate, but more likely the school teacher and the district nurse."[17]

CHOLERA

It was neither a drug nor any other form of medical intervention that allowed the modern industrialized world to become relatively free from plagues like cholera. It was a dedicated advocate of Hygeian principles named John Snow.

Between 1830 and 1896, the major cities of North America and Europe suffered four devastating pandemics of cholera. The death toll was high. In 1832, some 500,000 people died from the disease in New York City alone. When the 1849 epidemic hit St. Louis, 10 percent of the city's population succumbed to the disease in the first three months.[18]

It was not known at the time that the disease was caused by a bacterium that entered human bodies through contaminated food or water, nor that it got into water in the first place through the fecal waste of infected people.

When cholera ripped into London in 1849, John Snow was at work trying to understand how the disease was transmitted. Focusing his attention on a middle-class residential area of south-central London where the incidence was high, he began to suspect that the disease was waterborne. In one of the great moments in the health history of humanity, he removed the Broad Street pump, then the primary source of water for the cholera-ridden community—and the epidemic "miraculously" subsided.[19]

Medical authorities remained unconvinced, however, and so when another cholera epidemic hit London in 1853, Snow tried again to get his point across. He showed that water was now supplied to residents in the area by two companies which drew their water from different points along the Thames river. One got its water from the upper Thames, while the other drew from the lower Thames, which included human waste from upstream. If cholera was transmitted by water, he said, then the homes using water from the lower part of the river would experience more cholera than those getting water from the other company.

They did. Nearly ten times more.[20]

Unfortunately, Snow's magnificent demonstration still failed to convince authorities of the need to clean up water supplies. What finally got them to act was a phenomenon that came to be known rather pungently as "The Great Stink." As the quantity of human sewage dumped directly into the Thames increased over the years, the consequence, according to historians, was "an infinitely more powerful stimulus to legislative action than Snow's work on the transmission of cholera, or than the appallingly high death rates from the disease."[21]

A TIME OF GREAT HOPE

Thanks to the work of people like Ignaz Semmelweis, Thomas Crapper, and John Snow, and to the dedicated efforts of countless others whose names we don't know, the industrialized world had become, by the middle of the 20th century, relatively free from the great infectious diseases that had previously taken such a toll. The historic improvements in nutrition and hygiene were now in place, and had dramatically reduced the incidence and severity of almost all the great infectious diseases.

Then came the advent of antibiotics. For the first time in history, doctors had a really useful tool to combat those bacterial infections that remained despite the advances in public health. Thanks to antibiotics, the survival rate for pneumonia increased dramatically from 20 percent in 1937 to 85 percent in 1964.[22] The term *miracle drug* entered the language. The family doctor became a hero.

After World War II, Sir Alexander Fleming, the British discoverer of penicillin, toured the United States and was given a hero's welcome. A few years later, U.S. Secretary of State George Marshall told the Fourth International Congress on Tropical Medicine and Malaria that the conquest of all infectious disease was imminent.[23]

This was a time when it seemed that technology could conquer any problem. Many people believed that a bomb too terrible to ever be used again would prevent all further wars, and that nuclear energy was going to provide us with power "too cheap to meter." Chemotherapy was going to vanquish cancer. The green revolution, with its high-yielding hybrid seeds and its reliance on petroleum-based fertilizers and pesticides, was going to end world hunger. In 1962, Sir F. Macfarlane Burnet, the Australian immunologist and Nobel laureate, wrote that the late 20th century would see "the virtual elimination of infectious disease as a significant factor in social life." Infectious disease, he said, had almost "passed into history."[24] In 1967, U.S. Surgeon General William H. Stewart told a White House gathering of state and territorial health officers that infectious disease would soon be eradicated from the planet.[25]

It was in this mood of optimism that the world's health authorities would mount two ambitious campaigns to further eradicate pathogens from the planet. They would seek to eliminate human history's two most dreadful and murderous scourges.[26]

One campaign would represent the Asklepian approach, the other the Hygeian. According to medical writer Laurie Garrett: "One effort would fail so miserably that the targeted microbes would increase both in numbers and in virulence, and the Homo sapiens death toll would soar. . . . The other would succeed, becoming the greatest triumph of modern public health."

THE CAMPAIGN TO CONQUER MALARIA

Spread by mosquitoes, malaria has over the course of human history killed more people than any other disease except smallpox.

Though primarily a tropical disease, it has not overlooked the people of more northern latitudes. A million American soldiers suffered from the disease during the Civil War, and more than 500,000 GIs caught it during World War II.[27]

During the construction of the Panama Canal (1904–1914), the U.S. Army Medical Corps conducted the first successful campaign against malaria. By draining swamps, treating infected people with quinine, and killing mosquito larva floating in stagnant water, they managed, without the use of any pesticide, to virtually eradicate malaria from Panama.[28]

Today, there are other successful Hygeian approaches to malaria prevention, including building mosquito-proof housing, placing screens or mosquito nets in windows and doorways, cultivating fish that feed on mosquito larva, filling puddles, covering water containers, distributing mosquito coils, and planting trees to soak up water in low lying marsh areas where mosquitoes thrive. In Pudukkupam, a coastal village in southeastern India, malaria has been eliminated without the use of pesticides by transforming stagnant pits into prawn pools and introducing larva-eating fish into rice paddies.[29] Similar campaigns virtually eliminated the disease from the United States by 1950, though the disease had remained a major killer in the south as late as the 1930s.[30]

In the 1950s, however, world leaders were enormously impressed with the ability of a new chemical called DDT to kill mosquitoes and other insect pests on contact, and to go on killing for months or even years any insect that might alight on a surface that had been sprayed with the pesticide. The idea arose to use the poison on a massive worldwide scale, with the goal of extinguishing all malaria from the planet.

The concept caught the fancy of prominent Washington politicians, including Senators John Kennedy and Hubert Humphrey, and President Dwight Eisenhower. The president, always comfortable thinking in military terms, called for the "unconditional surrender" of the microbes.[31] Senator Kennedy predicted that children born in the 1960s would neither know nor fear the ancient scourge.

The decision was made to undertake the project. The United States alone would contribute more than a billion dollars.

The excitement was palpable, and the campaign was cranking up, when a middle-aged marine biologist at the Woods Hole Oceanographic Institute in Massachusetts challenged the whole project, saying that it was terribly miscast and would only lead to disaster. She said that massive spraying of DDT would have a devastating impact on the environment and human health, and that it would all be to no avail because mosquitoes would develop resistance to the pesticide. She also warned against widespread agricultural use of DDT and similar compounds, saying they would only increase general insect resistance to pesticides, further jeopardizing efforts to control not only malaria, but also typhus, African sleeping sickness, yellow fever, and encephalitis.

Her name was Rachel Carson.

In 1962, she published her seminal book *Silent Spring*, in which she wrote: "The world has heard much of the triumphant war against disease through the control of insect vectors of infection, but it has heard little of the other side of the story—the defeats and the short-lived triumphs that now strongly support the alarming view that the insect enemy has been made stronger by our efforts. . . . The whole process of spraying seems caught up in an endless spiral. Since DDT was released for civilian use, a process of escalation has been going on in which ever more toxic materials must be found. This has happened because insects, in a triumphant vindication of Darwin's principle of the survival of the fittest, have evolved super races immune to the particular insecticide used, hence a deadlier one has always to be developed—and then a deadlier one than that. It has happened also because destructive insects often undergo a 'flareback,' or resurgence, after spraying, in numbers greater than before. Thus the chemical war is never won, and all life is caught in its violent crossfire."[32]

The very year that Rachel Carson published *Silent Spring*, the United States and the World Health Organization officially undertook the massive and wholesale spraying of DDT to eradicate malaria from the earth. Health authorities spoke of "annihilating the enemy." It was the dominator approach to prevention—conquer the disease by obliterating the entire Anopheles mosquito population of the planet.

In country after country, an unfortunate pattern came to repeat itself. As spraying began, there was at first a dramatic decline in malaria incidence. But sooner or later, the mosquitoes always developed resistance to DDT, and the incidence of disease climbed. As time went along, developing countries were forced to spend ever larger sums fighting a problem that only grew bigger the more they struggled with it. In 1965, India devoted more than a third of its entire health budget to malaria control.[33] Poor Tanzania, with a per capita annual income of only $250, was spending 70 percent of its total health budget on the project.

Resistant mosquito populations appeared all over the world. As their numbers rapidly multiplied, the drug that had up until then been able to cure malaria—chloroquine—had to be used so much that it, too, now generated resistance in the microbes it attacked, and lost much of its efficacy.[34]

The campaign completely backfired. By 1975, the worldwide incidence of malaria had more than doubled since the campaign had begun in 1962. In many countries, the disease was totally out of hand. In China, where there had been 1 million cases in 1961, there were 9 million cases in 1975. India jumped in the same time period from 1 million to more than 6 million cases.[35]

There is no calculating how many birds and other animals were killed, how many species went extinct, and how many birth defects and cancers the world has known as a result of the massive use of DDT. Entire ecosystems were eviscerated. A campaign that had begun with the best of intentions, but had not understood the interconnectedness and wholeness of life, had led to tragedy.

By 1994, more than a million African children were dying from malaria every year.[36]

Sadly, Rachel Carson's predictions had come true.

THE SMALLPOX CAMPAIGN

If the campaign against malaria was Asklepios in its full dominator regalia, the campaign against smallpox was Hygeia in its deepest spirit of partnership. And it would succeed as spectacularly as the malaria campaign had failed.

In its long history, smallpox has killed and blinded more human beings than any other disease. In the year 165, the Roman Empire was so devastated that many towns lost a third of their population. India, China, Japan, Europe, the Americas—the whole world suffered continual blows from the heavy, heavy hand of smallpox.[37]

In what I consider to be one of the greatest shames in the history of Western culture, the European colonialists took advantage of the American Indians' goodwill, deliberately spreading the disease among Indians they wished to destroy under the guise of friendship. In 1763, Sir Jeffrey Amherst, commander in chief of all the British forces in North America, ordered blankets deliberately infected with smallpox to be given as gifts to the Pontiac Indians. Not only was the Pontiac tribe obliterated, but the disease quickly spread to the northwest where it killed huge numbers of Sioux and Plains Indians, eventually taking enormous tolls on tribes as far away as Mexico and Alaska.[38]

Cortez's capture of Mexico City with just a small army of exhausted Spanish soldiers was possible only because smallpox had destroyed the ancient Aztec culture. When Cortez reached the capital, there were only a few remaining Aztec soldiers able to fight.[39]

Smallpox utterly devastated the Native Americans. According to the official World Health Organization history of smallpox, the disease, along with several others brought from Europe such as measles, tuberculosis, and influenza, killed an estimated 56 million North American Indians. By the time the disease had played itself out, less than 2 percent of the original population remained alive.[40]

In 1958, smallpox was still killing 2 million people worldwide each year, and cases could be found in 33 countries. In India alone, there were more than 1 million blinded by the scourge. So many children died of smallpox in parts of northern India that the rivers could not run because they were so clogged with dead bodies.

That year, however, the Soviet Union went to the World Health Assembly and officially requested an international campaign to eliminate smallpox.[41]

Could it be done? There were several factors that made smallpox susceptible to a concerted campaign. There was a uniquely effective vaccine. The disease was easy to diagnose, even with no professional training. The disease was spread from person to person, by touch or respiration, so there was no need to control mosquitoes, rats, ticks, or fleas. And even though the virus spread rapidly, most people were infectious for only a few days, during which they were so sick that they could not walk about and infect large numbers of people.

The program formally began in 1967 under the leadership of the American physician Donald Henderson. At that time, though the disease was comparatively rare in the Northern Hemisphere, it was still thriving in most of Africa and Asia.

The smallpox campaign was a tremendous enterprise, involving a quarter billion vaccine doses per year, and entailing a sustained and incredibly thorough worldwide effort to reach every single human being who could be at risk for the disease—even those in the midst of war, famine, and/or natural disaster.[42]

It was the partnership model in action. Supported by laboratory science and sophisticated strategic planning, 100,000 grassroots health workers in India alone visited 150,000 villages every month. All in all, they made more than 2 billion housecalls.[43]

In order to convince people to be inoculated, health workers would inject themselves in order to show that it was safe. Some injected themselves many hundreds of times with smallpox vaccine over the course of the campaign.

Barely out of medical school, the French physician, Daniel Tarantola volunteered his services to a charitable group which arranged for him to perform primary health care in northern Bangladesh, and he soon became involved in the smallpox campaign. At one point, word spread of a murderer and his gang of robbers who bore the classic pockmarks on their faces and were spreading the epidemic throughout the countryside. Even the local police were terrified of the gang, and so Tarantola, without police protection, sought out the notorious killer in his hideout, where, with guns pointed at his head, he sought to convince the leader and the other outlaws to be immunized. Somehow, he succeeded, and the vaccinations proved critical to halting a local epidemic, and the eventual success of the entire campaign.[44]

On May 8, 1980, the World Health Assembly was able to formally announce: "The World and all its peoples have won freedom from smallpox."[45]

Tens of millions of people have been spared agony, blindness, and death. To Larry Brilliant, an American physician who spent a decade in India fighting smallpox, the triumph was one for the entire human community: "While the burden of nearly all diseases is borne unequally by the poor in the Third World, the only disease shared equally by all—black and white, rich and poor, First World, Second World, and Third World—is smallpox. This single disease is now shared equally, because it is no longer there to be shared."[46]

No one on this earth will ever see another case of smallpox.

TO VACCINATE OR NOT TO VACCINATE?

Justifiably impressed by the success of the smallpox campaign, and also by dramatic results in many parts of the world from other vaccines (most notably polio), the world health community now looks upon vaccinations, along with antibiotics, as the foremost weapons in the human arsenal against infectious disease.

And yet the issue of mandatory vaccinations is extremely controversial. There are many in America's alternative health community who question the safety of some of the vaccines that are currently employed in routine childhood vaccination programs.[47] They speak of concern for the children who have allergic or other toxic reactions, possibly due to viral contamination. They see cases of vaccine-damaged children, and they are afraid that vaccines may have long-term effects, possibly triggering developmental disorders and autoimmune diseases. They question if there could be a connection between certain vaccines and the poorly understood syndromes of chemical sensitivity and chronic fatigue. And they worry about what some of the vaccines do to the delicate immune systems of infants.

While prominent medical authorities from the Centers for Disease Control and Prevention to the Harvard School of Public Health promote preventive vaccines with an enthusiasm bordering on reverence, there are many parents who want to take personal responsibility for their decisions, and who are concerned that there might be potential dangers to their children from the current routine vaccination programs. They are not reassured when they see reports such as the one published in the AMA *Journal* in 1994, which said that children receiving the pertussis vaccine are six times more likely to develop asthma than those not receiving the vaccine.

I am often asked about my perspective on the subject. My answer follows from my guiding rule regarding the use of drugs:

In the first place, I do what I can to avoid needing any drug. When truly needed, I gratefully use Western medicines; but I do so with as much consciousness as possible about adverse effects in both the short and long term, and I always employ the minimum amount that is effective. Meanwhile, I do everything that I can to heal the underlying problem and make the medications unnecessary.

Some alternative health people say that they live a natural lifestyle, and trust their children's natural immunity to protect them from infectious disease. I agree that the healthier you are, the less vulnerable you are to microbes, but I also remember how decimated the Native Americans were by smallpox. They lived a natural lifestyle, yet their natural immunities were no match for this scourge.

There are others who say that they are protected by their positive thoughts and healthy diet. I have enormous regard for the power of our thoughts, and I'd be the last to shortchange the power of good nutrition to strengthen the immune system's ability to ward off infections, but I'd hate to have to depend only on a positive attitude and even the best diet in the world to protect myself or my family from microbes like the ones that are linked to diseases such as diphtheria or polio.

Remembering the tens of thousands of kids with polio we used to see in iron lungs and leg braces, and also having had a form of childhood polio myself, I have a healthy respect for the power of these tiny microorganisms. A small bacterium weighs less than one billionth of a gram; a blue whale weighs about 120 tons; yet a single bacterium can instigate a process that will kill a blue whale.

Opponents of vaccination point out that many of the diseases for which children in the United States are routinely vaccinated, including polio and diphtheria, are now exceedingly rare in this country. This is true, although whether they will remain so in the coming decades is not certain, particularly if vaccination levels drop, and if the levels of poverty and social despair continue to rise. It's hard not to notice that conditions in parts of some U.S. cities are already starting to resemble the Third World, with drug addiction, violence, alcoholism, pollution, hunger, and homelessness on the rise. Under such circumstances, increasing numbers of immunosuppressed people can come to resemble walking petri dishes.

This is one of the reasons that pertussis (whooping cough) has made a major comeback in the United States in recent years. The number of cases in 1993 leapt 82 percent beyond the 1992 incidence, and represented the highest annual number in 25 years.[48]

Diphtheria, a serious flulike disease that kills 10 percent of its victims, was almost unknown in the former Soviet Union only a few years ago. With the nation's breakup and social upheaval, however, vaccination levels dropped, and the disease roared back. In 1989, there were fewer than 1,000 cases in the entire country. By 1995, the number approached 200,000, and was rising rapidly.[49] The shortage of vaccines, disposable syringes and needles, vitamins, trained personnel, stethoscopes, and other basic medical equipment, coupled with a deteriorating environment, has produced a number of other epidemics, including polio. The very rivers that Russians depend on for life—the Volga, the Dvina, and the Ob—now harbor strains of cholera, typhoid, dysentery, and viral hepatitis.[50]

For people considering vaccinating their children in the United States today, the dilemma is this: we do not know what the future holds, and whether our public health safeguards will remain viable in future years. But we also do not know the long-term effects of many current vaccinations.

To my eyes, therefore, the vaccination issue comes down, as so many things regarding health do, to a personal decision. As Peggy O'Mara, editor of *Mothering* magazine writes, "Whatever family health decisions we make, I know we feel better in the future when they are informed, personal, and well thought out."[51]

I do not agree with the prevailing assumption that parents who don't get their children vaccinated are necessarily negligent or ignorant. Some are thoughtful and concerned parents who want the best for their children. It is certainly possible that for people who are fortunate enough to be well fed, and to live under conditions of satisfactory sanitation and hygiene, the routine "baby shot" vaccinations are not necessary. I also do not think it wise to vaccinate children when they are suffering from any illness, no matter how seemingly minor. And I do not agree with the current push to vaccinate infants at earlier and earlier ages. For these reasons, and because I dislike coercion as a matter of principle, I am not a supporter of mandatory vaccinations. In many nations with better health records than the United States, including Switzerland, England, Germany, and Austria, vaccines are optional.[52]

At the same time, I recognize that the majority of human beings on this planet live in situations where the use of vaccinations can alleviate an enormous amount of suffering. Half a million unvaccinated children in West Africa will die this year from measles, and many millions more will survive the disease but suffer mental retardation. Although high doses of vitamin A over short periods of time can be extremely helpful when poorly fed children get measles, it remains the case that many times the children's malnourished immune systems simply can't handle the infections, and permanent brain damage, if not death, results.

In such situations, vaccines are unquestionably a great blessing, but I do not believe they are a panacea. To vaccinate underfed people who are living in overcrowded squalor and poverty may save them from the particular disease involved, but they will remain susceptible to a host of other problems. Though international vaccination programs have saved countless lives, it is unfortunately the case that most of these people in turn succumbed to other devastating diseases born of poverty, malnutrition, and unsanitary living conditions.

People who enjoy the benefits of advances in nutrition and hygiene, but do not have access to medical technology, fare infinitely better than those who receive vaccinations and other medical interventions, but live in unhealthy conditions. In those parts of the world blessed with adequate and safe food, clean water, and sanitary living conditions, wrote the medical historian Thomas McKeown, "Infectious deaths fell to a small fraction of their earlier level without medical intervention, and . . . had none been available they would have continued to decline."

The best vaccine is a good diet, clean water, and a decent living situation.

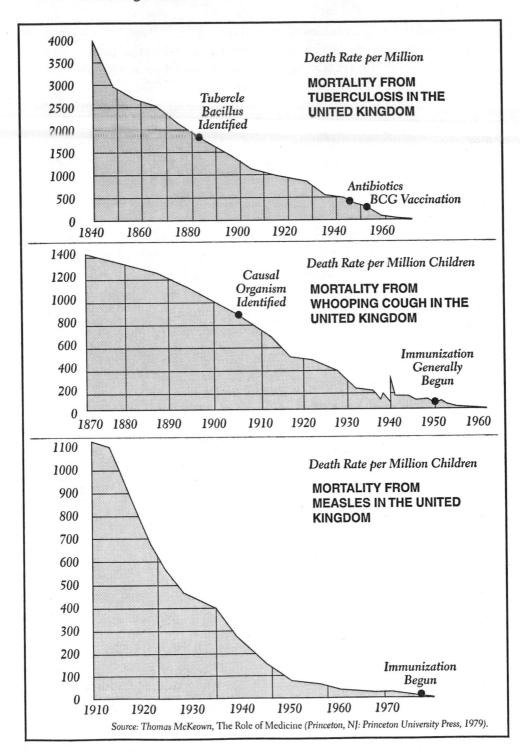

Source: Thomas McKeown, The Role of Medicine (Princeton, NJ: Princeton University Press, 1979).

THE WISE USE OF
WESTERN MEDICINE—
WHAT ABOUT ANTIBIOTICS?

In my younger days, while traveling in India, I developed a tropical disease that was never accurately diagnosed. Although I was extremely careful about the food I ate and the water I drank, I ended up with horrendous stomach cramps and a fever of higher than 106 degrees for more than a week. I do not know whether I would have survived without antibiotics.

Antibiotics are lifesavers in some emergencies, and can be extraordinarily helpful in other serious situations. Their appropriate and judicious use, coupled with a combination of natural methods (including the use of immune enhancing herbs, a wholesome diet to reduce vulnerability to microbes, and the replenishing of intestinal flora) is a fine example of a partnership approach, combining the best of Asklepian and Hygeian methods.

Unfortunately, antibiotics, like most conventional medicines, have been vastly overused, particularly in the United States.

A case in point is childhood ear infections. While otitis media (middle ear inflammation) can occasionally lead to mastoiditis or meningitis (emergency situations requiring immediate medical attention), it is not usually serious.

Today, however, nearly 90 percent of children diagnosed with otitis media receive antibiotics. To what avail? In 1990 the *British Medical Journal* published a study of 3,660 children in nine countries that found antibiotics had little impact on the rate of recovery from otitis media.[53] A *Lancet* study found that children receiving antibiotics for the condition fared no better in terms of pain, level of hearing, recurrence of inflammation, fever, or healing time than did children left untreated.[54] Other studies have found that when antibiotics are used early and frequently, the rate of recurrence is markedly *higher* than when the drugs are delayed or not used.[55]

Bottle-fed infants have far more ear infections than those who are breast-fed, particularly if they are fed while lying on their backs. A 1990 study in *Otolaryngology Head and Neck Surgery* studied children with chronic earaches who undertook elimination diets, and found that 100 percent of the youngsters responded with resolution of their earaches and improvement in their hearing.[56] A 1994 study at Georgetown University School of Medicine found that 78 percent of children with chronic ear infections had food sensitivities. Some 86 percent of the time, infections cleared when the problem food was eliminated for a period of several months, and the infections nearly always reoccurred upon resumption of the former diet. Milk was by far the most frequent culprit, followed by wheat, eggs, and peanuts.[57]

Parents may balk at the thought of undertaking an extensive project in the hope of discovering a specific food sensitivity. But in many cases it's not necessary to become a research scientist and adopt a full-scale elimination diet. Michael Schmidt, M.D., author of *Childhood Ear Infections: What Every Parent and Physician Should Know*, summarizes many studies in the medical literature by saying that "children with recurrent earaches often improve simply by switching to a whole foods diet and eliminating junk food."[58]

There are many good reasons to try dietary and other natural approaches before resorting to antibiotics. One that is often overlooked is that these drugs disrupt the microbial balance in the intestinal tract.

Only a small fraction of the bacteria that exist are dangerous to human beings. Most are harmless, and some are actually quite helpful. A number of bacteria, including Lactobacillus acidophilus and Bifidobacterium bifidus, manufacture B vitamins, play crucial roles in digestion, and help protect against the invasion of parasites. Unfortunately, antibiotics kill off the good bacteria as well as the bad. By altering the balance of internal flora, they can compromise the immune system, often setting the stage for bladder infections and other problems.

While antibiotics kill bacteria, they do not kill yeasts. In women particularly, proliferation of yeast growth and outbreaks of yeast infections are common after antibiotic use, and often become chronic.

ANTIBIOTICS TOMORROW?

Antibiotics have saved millions of lives, and their discovery ranks with the great medical achievements of history. But even Sir Alexander Fleming, the man who first discovered penicillin, warned that overuse of the drug would lead to bacterial resistance.

Unfortunately, his voice was not heeded. When Fleming spoke, no

Staphylococcus aureus were resistant to penicillin. Today, more than 95 percent worldwide are resistant.[59]

Human beings reproduce and cycle through a generation every 20 *years* or so, but bacteria take only 20 *minutes*. They evolve 500,000 times faster than we do.[60]

The speed with which bacteria can develop and spread resistance, coupled with the overuse of antibiotics, has not created the brightest of scenarios.[61] According to Jeffrey Fisher, M.D., a pathologist and consultant to the World Health Organization on emerging health technology, "The pendulum has incredibly begun to swing back to the 1930s. Hospitals are in jeopardy of once again being overwhelmed with untreatable infectious diseases such as pneumonia, tuberculosis, meningitis, typhoid fever, and dysentery. . . . Just by being in a hospital today, we are at risk of contracting one of these deadly diseases. . . . When we go into the hospital, we expect to get well, not sick. We expect that conditions there will be far more antiseptic than in our own homes, not contaminated with dangerous bacteria. Appallingly, the situation is exactly the opposite."[62]

Not that long ago, I was so impressed by the sophisticated instruments and vast array of pharmaceutical and other forms of technology that characterize modern hospitals that I simply assumed the hospital environment was hygienic and sanitary. But I've come to recognize that virulent microbes often lurk in these Asklepian cathedrals. In fact, our hospitals have become perfect environments for new diseases to evolve. Marc Lappe, M.D., a University of California toxicologist, says, "In some hospitals the odds are one in ten of getting an infection you've never had before. What you will get in the hospital will be much worse than what you would have been contaminated with at home. They are the most tenacious organisms you can imagine. They can survive in the detergent. They can actually live on a bar of soap."[63]

Hospital brochures don't usually mention this, but the number of Americans who die each year from infections they picked up in a hospital is greater than the number who died in either the Korean War or the Vietnam War, and more than four times the number killed in automobile accidents each year.[64]

We are trapped in a vicious cycle. The levels of resistant bacteria in hospitals are accelerating at a spell-binding rate. Trying to cope, hospitals are using higher doses and employing ever more antibiotics, particularly the broad-spectrum types. But this only accelerates the development of

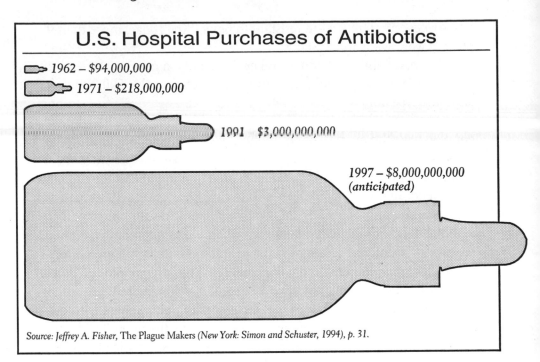

U.S. Hospital Purchases of Antibiotics

1962 – $94,000,000

1971 – $218,000,000

1991 $3,000,000,000

1997 – $8,000,000,000
(anticipated)

Source: Jeffrey A. Fisher, The Plague Makers *(New York: Simon and Schuster, 1994), p. 31.*

resistance, so then even more drugs must be used. In 1962, United States hospitals purchased $94 million worth of antibiotics. Today, the figure is nearly 100 times higher.[65]

It hasn't helped matters that many physicians routinely prescribe antibiotics for the common cold. Colds, like all viral infections, are completely immune to antibiotics. And yet in 1991 four million prescriptions were written for antibiotics in the United States for colds and related upper respiratory viral infections.[66] Most of these prescriptions were futile, unnecessary, and contributed to the increasing development of antibiotic-resistant bacteria.

Nor has it helped that we've been feeding more than half of our nation's entire production of antibiotics to livestock in factory farms. Most of today's cows, hogs, and chickens are fed the drugs in every meal they eat. The conditions in which these creatures are housed, and the diets they are fed are so unnatural, cruel, and disease producing that a steady supply of these drugs is needed to keep the animals alive. This use has contaminated the food chain with drug residues, and contributed enormously to the development of antibiotic resistant bacteria. England, Canada, Germany, and other European countries do not permit antibiotics to be routinely fed to livestock, but in the United States the meat industry has fought successfully to retain that right.

We've gotten used to being able to treat pneumonia and other bacterial diseases successfully with antibiotics. Yet in 1990, Jim Henson, the puppeteer-inventor of the Muppets, died of a common, up-until-then curable, bacterial infection in a New York hospital. Unfortunately, his death was not an isolated incident.

"We're running out of bullets for dealing with a number of these infections," warned Nobel laureate Joshua Lederberg, M.D. "Patients are dying because we no longer in many cases have antibiotics that work."[67]

Mitchell Cohen, M.D., an infectious disease specialist at the Centers for Disease Control and Prevention, coined a term to describe what he believes looms on the horizon. "The 'post-anti-microbial era,'" he wrote in 1992, "may be rapidly approaching in which infectious disease wards housing untreatable infections will again be seen."[68]

It can be frightening to contemplate antibiotics being rendered ineffective, given how many lives they have saved, and how dependent Western medicine has become on them. But to my eyes the situation also presents a challenge—to restore our commitment to replace the conditions that lead to disease with the conditions that generate and protect health.

If we are going to find ourselves less able to treat diseases, then all the more reason to focus on preventing them in the first place.

The development of bacterial resistance to antibiotics, and the resultant loss of these drugs as reliably effective, makes it all the more imperative that our medical system come to include the Hygeian approaches in a full medical partnership. The Hygeian way is far more prevention oriented, far more able to keep people healthy so that the diseases we have grown dependent upon treating with antibiotics will less often arise.

The Asklepian model has risen to prominence primarily on the back of antibiotics. It has been the power of these drugs to defeat many kinds of bacterial disease that has made many Americans feel as if doctors were gods.

With their decline, we are going to need Hygeia more than ever.

PARTNERSHIP MEDICINE—
INTEGRATING THE TWO LINEAGES

When it comes to treating various kinds of disease, a partnership model would allow patients to have access to the best ideas and practices of both

worlds. Although I believe that all of Asklepian medicine, not just antibiotics, tends to be overused, there are instances in which it can be vital.

For example, I am an unabashed advocate of a high-fiber, low-fat vegetarian diet—a Hygeian approach—because I believe that following a
healthy vegetarian diet is probably the most important single thing most
people can do to take charge of their health. And yet if someone were having a heart attack, I would not choose that particular moment to lecture
him or her about the advantages of healthy food choices. There are times
when drugs and surgery can be lifesaving.

What kinds of problems are well suited for today's standard allopathic
medicine, and what kinds are not? Andrew Weil, M.D., is the director of
the Program in Integrative Medicine at the University of Arizona in Tuc-
son, and one of the leading voices in American medicine calling for a partnership paradigm. He says the areas where conventional medicine can
shine are in its ability to:

- Manage trauma better than any other system of medicine.
- Diagnose and treat many medical and surgical emergencies.
- Treat acute bacterial infections with antibiotics.
- Treat some parasitic and fungal infections.
- Prevent many infectious diseases by immunization.
- Diagnose complex medical problems.
- Replace damaged hips and knees.
- Get good results with cosmetic and reconstructive surgery.

On the other hand, he says that even at its best, conventional medicine
cannot:

- Treat viral infections.
- Cure most chronic degenerative diseases.
- Effectively manage most kinds of mental illness.
- Cure most forms of allergy or autoimmune disease.
- Effectively manage psychosomatic illness.
- Cure most forms of cancer.[69]

If I had a broken leg, a badly inflamed appendix, or a fractured skull,
or if I were injured in a serious accident, I would want the best of orthodox care and would be glad such services were available. If I required hos-

pitalization, however, I would want to have an advocate with me, someone aligned with my values and knowledgeable about the medical system, to support me through the process, to help me make decisions, and to help see to it that my needs were met. Once the acute emergency was over, I would want to return home as soon as possible, and continue my recovery process in the company of family and friends, perhaps aided by the services of an acupuncturist, massage therapist, or other alternative healer.

I look upon conventional medicine as "crisis medicine."

While I think it is a mistake to look to alternative medicine for conditions that conventional medicine is well equipped to handle, for most chronic and persistent conditions, it seems wise to work first with lifestyle changes, and then, if necessary, to consult alternative practitioners. In all cases, reading and other forms of education can be of great value—in order to become as knowledgeable as possible about health and healing. Self-knowledge is a major part of self-care.

HEALTH INSURANCE AND HMOS

How does all this translate into a practical decision on health insurance? For residents of the United States who do not want to be overly dependent on Asklepian medicine, there is a financially viable option. If you are going to purchase health insurance, you can seek a policy with the highest possible deductible. That way, you will be covered in the event of a serious accident or emergency (where conventional medicine has much to offer), but will not have to pay the much higher premiums you would with a lower deductible. If you get a major illness or are involved in a serious accident, you won't be destroyed financially.

If your deductible is, say, $5,000, you can put the considerable amount of money you save on lower premiums into a special account, and in a short time the savings will add up to $5,000. Then you can leave the money there, accruing interest, and having it available if you should ever have a major emergency and need to use it to cover the deductible on your policy. From that point on, you can use the money you are saving with your far less expensive policy to buy supplements, healthy foods, time off, yoga classes, or whatever health building activity you might want. That way, you will get a real return on your dollar, and will be purchasing true "health insurance"—rather than "disease insurance," which is what insurance policies actually are.

There is another advantage to this approach. When you wish to utilize the services of a practitioner for day-to-day care, be it Asklepian or Hygeian, you will be paying directly and so will be in control, rather than placing yourself at the mercy of the insurance company bureaucracy and its coverage policies. You can choose with whom you work, and employ those methods you find appropriate and helpful. You will no longer be a prisoner of your benefits.

To my eyes, our culture has gone a little crazy regarding health insurance. If you have automobile insurance, you don't expect it to cover every purchase of gasoline, or each time you need a tune-up. Why do we expect health insurance policies to cover our day-to-day needs?

These companies are not in business for your health. In 1995, *Lancet* reported that the Prudential Insurance Company had $248 million invested in tobacco stocks. Meanwhile, Cigna, Travelers, MetLife, and Aetna—all heavily involved in the health-care industry—were also big investors in tobacco.[70] I would understand if you didn't feel entirely comfortable trusting these organizations to make your health decisions for you.

Health insurance companies pay out an average of only about 70 cents for every dollar they receive. If you are taking good care of yourself and needing fewer medical services than the average person, you get even less return for your money. Buying a standard policy is like playing against the house in Las Vegas. The casino will always win. That's how it's arranged.

In 1995, United States health insurance companies lobbied aggressively for national legislation that would place a lifetime cap of $250,000 on injury awards for pain and suffering. Meanwhile, many of their CEOs made that amount in two weeks. Maurice Greenberg, the CEO of American International Group Insurance Company, a leading advocate of the legislation, made $12,080,000 in 1994, or $232,308 every week.[71] It would appear that he considers six working days of his time to be worth more money than a lifetime of pain and suffering is worth to the people whose premiums pay his salary, people who may have been harmed by the very cost-cutting measures which produce the huge profits for which he is so amply rewarded.

On the other hand, maybe Greenberg feels poor by comparison to his peers. After all, S. I. Weill, chairman and CEO of Travelers, another of the insurance companies deeply invested in tobacco stocks, received a total of more than $52 million in compensation in 1993.[72] That's $200,000 per day.

What about joining managed care and health maintenance organizations (HMOs)? These corporations are if anything even more notorious for their penny-pinching. They often do not pay for hospital emergency room treatments, and seem to be uniquely talented at making both health care professionals and patients feel like frustrated pawns in impersonal systems.[73] Even those physicians who want to spend time with their patients and treat them as individuals are forced to adopt an assembly line mentality. Physicians working for HMOs are often paid to withhold care from their patients, and are put in a position where their own financial interests are in direct conflict with their patient's medical needs. This is a great way to pit patients and physicians against each other. I predict that in the years to come we will see increasing numbers of lawsuits against HMOs and HMO physicians for incompetence and malpractice.

As profit-making machines, however, they're not doing too shabbily. In 1995, the nine largest publicly traded HMOs had amassed enough cash, said the *Wall Street Journal*, "to buy every minute of ad time on Superbowl telecasts to run commercials for the next 136 years." The cash and stock awards to their chief executives averaged $7 million a year.[74]

There are probably not too many of us who like the idea of our health care being governed by rules that are designed to generate such numbers.

Like chefs who do not eat the food they prepare, many HMO and insurance company top executives do not get their own health care through the organizations over which they preside. What would happen if they were required by law to do so? Would patients receive better treatment?

HELPING PEOPLE LIVE HEALTHIER LIVES

There are currently many people in the United States who do not have health insurance, and much more importantly, who have little access to any type of health care. It is painful to see their plight, and to see at the same time such sums being tucked away by a greedy few. Thomas F. Frist, M.D., CEO of the Hospital Corporation of America, took home compensation in 1992 totaling more than $127 million. That's more than $500,000 per working *day*.

Our fixation on the Asklepian approach costs us dearly. It leads to dangerous $35,000 bypass surgeries performed on overweight and overburdened people who do not make corresponding dietary changes. It leads to people with headaches being sent for MRI scans rather than being taught relaxation and stress management techniques. It leads to an aging alcoholic former baseball star, Mickey Mantle, being given a $200,000 liver transplant only to die weeks after the operation, while increasing numbers of children are suffering from malnutrition and many of the other health problems that stem from poverty.[75] It leads to escalating costs, and declining health. It leads to increasing numbers of people being left out.

What would happen if, instead of investing our money in fetal monitors, chemotherapy, artificial hearts, and other dubious high-tech procedures and their attendant bureaucracies, we invested our resources in educational and low-tech community-based health supporting approaches? Such things as:

- Community health clinics;
- Subsidizing whole wheat bread, brown rice, fresh fruits and vegetables, and other wholesome staples to make them easily affordable;
- Improving air and water quality;
- Safe low-cost housing;
- Healthy school lunch programs;
- Basketball and volleyball courts, bicycle lanes, jogging tracks, parks, and other recreational facilities;
- Community centers and community gardens;
- Family planning services;
- Prenatal services;
- Breastfeeding and new parent support groups;
- Parent effectiveness trainings;
- Nutrition education;
- Conflict resolution trainings;
- Life skill and job training programs;
- Support for organic and other forms of low-input sustainable agriculture;
- Subsidizing of vitamins and other essential nutritional supplements;
- Public libraries;
- Programs to deal with illiteracy.

How would our lives be different if we made sure that all pregnant women had access to prenatal care and adequate nutrition? Would we have fewer low birth weight and extremely premature babies? Would we less often need to spend an average of $200,000 to keep extremely premature babies alive, babies who live only a few years in most cases and even then are troubled by severe brain damage? What if instead of spending 20 percent of our health-care dollars during the last few months of people's lives, we respected the requests of the terminally ill not to be hooked up to machines that only prolong their agony?

What would happen if we banned tobacco and alcohol advertising? What if we taxed tobacco and other products that are damaging to health far more heavily? What if we stopped subsidizing high-fat meat and dairy products? What if we based our health-insurance programs on wellness instead of illness?

What if we started using more of our resources to help people live healthier lives? Our high-tech, interventionist, Asklepian approach to health care consumes more than 14 percent of the gross national product of the United States, and costs more than a trillion dollars a year.

A more partnership and preventive approach would support better health for all and save hundreds of billions of dollars.

16
The Health
of Humanity

As one species, we share a common vulnerability to [infectious] scourges.
No matter how selfish our motives, we can no longer be indifferent to the
suffering of others. The microbe that felled one child in a distant continent
yesterday can reach yours today and seed a global pandemic tomorrow.
— Joshua Lederberg, Nobel laureate in medicine

O UR ENTHUSIASM FOR TREATMENT instead of prevention, for Asklepios at the expense of Hygeia, has unfortunately spread to the rest of the world. In 1991, *WorldWatch* reported that the world's 36 least developed countries were spending 60 to 80 percent of their entire public health budgets on urban hospitals, even though the vast majority of their populations lived in rural areas.[1]

As the world's nations have followed the American lead and begun to favor high-tech medical intervention over community-based public health and prevention, the results have not been pleasant. The world's coastal waters have become increasingly polluted by enormous quantities of raw sewage, fertilizers, pesticides, and other chemical waste. In Tokyo, less than 40 percent of the city's housing is connected to functioning sewage systems, with the decidedly unhygienic result that vast quantities of untreated human waste end up in the ocean.[2] Taiwan has sewage service for only 1 percent of its population. Hong Kong dumps one million tons of raw human waste directly into the South China sea every day.[3] In 1993, a World Bank marine biologist, Jan Post, declared none-too-happily: "The ocean today has become . . . mankind's ultimate cesspool, the last destination for all pollution."[4]

The conversion of coastal marine ecospheres into microbial soup has immediate health significance. Hepatitis, polio, and a host of other pathogenic microbes have been turning up in shellfish in the world's coastal waters. Strange microbes have appeared which burn through the shells of mollusks, kill off salmon, and cause lobsters to lose their sense of direction.[5]

It was as a direct result of ocean pollution that cholera exploded in Peru in 1991. Vast numbers of people in coastal towns were infected by eating a popular mixture of raw fish in lime juice, but the contamination spread primarily through the water supply. In the Peruvian capital of Lima, 40 percent of the population has no access to clean, piped water. As medical writer Laurie Garrett explains, "The majority of Peru's cholera microbes were transmitted straight into people's homes, dripping from their water faucets."[6]

John Snow must have been turning over in his grave. It had been nearly 150 years since he had shown that cholera was waterborne. Now, as if to demonstrate the degree to which the world's oceans are one vast ecosystem, an Asian strain of the disease had arrived in Peruvian waters in bilge water carried by a Chinese freighter.[7]

In the absence of safe water supplies, the disease spread rapidly from one Latin American port to another. By 1993, nearly a million cases of cholera had been reported. Startling as it is, this figure clearly represents only a shadow of the true epidemic, because the vast majority of cases were not reported.

Peru was forced to spend hundreds of millions of dollars in emergency medical care to try to abate the crisis. This same expenditure could have provided low-cost clean water and sanitation to millions of the country's disadvantaged, not only preventing this cholera epidemic from developing, but also preventing countless other infectious diseases in the future.

LOW-TECH, NON-POLLUTING ANSWERS

Cholera outbreaks, like those of almost all waterborne diseases, can be curtailed by providing people with access to clean water. Presently, though, more than 1 billion people on this earth do not have safe water to use for drinking or washing.

The medical consequences are staggering. Waterborne diseases account for an estimated 80 percent of all illnesses, worldwide. More children today die from diarrheal diseases, caused by the lack of clean water supplies, than from any other cause. Half a billion people are afflicted by waterborne trachoma, a principal cause of blindness. In India, a child dies every 20 seconds from dirty water.

How can this be prevented? Chlorination is typically used in developed countries to disinfect water, but water in the Third World is often contaminated with bacteria, viruses, and parasites associated with human waste that are resistant to chlorine. Boiling water is the most common method of killing bacteria, but the fuel needed for boiling is often too scarce or too expensive for the world's poor.

Fortunately, there are other solutions, one of which is the use of solar-powered water pasteurizers. These devices, capable of heating water to high enough temperatures to destroy pathogenic waterborne microbes, are currently being tested extensively at the University of Hawaii. The units are produced in three sizes, with the smallest providing up to 30 gallons of pasteurized water per sunny day, and the largest 240 gallons. The cost of the devices is at present too high for poor families to purchase individually ($300 for the smaller unit), but the price will come down considerably with mass production, and the idea is to provide units to women selected by local women's organizations, who will then sell water to their neighbors, providing both a livelihood and a means of paying back the cost of the unit. The project is empowering to women, community-building, and the solar-powered water pasteurizers have the additional benefit of being entirely unpolluting, unlike the burning of wood or coal to boil water, or the use of chlorine.[8]

THE PLAGUE

The outbreak of cholera in Peru, like other mass epidemics, was frequently referred to as a "plague." The word *plague* is often used to mean any kind of disastrous pestilence, though it originally referred to a specific disease— the bubonic plague—the source of which are bacteria *(Yersinia pestis)* that are carried by fleas residing on rats. Our word *pestilence* derives from this species of microbes, who have utterly decimated humanity on a number of occasions.

In the 13th century, the plague killed half the population of China.[9] From there, it was carried on rats aboard ships to Europe and North Africa, where it produced what became known as the Black Death. The city of Strasbourg dealt with the situation none-too-admirably by blaming its

Jewish residents for the pestilence, and then proceeding to kill all 16,000 of them.[10] Not to be outdone, the town leadership in Basel voted "to kill all Jews, destroy their homes, and ban Jews from entering the city for another two centuries."[11]

Meanwhile, the physicians of the time were teaching that bathing was dangerous, and so the population rarely washed, creating ideal conditions for fleas to proliferate. Laurie Garrett observes: "The terrorized European population did everything save what might have spared them— ridding their cities of rodents and fleas."[12]

Between 1346 and 1350 more than one-third of Europe's total population perished from the plague. Another epidemic hit Europe during the 17th century, once again killing enormous numbers of people in short periods of time. In 1665 alone, more than half of London's population succumbed to the disease.

Once again, the terrorized population displayed something less than the pinnacle of enlightenment, this time often burning, not only Jews, but also homosexuals, witches, and cats, and blaming them all for the pestilence. Decimating the cat population in this manner did not exactly help matters. In fact, it had the effect of increasing the rat and mouse population, thus further spreading the disease.

It is not commonly recognized, but cats, by virtue of their skills in rodent control, have played a unique role in human health history. During the 1960s, when the campaign to extinguish malaria came to Bolivia, the heavy DDT spraying produced what was called "feline die-off," and the numbers of mice and rats in many areas soared.[13] It wasn't long before the country experienced an outbreak of a terrifying viral disease (Bolivian hemorrhagic fever) that swept rapidly through entire villages, killing as many as 50 percent of their human inhabitants.[14] So much panic broke out that the Bolivian government declared martial law in the worst hit area, and flew in 55 soldiers to maintain order. Some 37 of these soldiers eventually contracted the disease. When the problem was finally traced to a virus which spread through mouse urine, national radio sent out a plea for donated cats to be sent to the afflicted area. The epidemic was halted by the airlifting of hundreds of cats.[15]

The idea of cats being flown in to combat a lethal epidemic may seem a bit surreal, spawning visions of thousands of little parachutes descending from the sky bringing a brigade of "purr-atroopers" to the rescue. But what happened in Bolivia was quite serious, and reflects the role cats have long played in keeping rodent populations in check. Today's "house-cats" are descended from animals bred by the Egyptians to protect their grain stores. In the great sweep of history, there have been times, I suspect, when cats may have done more to protect human health than physicians.

Currently in the United States, while spending on high-tech Asklepian medicine exceeds a trillion dollars a year, cities throughout the nation are experiencing severe budgetary restraints, leading to dramatic reductions in rodent-control programs and garbage collection. The medical consequences have yet to be measured. Urban centers have a unique ability to breed microbes that are pathogenic to human beings, and rodents are one of the means by which these microbes spread. In 1992–1993, after city budget cuts left plastic bags of garbage sitting on sidewalks, New York City experienced a 70 percent increase in reported incidents of rats biting people.[16]

Could plague resurface today? Infectious disease experts are concerned that it could. In 1994, a deadly outbreak of plague struck India, forcing the stoppage of all air travel to and from the nation. Nearly half a million people fled the city of Surat, where the epidemic originated, and 900 million Indians feared the worst. The outbreak occurred after dramatic budget cuts in rat catching and trash collection.

As media hype inflamed the crisis, estimates of what the epidemic cost India ranged as high as $10 billion.[17] **That same amount of money, spent on rodent control and garbage collection, could almost certainly have prevented the outbreak—with enough left over to provide food and basic health care for the tens of millions of Indian children who die from diseases caused by poverty and malnutrition annually.**

EBOLA AND AIDS—
THE WORLD AS MICROBIAL SUPERHIGHWAY

In the United States, the possibility of widespread infectious disease epidemics has seemed remote until recent years. But in 1996, the AMA *Journal* announced that deaths from infectious diseases, formerly on the decline, rose 58 percent between 1980 and 1992, leaping from the fifth to the third leading killer.[18] Recognizing the seriousness of the threat, the *Journal* devoted the entire issue to calling attention to the growing danger posed by microbes. Meanwhile, the American public was becoming fascinated by the real threat of old diseases resurfacing, or new ones emerging. Popular movies were being made on the subject with titles like *Outbreak* and *Virus*.

In 1995, a nonfiction book titled *The Hot Zone*, by Richard Preston, became a number one best-seller. It accurately described how an extraordinarily lethal virus known as Ebola reached Western civilization from the same remote African rain forest where HIV is thought to have originated. Complete with gruesome descriptions of how the virus rapidly liquefies human flesh into viral soup, the book explained how the virus ate through a population of captive monkeys in a suburb of Washington, D.C., in 1989, only to be finally contained by a secret U.S. Army operation. At the time, there was tremendous fear, and some suspicious evidence, that the virus had mutated, become airborne, and leapt to human hosts. Had it actually done so, the damage would have been incalculable.

Though the book was written as a popular thriller, it was accurate about the events that occurred, and there were sober thoughts in its conclusion. After noting the widely held belief that both the Ebola virus and HIV emerged into civilization as a consequence of environmental destruction, Preston added that "AIDS is arguably the worst environmental disaster of the 20th century. . . . The emergence of AIDS, Ebola, and any number of other rainforest agents appears to be a natural consequence of the ruin of the tropical biosphere. The emerging viruses are surfacing from ecologically damaged parts of the earth."[19]

As human activity invades parts of the world never before inhabited on a large scale—including the jungles and rainforests of equatorial Africa and South America—we encounter hitherto unknown viruses. But we don't just encounter them, we then bring them back with us and rapidly spread them to the rest of civilization. The world has become, in the words of virologist Stephen S. Morse of Rockefeller University in New York City, a "microbial highway."

With modern transportation, viruses can hitch a ride inside an infected person, animal or insect. In a matter of hours, they can infect people thousands of miles away. What we are seeing today is the globalization of disease.

AIDS is a clear example. Of the 1,200 cases of AIDS identified in the world by March 1983, virtually all were in the United States and Haiti.[20] But by 1995, 8.5 million people worldwide had developed full-blown AIDS, and more than 80 percent were in sub-Saharan Africa.[21]

Every area of the globe has now become involved, even countries previously unscathed. Very few people were HIV-infected in Asia prior to 1990, but by 1995 the number of HIV-infected people in Southeast Asia alone was estimated to be 4.5 million, more than twice the total number of HIV-infected people in the entire industrialized world.[22]

Though there is increasing evidence that HIV is not the sole cause of AIDS, and that the virus may require the presence of other organisms and infections in order to become virulent, the correlation between HIV and AIDS remains strong. In order to halt the spread of AIDS, people must understand the routes by which HIV is transmitted (sexual intercourse, blood contact, and mother-to-fetus or newborn). Condoms must be available that are affordable and of good quality. Testing services must be confidential, accurate, and accessible. Every nation's blood banks must be free of HIV. Sterile syringes must be readily available.[23]

But there is one more key that may be the most important of all, according to Jonathan Mann, founding director of the World Health Organization's Global Program on AIDS, and director of the International AIDS Center. "Discrimination simply drives AIDS underground," he has said repeatedly. "The epidemic doesn't go away; it simply becomes harder to see, more alienated from public health. If you drive it underground, you guarantee its spread."[24] The last 15 years have shown, he says, that the marginalization and stigmatization of those who are at risk insure that the disease will spread. "The failure to realize human rights and respect human dignity has now been recognized as a major cause—actually, the root cause—of societal vulnerability to HIV/AIDS."[25]

Is it a coincidence that it is in those very parts of the world where human rights are least respected, where women are regarded as beasts of burden, playthings, or childbearing machines, that AIDS is spreading the fastest? Where women are denied participation in the economic system, and have few ways of earning income, some must resort to prostitution to support themselves. In Bombay, the rate of HIV infection among female prostitutes is nearly 40 percent.[26] The director of the Indian Medical Research Council , Dr. A. S. Paintal, estimates that 100,000 sexual acts are performed with HIV-positive female prostitutes in the city every day.[27] In parts of Africa, the infection rate among prostitutes is even higher, reaching above 75 percent in several Tanzanian cities, and 85 percent in Nairobi.[28]

But it's not only the women who become prostitutes and their clients who are at greater risk in societies where women are treated as second-class people. In East Africa, Mann says, "even if a woman knows that her husband is HIV-infected, she cannot refuse unwanted or unprotected intercourse for fear of being beaten, without civic recourse, or for fear of divorce, which translates into civil and economic death for the woman. Therefore, even though knowing about HIV/AIDS and despite condoms being available in the marketplacc, these women cannot protect themselves. They lack the equal rights that alone would enable translation of knowledge into protection."[29]

How otten does this happen? In East Africa, says Mann, "being [a] married and monogamous [woman] is now considered a risk factor for HIV infection."[30]

Since the beginning of the epidemic, the world has looked to the United States, home to the first wave of reported AIDS cases, and the country leading the world's AIDS research efforts, for direction. Unfortunately, people in positions of power during the Reagan administration did not always model the virtue of clear-headed compassion. In fact, their antagonism toward the homosexual community was so great that for more than five years Surgeon General C. Everett Koop was forbidden to publicly discuss the disease.[31]

When Pat Robertson, founder of television's Christian Broadcasting Network, ran for the Republican presidential nomination in 1988, he repeatedly called the disease "the gay plague," and said that scientists were "frankly lying" when they claimed that HIV could be transmitted heterosexually. Condoms, he said, were useless to prevent infection.[32]

The Americans did not have a monopoly on ignorance. In 1987, the president of the German Federal Court of Justice, Gerd Pfeiffer, announced that it might "soon prove necessary to tattoo and quarantine people infected with the virus."[33] This was a terrifying thought, given what happened the last time a German government saw fit to "tattoo and quarantine" those people it found socially undesirable, but the idea was also being entertained in the United States. That same year, the chairman of a powerful right-wing group with influence at the White House, Howard Phillips, announced that "quarantining is something we have to consider."[34]

How counterproductive such ideas are when put into practice was seen in India in 1991. After several hundred HIV-positive people were placed in "permanent seclusion," chained to their beds, and barred from further social interaction, the numbers of people in the area willing to be tested dropped almost to zero.[35] Potentially infected people went underground, wanting no part of the public health system.[36]

While the dominator mentality has responded to the AIDS epidemic by demanding harsher restrictions on the rights of high-risk groups and proposing actions that would further stigmatize those infected with HIV, there have been other voices calling for campaigns to educate people in order to prevent the spread of the disease. When he was finally allowed to speak about AIDS, Surgeon General Koop was one of these voices. He advocated the frank discussion of the AIDS epidemic and sexual activities in American society, including its schools. There is no calculating the number of lives saved by his willingness to speak out, and by the health and safe sex education his courage inspired.

What are we learning in the age of AIDS? We are seeing that few things favor the spread of the disease so much as stigmatism and panic-driven repression. Scapegoating is cruel, which is reason enough to avoid it. But there is an additional reason: It diverts attention away from effective answers. Compassion is not only kind; it is a critical ingredient in any true solution to the problem.

A partnership attitude toward those who are most at risk not only saves lives and prevents magnitudes of suffering. It also saves enormous amounts of money—in the long run more than would be required to provide adequate food, clean water, basic education, and decent housing to all the world's poor.

We are learning something too, in this age of AIDS, about global interdependence. When the World Health Organization was formed after World War II, a not entirely forward-thinking official of the AMA denounced the idea as "the work of a bunch of star-gazers, social uplifters, and advanced one-worldists."[37] **But today, a health problem anywhere in the world can quickly become a health problem everywhere. To pathogenic microbes, it truly is one world. Viruses, parasites, and bacteria do not recognize the artificial boundaries erected by human beings.**

When Martin Luther King, Jr., said, "We will either learn to live together as brothers [and sisters], or we will perish together as fools," he could have been speaking as a modern immunologist.

AND ONCE AGAIN, THERE ARE ALTERNATIVES

We have today the knowledge of how HIV is transmitted—and the realization that with a combination of abstinence, safe sex, clean needles, and a safe blood supply, we can prevent it from spreading. But when it comes to finding a cure, conventional medicine has so far come up empty-handed.

In the United States, AIDS is now the leading killer of people between the ages of 25 and 44.[38] Two-thirds of those who have been diagnosed with AIDS have died, and conventional medicine fully expects the remaining third to follow them shortly. Though the field is changing rapidly, the exclusive reliance on drugs like AZT (a reverse transcriptase inhibitor), and even the newer drugs like ritonavir and saquinavir (protease inhibitors), has so far been of only limited usefulness.

As with cancer, though, there are numerous practitioners of alternative approaches who are claiming success in treating HIV/AIDS. Though many of these claims are no doubt exaggerated, it remains a fact that there are thousands of people who have been HIV positive for ten to fifteen years and who are not only still alive but showing no signs of AIDS. Many have used alternative therapies that represent the Hygeian lineage.

Jon Kaiser, M.D., is a primary-care physician in San Francisco who has been working with AIDS patients for more than ten years. Seventy percent of his patients are HIV-positive. "When I think back to medical school, I was taught two things," he says. "First, look for the infection or tumor and try to kill it. Second, if the patient's body has symptoms, find a drug that suppresses the symptoms."[39]

Kaiser now takes a different approach, one that is truly holistic and inclusive. He is not opposed to the use of conventional medicine when it is helpful. In fact, he says that "the intelligent and effective use of standard medical therapies will always play an essential role in the treatment of HIV." But he bases his treatment of HIV/AIDS on a comprehensive system of natural therapies. The result? With his natural therapies program, when drugs are needed, far lower dosages accomplish the desired result.[40] The corresponding decrease in side effects is a tremendous gain, because the side effects themselves can be not only brutal, but are sometimes fatal.

I consider Kaiser's work with HIV/AIDS to be an exquisite example of partnership medicine at its best, and his results are vastly superior to any achieved by conventional medicine alone. During a recent surveillance period of four years, Kaiser's statistics were nothing short of magnificent. His treatment program, based on a natural foods diet, extensive use of vitamins and other supplements, Chinese herbs, exercise, stress reduction, and the cultivation of a positive attitude, produced "a stability rate of 90 percent, meaning that these patients either improved or did not further decline in their diagnosis. The survival rate during that same period was

98 percent. There were only 3 deaths out of 134 HIV-positive patients, including 30 who had full-blown AIDS symptoms."[41]

These numbers are staggering in a medical system that considers HIV to be a death sentence. Their significance can hardly be exaggerated.

But Kaiser is not alone in making remarkable progress by using the methods of Hygeia alongside those of Asklepios. Joan Priestley, M.D., of the Omni Medical Center in Anchorage, Alaska, is another internationally recognized expert in AIDS management who is willing to employ drugs and make use of other tools of conventional medicine when she feels they will truly help, but bases her approach on natural treatments. In 1994, she gave sworn testimony to a U.S. Senate subcommittee. "Since 1986," she said, "I have used an array of natural products to treat over 700 AIDS patients. The vast majority of my clients maintain excellent health and lead productive lives."

One of Dr. Priestley's patients, Sharon Lund, is well known throughout the United States and internationally as an AIDS educator, and has appeared on many television programs. When she testified before the Congressional Hearings on Dietary Supplements, as both an expert on AIDS and a person afflicted with the disease, she received a standing ovation from the congressional delegation.

More than a decade previously, Sharon almost died from AIDS. With death looming on the horizon, Sharon prepared her will, and made the difficult decision as to who would assume custody of her 12-year-old daughter when she died. Then she became one of Dr. Priestley's AIDS patients. Rather than take AZT, she chose to take various herbs and dietary supplements, and receive acupuncture treatments, to support and bolster her immune system.

Within only a few months, virtually all of Sharon Lund's symptoms disappeared. Her diarrhea ended, her memory improved, she no longer had to have her daughter change her sheets three times a night due to night sweats, and she could function on 8 hours of sleep, not 18 to 20, as had been the case before.

Five years later, her insurance company stopped paying for the cost of her supplements and acupuncture treatments. Unable to afford them, her health immediately declined. In a matter of weeks, she lost substantial weight, and again her prognosis was poor. Fortunately, she was able to raise enough funds to get back on the supplements and resume the acupuncture treatments, and in months her health returned.

It has been my privilege to spend time with this remarkable woman, and to see why Sharon Lund is one of the many AIDS patients whose long-term survival provides a beacon of hope to those suffering from the disease.

In October 1994, the Office of Alternative Medicine of the National Institutes of Health awarded Bastyr University in Seattle a landmark $840,000 three-year grant to study the use of alternative medicine in the treatment of HIV/AIDS. In 1996, the president of Bastyr University, Joe Pizzorno, told me that more than 50 percent of people with AIDS in the United States are now using some form of alternative medicine.[42]

HANTAVIRUS

AIDS and Ebola have roots in environmental destruction. But they are not alone. The list of connections is sobering to contemplate: The depletion of the ozone layer, and skin cancer; air pollution, and respiratory disease; acid rain, damaged crops, and malnutrition; lead and other heavy metals, and central nervous system poisoning; pesticides, other toxic chemicals, and nuclear radiation, and increasing rates of birth defects, cancer, and autoimmune diseases.

Now, scientists studying the relationship between ecology and public health are saying that if we continue creating imbalances in the biosystems of the planet, we will experience yet another dimension to the problem. Global warming, they are saying, would expand the range and activity of a variety of creatures that can carry pathogenic microbes — including mosquitoes, flies, ticks, mice, and rats. This would present a number of not particularly pleasant scenarios, including the spread of tropical diseases into areas of the world that have up until now been protected from them by their colder climates. Even a slight rise in temperature, for example, would allow the mosquitoes that carry malaria, dengue fever, and yellow fever access to much of the United States and southern Europe.[43]

Apparently, the medical consequences of climate change are already entering the American experience. In 1993, there was a serious outbreak of an unknown but swiftly fatal disease in the American southwest. The first victim was Merrill Bahe, a long-distance runner who, while driving to his girlfriend's house, was suddenly overcome with fever, headache, and difficulty breathing. His grief-stricken relatives watched helplessly as the athlete gulped desperately for air. Minutes later, he was dead.

In the next few weeks, dozens of people in the area experienced similar tragedies. Most cases began with flulike symptoms, including fever, muscle aches and headaches. After a few hours, coughing would set in. The capillary network feeding the lungs would spring leaks, and fluid would begin seeping into the lungs. Within a matter of minutes or hours, the afflicted people would begin having trouble breathing, a situation that would grow desperately worse as their lungs filled with fluid and became unable to absorb oxygen. Hypoxic and starving for oxygen, they would gasp in agony until they finally died, either from heart failure or pulmonary edema.

As the epidemic spread, with mortality rates running appallingly high, local people began to panic and point the finger, creating a situation that seems all too sadly familiar when disease epidemics strike. With many of the outbreaks taking place on a Navajo reservation, people started calling it the "Navajo disease," and scapegoating the Native Americans. Schoolchildren from the Navajo nation were denied a planned field trip to California. Waitresses began wearing rubber gloves when serving Navajo customers. Local people driving across the Navajo mesas began wearing surgical masks.[44]

Scientists at first believed the disease was pneumonic plague, but sophisticated lab tests at an extraordinary New Mexico plague laboratory enabled them to discount that possibility.[45] Eventually, they were able to identify the pathogen—the Hantavirus (named after the Hanta River in Korea where it was originally discovered)—and trace its mechanism of transmission.[46] It spreads through the feces and urine of a particular deer mouse, a brown, big-eared rodent with a white belly and tail, and huge black eyes. The mouse had in recent months mysteriously appeared in great numbers, leaving its droppings in kitchens and playgrounds.

Scientists now had a crucial piece of the puzzle. But to prevent the scourge from spreading, they needed to know why this normally reclusive deer mouse had suddenly shown up in human habitations. The stakes were high, and a full understanding of the ecology of this disease especially critical, because this deer mouse can be found, with the exception of a few southern states, throughout the continental United States and Canada. Already there were suspected outbreaks in California, Nevada, Oregon, Louisiana, Arizona, Utah, and Idaho. By 1995, the disease would surface in 23 states.[47]

In a beautiful example of partnership medicine in action, the scientists asked the help of the Navajo medicine men. The medicine men pointed out that there had been severe drought in the area for the previous five years. But record amounts of snow had fallen in the winter of 1992–1993, and the spring of 1993 had been wet. The rain, combining with the melting snow flowing down into the valley had produced an abundance of pine nuts on pinon trees, and also an abundance of grasshoppers —both food for the deer mouse. Gorging on this extraordinary harvest, the deer mouse population had increased ten-fold in a matter of months.

Then more rain had come, flooding the mice's burrows, and forcing the rodents above ground. Looking for food and shelter, they had sought out human habitation.

Together, the scientists and the medicine men were now able to understand more fully how, in the interconnectedness of all life, the Hantavirus had spread. By joining forces, they had taken a step forward in understanding the ecology of this disease.

GLOBAL HEALTH, THE POPULATION EXPLOSION, AND THE STATUS OF WOMEN

At the center of all of the earth's environmental problems there stand two of the most dogged realities of the modern world—unsustainable population growth and unsustainable levels of consumption.

At present growth rates, the world's human population will double in the next 40 years. How will we be able to continue to feed a growing population, when every year more arable land is lost to soil erosion, desertification, acid rain, and urban growth—not to mention the decline in world food production that could occur with climate change? According to WorldWatch Institute, world grain carryover stocks for 1996 were already at the lowest level on record.[48]

In 1994, representatives from 189 nations convened in Cairo to launch what may have been the boldest initiative ever undertaken by the United Nations—the attempt to deal directly with the issue of population. The nations agreed on the need to provide family planning services to the 120 million women who are wanting to limit the size of their families but lack access to the services needed to do so. And they understood that achieving a sustainable population is not merely a matter of airlifting condoms to Africa; it means improving educational and employment opportunities for the poor, and ensuring women's equality in all areas of life.

Gender inequity, they agreed, is one of the principal causes of high fertility. The population explosion, they said, with its enormous implications for the environment and for human health, is linked directly to the status of women in the world.

The conference culminated in the World Population Plan of Action, which called for humanity's resources to be directed toward the education of girls, for it was recognized that the more education women have, the more social and economic choices will be available to them, and the fewer children they will bear.[49] This realization had been prophetically foreseen by Riane Eisler in *The Chalice and the Blade*, when she predicted that the problems caused by the population explosion could only be solved within a partnership paradigm. "If population planning is to succeed," she wrote, "creating satisfying and socially rewarded roles for women other than those of wives and mothers is even more important than the availability of birth control education."[50]

In most of the Third World, poverty seems so indelibly associated with rapidly increasing population numbers that many world leaders have come to believe that there is no way a society can curtail population growth without becoming more affluent and raising its level of resource consumption. But since environmental degradation is a product of both population growth *and* unsustainable levels of consumption, lowering the birth rate by raising the consumption rate only seems to create a different kind of destabilization. The wealthier nations of the world consume far more resources, generate far more pollution, and create far more toxic waste per capita than the poorer nations. The puzzlement has been this: It has not seemed feasible to achieve stable population numbers and a healthy society without a level of consumption that is environmentally destructive.

Stunningly, there are a few societies who, even with extremely low levels of consumption, have been able to stabilize their numbers at sustainable levels, and also to achieve outstanding levels of health for their people.

How do they do it? These cultures devote their limited resources to public health rather than high-tech treatment. Their wealth is not concentrated primarily in the hands of the few, and they provide universal access to both education and contraception. Most importantly, women are afforded full rights and equal status.

They are partnership societies.

In southern India, the state of Kerala is home to 30 million people—as many as live in the state of California. **This society has achieved universal health care and education, and a birth rate as low as almost any**

Kerala: First World Quality of Life and Zero Population Growth Despite Third World Poverty

	U.S. and Canada Combined	Kerala	India
Fertility Rate (children born per woman)	2.0	2.0	3.9
Infant Mortality Rate	8	17	91
Life Expectancy, Male	72	70	58
Life Expectancy, Female	79	74	59
Literacy, Male	99%	94%	64%
Literacy, Female	99%	86%	39%
GNP per capita	$22,430	$365	$350

Source: GAIA Ecological Perspectives in Science, Humanities, and Economics, 1994, 3(4), 211.

nation in the world, on a per capita income that is only one-sixteenth of what would be considered poverty level in the United States.[51] No coercive family-planning schemes, no forced sterilizations, no heavy-handed tactics are involved. Only a few abortions are performed every year.[52]

The accomplishments of Kerala are spectacular. Fertility, infant mortality, and life expectancy statistics in this Third World community are comparable to the industrialized world, rather than to the other Indian states. The average Indian lives to the age of 59; the average Keralan to 72. This, Kerala achieves on a per capita income of only $365 a year.

Even with very little income, this state has achieved a stunning quality of life. Kerala stands as a model, because it is a society that is succeeding in living healthfully with no population growth, and yet does not depend on an environmentally destructive level of consumption. You might think that the only way this could be achieved is through a benevolent dictatorship. But no, Kerala is a thriving democracy, where 90 percent of the electorate votes.

What, then, has enabled Kerala to achieve such outstanding results for its people? The state places an unusually high value on public health, education, and the status of women. There is strong governmental support for breastfeeding, and state supported nutrition programs for pregnant women and new mothers. While the overall female literacy rate in India is 39 percent, in Kerala it is 86 percent and rising rapidly. In fact, Kerala

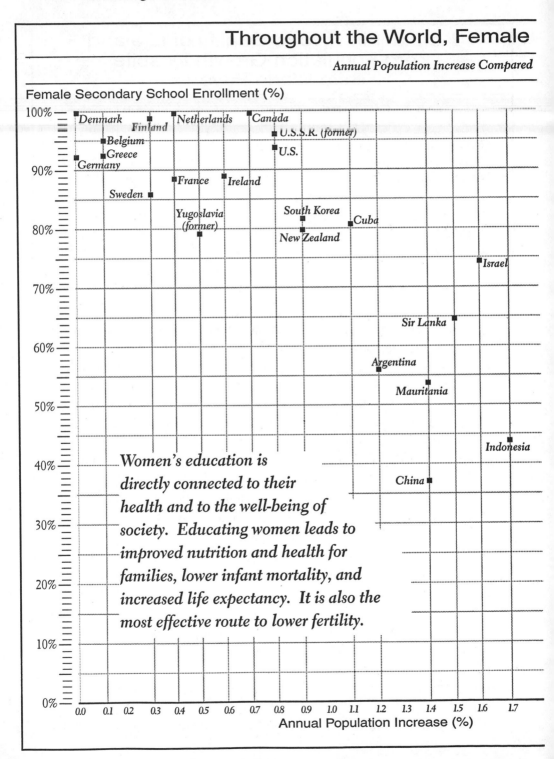

Throughout the World, Female

Annual Population Increase Compared

Female Secondary School Enrollment (%)

Denmark Finland Netherlands Canada
U.S.S.R. (former)
Belgium
Greece U.S.
Germany

France Ireland

Sweden

Yugoslavia (former) South Korea Cuba

New Zealand

Israel

Sir Lanka

Argentina

Mauritania

Indonesia

China

Women's education is directly connected to their health and to the well-being of society. Educating women leads to improved nutrition and health for families, lower infant mortality, and increased life expectancy. It is also the most effective route to lower fertility.

Annual Population Increase (%)

Education Is a Key to Birth Control.

to Female Secondary School Enrollment

In 1993, more than 600 of the world's most distinguished
scientists, including a majority of the living Nobel laureates in
the sciences, issued the World Scientists' Warning to
Humanity. It read, in part: "The earth is finite. Its
ability to provide for growing numbers of people is
finite. Current economic practices which damage
the environment, in both developed and
underdeveloped nations, cannot be continued
without the risk that vital global systems
will be damaged beyond repair....
Pressures resulting from
unrestrained population growth
put demands on the natural
world that can
overwhelm any effort
to achieve a
sustainable
future."

Chile

Jamaica   ■ Mexico

Guiana
■ Colombia

Vietnam

Tunisia ■   ■ Costa Rica
   ■ Iraq

Turkey ■   Bolivia

■India   Morocco

Laos
Cambodia   Nigeria ■   ■Madagascar
   Haiti
   ■Nepal   Congo Zaire
Bangladesh   Ethiopia ■
   Senegal ■   Pakistan
   Afghanistan   Angola   Rwanda ■   Yemen
   Malawi ■   Tanzania

| 1.8 | 1.9 | 2.0 | 2.1 | 2.2 | 2.3 | 2.4 | 2.5 | 2.6 | 2.7 | 2.8 | 2.9 | 3.0 | 3.1 | 3.2 | 3.3 | 3.4 | 3.5 | 3.6 | 3.7 |

Source: Chart compiled by the author from data provided by Population
Crisis Committee and World Health Organization, 1992.

is expected to soon achieve both a 100 percent female literacy rate and a zero population growth rate.

Dr. C. R. Soman, professor of nutrition at the medical school in Kerala's capital city, Trivandrum, was asked how, in a world where poor nations almost invariably have frighteningly high birth rates, such a poor society could manage to stabilize its population. His answer was simple: "The most enduring contraception is female education."[53]

"MY WAITING ROOM EXPANDED
TO INCLUDE THE WHOLE PLANET"

The experience of Kerala provides a model from which we can learn a great deal about how to deal effectively with the population explosion, and thus save enormous health and environmental suffering. But from a dominator perspective, other cultures are only resources to exploit, not communities from which we can learn. It's the ascendancy of the dominator impulse in American medicine that has led to our universities and medical schools having virtually no classes in international health, and to organized medicine in the United States only feebly (if at all) supporting the World Health Organization and other global efforts concerned with the health of humanity.

If our physicians had a better understanding of global health issues, they would not only be better prepared to play a role in the world health community, they would also have an enlarged perspective that would enable them to function in their own communities with more open-mindedness and efficacy. They might realize the significance of the fact that while in New York City, 10.8 infants out of 1,000 die before their first birthday, the rate in Shanghai, China is only 9.9.[54] Life expectancy at birth in Shanghai is now 75.5 years, compared to a life expectancy in New York City of 73 years for whites and 70 years for people of color.[55] If our medical authorities had the advantage of a more international perspective, they might ask how Shanghai, a dilapidated Third World metropolis in a country with a per capita income of $350, can generate a better health record than New York City. Recognizing that China spends just $38 per person annually on medical care, compared to more than $3,000 in the United States, they might understand how much is to be gained from channeling funds toward prevention and basic care.

There's more. If our physicians understood the critical importance of female education and empowerment to the living web of global health, they might be more inclined to inform women rather than dictate to them. If they knew that in the Netherlands 35 percent of births take place at home, with vastly better results than we obtain in hospitals, they might be more supportive of home birth. If they were aware that all of the many countries with lower infant mortality rates than our own employ midwives as the principal birth attendants, they might be more respectful of midwives. If they knew that in Ostend, Belgium, Herman Ponette, M.D., has safely delivered more than 2,000 babies in water, including breeches and twins, with statistics that show water birth to be thoroughly safe, they might be more supportive of the practice.

The rampant overuse of antibiotics in the United States, and the consequent proliferation of antibiotic-resistant bacteria, might be checked by the realization that the other industrialized countries use far fewer antibiotics. In the United States, more prescriptions are written for antibiotics than for virtually any other class of drugs. In West Germany, by contrast, there are no antibiotics in the top 20 drug classes.[56]

The rush to remove women's wombs might be slowed by the realization that the Europeans do far fewer hysterectomies, with more healthful outcomes. Similarly, American physicians' penchant for treating menopause and aging as a disease might be tempered by the understanding that many traditional peoples honor the transition and revere elder women. Before prescribing estrogen to prevent osteoporosis, they might recall that this disease is only a problem in nations who base their diets around animal products. And that vegetarians have far stronger bones and less osteoporosis than meat-eaters.

Instead of believing that cancer prevention is primarily a matter of mammograms and other tests, our doctors might recall that Israel, the only nation in the world to reduce the incidence of breast cancer, did so by banning a number of organochlorine pesticides. They might recognize that nations whose diets are lower in meat and fat than ours consistently have lower rates, not only of cancer, but of heart disease and diabetes as well.

We would no longer have medical schools that ignore nutrition, or the medical consequences of environmental deterioration. There would be more doctors like Michael Klaper, M.D., founder of the Institute for Nutrition Education and Research, who teaches other physicians about the latest advances in nutrition, and the impact of human activities on the environment. "My waiting room," he explains, "expanded to include the whole planet."

If American physicians were more aware of the impact of social and environmental factors on health, they would be less fixated on drugs and surgeries as the primary answers, and more committed to prevention. Less imprisoned in the biases of a cultural trance, they would be aware that the single-payer health care systems of many other countries do a better job for far less money, and generate far fewer malpractice problems. They'd realize that the United States, the only nation which actively excludes alternative medicine, spends far more per capita for health care than any other nation in the world, and is the only country in the industrialized world that does not guarantee minimum health care to every single citizen. Freed and humbled by a more global perspective, they would be more likely to treat their patients with understanding, and more inclined to appreciate the need for a partnership in medicine.

HEALING MEDICINE

A true partnership in medicine would integrate the best of standard and alternative approaches to the treatment of disease, and create clinics in which Asklepian and Hygeian practitioners worked in tandem. Rather than waiting to fight illness when it descends, they would actively strive to promote wellness through healing practices that stimulate the body's own defenses, catalyze the immune system, and support the body's natural wisdom. They would welcome unconventional approaches that had merit, and would gladly relinquish the use of harmful interventions when safer and less costly approaches were available and effective.

But grounding our medical system in partnership would do more than create a blend of orthodox and alternative medicine. It would bring our society closer to the recognition that all of us are partners in the fate of our world.

Recognizing that each of our personal health destinies is inseparable from those of our fellow human beings, our medical system would work for the healing of the world's communities. Realizing that the health of all nations, all races, all classes, and all members of both genders is intimately and equally dependent on the health of the global biosystems, it would commit itself to the healing of the biosphere. Appreciating that the ecological assault on the planet is intimately interwoven with the degradation of women, it would seek to restore balance both to planetary ecosystems and to the ecology of human relations. Maybe our government would stop subsidizing the export of tobacco products, and instead subsidize the export of solar water pasteurizers and solar cookers.

A partnership basis to medicine would also bring about a change in the way many health professionals relate to patients. Their interactions would no longer be ones of dominance and submission, but would become collaborations between coworkers with a common goal. Doctors would not have to carry the burden of playing the all-knowing potentate, but could befriend their patients, support them in claiming their integrity, and help them to take responsibility for their lives and choices.

A shift in a partnership direction would alter the way we see and experience our bodies. It is dominator thinking that views the human body as a machine beset by the propensity to break down and cause problems, and sees the female body as particularly flawed and prone to malfunction. A more enlightened approach would recognize that each human body is extraordinary, and that every single human being is a miracle. It would help people to respect the exquisite intelligence their bodies possess. It would teach that the body can be an ally and a teacher, and is naturally blessed with marvelous healing capabilities. Such a medical system would help people to honor the wisdom of their bodies.

A more partnership-oriented perspective would also change our relationship to birth. To a dominator mind, birth is fraught with danger, at all times demanding close medical supervision and the full and immediate availability of invasive technologies. More partnership-oriented eyes, however, would see birth as a natural process of deep mystery and power, and an expression of the developing connection between mother and child. We would understand that the place for medical technology is as a backup, to be used only in those rare times when it is truly needed. By developing midwifery care, demedicalizing childbirth, and encouraging breastfeeding, we would dramatically reduce infant mortality, strengthen the bonds between mothers and children, and save $20 billion a year.

In a medical technocracy governed by dominator thinking, death is seen as a failure, and hundreds of billions of dollars are spent artificially keeping people alive even when the added time brings only pain and agony. In a system oriented more toward partnership, death would be embraced as part of the human experience, and known to be as natural as life itself. Dying people would be allowed to die when their time has come with dignity and without unnecessary pain. They would not be manipulated and controlled; they would be cherished.

Moving in a partnership direction would change our very definition of health. To a dominator viewpoint, health is simply the absence of symptoms sufficiently disabling to prevent an individual from functioning normally. A society and a medical community more imbued with a partnership perspective would see health as the presence of vitality, harmony, and balance; as the ability to understand one's own individual part of the common universal journey; as the capacity to function with a growing level of awareness, and a deepening level of joy.

RECLAIMING OUR HEALTH, RECLAIMING OUR LIVES

The same forces and tensions that are at work in our medical system are active in every aspect of society, and in each of our individual lives. Wherever they appear, the dominator and partnership tendencies bespeak an ancient and ongoing dialogue between fear and love.

It is not only our medical choices which can be pivotal in the swing toward a society more deeply rooted in compassion. We are part of this great work whenever we bring more respect and love into our relationships, whenever we are able to bring our lives into harmony with our humanity. We are part of this movement as we learn to respect ourselves and our fellow human beings, as we learn to honor the sacred magic of life.

It would be hard, at this date, for any of us not to feel a degree of pain for the world. And yet as paradoxical as it may seem, I find a beauty in this pain, because our planetary anguish speaks of our connection with each other, and brings with it the impetus to act. We have cause for hope, since we have the tools and the understanding to create a healthier, more just, and happier life for the vast majority of human beings. And we have grounds for gratitude, because we are given today an opportunity to participate in an historic transformation. Each of us, wherever we live and in whatever circumstances we find ourselves, is blessed with countless opportunities, in our relationships and in the way we live, to bring more love and healing into this world.

If we are aware of the perils that face us, and also of the promise and courage inherent in the human heart, then the great problems of our time become not a precursor to global disaster, but a call to compassionate action.

When I see how many people in our world are ill and suffering, I am always reminded that health is a precious gift, and one that I want to enjoy and to share. With life, there comes responsibility—the responsibility to nurture and care for our bodies, and also a responsibility to work for the health and wholeness of the planet and all the life it holds.

Dominator thinking has produced a society that defines responsibility in terms of compliance. It has yielded a medicalized society where parents who feed their children junk food and then take them for yearly checkups are considered to be doing the right thing. And where people who eat bacon and eggs for breakfast and then take cholesterol-lowering pills are viewed as responsible. Every day in our society, women who have obediently followed the rules say to their doctors, "I can't understand how this happened to me; I've come in for exams every year; I've had regular mammograms; and yet now I've got cancer." Meanwhile, more than half of two-pack-a-day smokers have never been advised by their physicians that their smoking is endangering their health.

If we are to create a society dedicated to supporting and maintaining health for all peoples, then it is up to us to do everything we can to place genuine responsibility for our lives into our own hands. **The medical establishment will only get off its pedestal when we get off our knees.**

If we are to take back our lives from the institutions that have lost their sense of commitment to the common good, we need to release ourselves from the belief that our health is primarily dependent on medical technology, and restore our faith in ourselves, in our own minds and hearts, and in the activities that truly generate and protect health. Wherever we are in our lives, each of us can always ask, "How can I take more responsibility for my health? In what ways can I help create a world with less suffering and more health, with less violence and more cooperation?"

Each of us is granted repeated opportunities to shift our lives—and our world—in a healthier and more beautiful direction. Though there are always factors that influence our lives and our health over which we have little control, there are also other factors that lie within our personal sovereignty. We can always ask, "What steps can I take to bring more love and healing into my life and into the world?"

It would be a wonderful medical system that reminded us that we each carry a piece of a great and sacred dream inside us. But in the meantime, it is always true that by caring for ourselves and others, we do the essential work of our time: We enhance our connection to all of life, and our ability to serve all of life. By cherishing ourselves and others, we help to fulfill one of the human spirit's most ancient and beautiful prayers.

We help awaken our world from the grip of fear into the celebration of love.

May all be fed. May all be healed. May all be loved.

To Contact
John Robbins

To contact John Robbins and/or to receive information about resources and projects, please write:

> EarthSave International
> 620 B Distillery Commons
> Louisville, KY 40206

People who write will receive the following:

- Information from EarthSave International, the nonprofit organization founded by John Robbins, about the benefits of a plant-based diet for our health and a more compassionate world.
- Quantity discounts for *Reclaiming Our Health*, available from EarthSave.
- Notification of upcoming John Robbins lectures and special events in your area.
- Information about workshops, river-rafting trips, video tapes and audiotapes, and other resources and activities.

Resource Guide

Natural Childbirth and Midwifery: Journals

Birth Gazette, 42 The Farm, Summertown, TN 38483-9626; 615-964-3798
(provides a list of midwifery schools and education programs).
Informed Homebirth, P.O. Box 3675, Ann Arbor, MI 48106;
313-662-6857.
Midwifery Today, P.O. Box 2672-405, Eugene, OR 97402;
541-344-7438.

Natural Childbirth and Midwifery: Organizations

American College of Nurse-Midwives, 818 Connecticut Ave., NW, Suite 900,
Washington, DC 20006; 202-728-9860.
Association for Pre- and Perinatal Psychology and Health, P.O. Box 994,
Geyserville, CA 95441; 707-857-4041.
Association of Labor Assistants and Childbirth Educators, P.O. Box 382724,
Cambridge, MA 02238; 617-441-2500.
Birth Works Childbirth Education, P.O. Box 2045, Medford, NJ 08055;
609-953-9380.
California Association of Midwives, P.O. Box 417854, Sacramento, CA 95841;
800-829-5791.
Doulas of North America, 1100 23rd Ave. East, Seattle, WA 98112;
206-324-5440.
Global Maternal/Child Health Association, P.O. Box 1400, Wilsonville, OR
97070; 503-682-3600 (a superb source of information and resources
regarding water births).
International Cesarean Awareness Network, P.O. Box 152, Syracuse, NY 13210;
716-244-2143.
International Childbirth Education Association, P.O. Box 20048, Minneapolis,
MN 55402; 612-854-8660.
Midwives Alliance of North America, P.O. Box 175, Newton, KS 67114;
fax: 316-283-4543.

Natural Childbirth and Midwifery: Recommended Books

A Good Birth, A Safe Birth: Choosing and Having the Childbirth Experience You Want, Diana Korte and Roberta Scaer (Cambridge, MA: Harvard Common Press, 1992). A thoughtful, informed, and balanced book, particularly useful for anyone who is going to have a hospital birth and wants to know how to make the best of it.

Birth Reborn, Michel Odent (Medford, NJ: Birth Works Press, 1994). Originally published in 1984, this classic has shown the world what maternity care can be.

Gentle Birth Choices, Barbara Harper (Rochester, VT: Inner Traditions, 1994). Contains an amazing chapter on water labor and birth.

Getting an Education: Paths to Becoming a Midwife (Eugene, OR: A Midwifery Today Publication, 1996). Includes a comprehensive directory of midwifery training programs.

Immaculate Deception II: A Fresh Look at Childbirth, Suzanne Arms (Berkeley, CA: Celestial Arts, 1994). A beautifully written overview of today's birth options.

Open Season: Survival Guide for Natural Childbirth and VBAC in the 90s, Nancy Wainer Cohen (New York: Bergin and Garvey, 1991). A dynamite book that I highly recommend for anyone considering a vaginal birth after a previous cesarean.

Spiritual Midwifery, Ina May Gaskin (Summertown, TN: The Book Publishing Company, 1990). A classic. Full of inspiring birth stories from The Farm.

Natural Childbirth and Midwifery: Recommended Videos

Babies Know More Than You Think. With David Chamberlain, Ph.D., and Suzanne Arms. Explores the capacity and consciousness of new human beings. This program will transform how you relate to babies, children, and to yourself! Length: 60 min. $24.95. Available from Touch the Future; 310-426-2627.

Gentle Birth Choices. This outstanding production combines art, education, and politics, graphically illustrating why it is vital for women to be in charge of their birth experience. Filmed at a birth center and at a variety of home births. You witness six actual births, including a VBAC, two water births, a squatting birth, and a woman birthing on her hands and knees. Winner of a national Telly award. Length: 47 min. $39.95. Available from Global Maternal/Child Health Association; 800-641-BABY.

Pregnancy, Birth, and Bonding. A dynamic presentation by Joseph Chilton Pearce, author of *The Magical Child*. Length: 60 min. $24.95. Available from Touch the Future; 310-426-2627.

Women's Health: Recommended Books

A Cooperative Method of Natural Birth Control, Margaret Nofziger (Summertown, TN: The Book Publishing Company, 1992). Simple and direct, the ABCs of fertility awareness.

A Woman's Worth, Marianne Williamson (New York: Ballantine Books, 1993). A rhapsody of the female spirit. Uplifting, real, and exquisitely beautiful.

Conscious Conception, Jeannine Parvati Baker and Frederick Baker (Freestone Publishing Co., North Atlantic Books, 1986). A look at issues of conception in terms of women's spiritual and sexual wholeness.

Take Charge Of Your Body, Carolyn DeMarco (Winlaw, B.C., Canada: Well Women Press, 1994). A guide to many women's health issues.

The Menopause Industry: How the Medical Establishment Exploits Women, Sandra Coney (Alameda, CA: Hunter House, 1994).

What Your Doctor May Not Tell You About Menopause: The Breakthrough Book on Natural Progesterone, John Lee, M.D., with Virginia Hopkins (New York: Warner Books, 1996). Provides the in-depth story of this intriguing natural hormone.

Women's Bodies, Women's Wisdom: Creating Physical and Emotional Health and Healing, Christiane Northrup (New York: Bantam Books, 1994). Insightful, thorough, and inspiring, this book is destined to be a classic. A truly outstanding guide to virtually all women's health issues.

Women's Health: Organizations and Services

Anna Keck, R.N, F.N.P., is the Founder of Wellcare Associates—Soquel Therapy Center, 5030 Soquel Drive, Soquel, CA 95073; 408-685-1636. She is a knowledgeable and caring clinician who can provide a comprehensive assessment of midlife issues, and fine-tune hormone and other treatment choices in a holistic way. She teaches women how to safely monitor their own bodies as they go through menopause, and can work effectively via phone and mail. The service she offers is especially useful for women who do not wish to overly medicalize menopause, yet want support in making choices that will optimize bone, breast, and heart health.

The Women's International Pharmacy; 800-279-5708. Information about natural progesterone, and referrals to health professionals familiar with it.

Cascade Health Care/Birth and Life Bookstore, 141 Commercial NE, Salem, OR 97301; 800-443-9942. An excellent source for mail order women's books, they also sell midwifery and birth supplies, herbal remedies, homeopathics, etc.

Women's Health: Fertility Testing, Microscopes, and Related Resources

Around the Moon, P.O. Box 3325, Applegate, OR 97530; 541-846-6677.

FemmeNet International, P.O. Box 879, Ojai, CA 93924 (The Natural Rhythm Fertility Tester).

Fertility Awareness Services, P.O. Box 986, Corvallis, OR 97339; 503-753-8530.

Jeannine Parvati Baker, P.O. Box 111, Junction, UT 84740; 801-326-4256.

Parenting and Schooling

Journal of Family Life (A Quarterly for Empowering Families), 72 Philip Street, BG, Albany, NY 12202; 518-432-1578.

Mothering, P.O. Box 1690, Santa Fe, NM 87504; 505-984-8116. A heartful and wide-ranging quarterly journal dealing with all kinds of mothering issues.

The Compleat Mother, P. O. Box 209, Minot, ND 58702; 701-852-2822. The only consumer magazine with a focus on breastfeeding, and very affordable.

The Doula (Mothering the Mother), P.O. Box 71, Santa Cruz, CA 95063-0071; 408-464-9488. Support for pregnant women and new mothers.

The Waldorf School Association of North America, 916-961-0927. Private schools (K–12) that cultivate wonder for life, enthusiasm for learning, and responsibility for the earth.

Healthy Diets and Lifestyles

Diet for a New America: How Your Food Choices Affect Your Health, Happiness, and the Future of Life on Earth, John Robbins (Tiburon, CA: H J Kramer, 1987). The runaway best-seller that launched EarthSave, and has empowered hundreds of thousands of people to make more compassionate, health-giving, and ecologically friendly life choices. To order, call 800-DNA-DO-IT.

EarthSave, 620 Distillery Commons, Louisville, KY 40206; 502-589-7676. Founded by John Robbins, EarthSave promotes the benefits of plant-based food choices for optimal health, environmental preservation, and a more compassionate world. Programs include the Healthy School Lunch Program, YES! (Youth for Environmental Sanity), and local action groups. Offers a quarterly newsletter and a catalogue of resources and materials to support healing our bodies, our lives, and our world.

The Feingold Association of the U.S. P.O. Box 6550, Alexandria, VA 22306.

Natural Health, 17 Station St., P.O. Box 1200, Brookline Village, MA 02147; 617-232-1000. A monthly magazine with ideas and guidelines for a natural and healthy lifestyle.

Natural Hygiene Society, P.O. Box 30630, Tampa, FL 33630; 813-855-6607. Publishers of *Health Science* magazine.

New Century Nutrition (formerly *The Nutrition Advocate*), P.O. Box 4716,
    Ithaca, NY 14852; 800-841-0444. An outstanding newsletter, informed
    and reliable.
Vegetarian Times, P.O. Box 570, Oak Park, IL 60303; 708-848-8100. A monthly
    magazine with recipes plus informative and inspiring articles.
Yoga Journal, 2054 University Ave., Berkeley, CA 94704; 510-841-9200. A bi-
    monthly magazine with many fine articles on holistic health and healing.

Alternative Physician Organizations

Doctors Without Borders, 11 E. 26th St., Ste. 1904, New York, NY 10010;
    212-679-6800. Offers assistance to populations in distress, to victims
    of natural or human-caused disaster, and to victims of armed conflict,
    without discrimination, irrespective of race, religion, creed, or political
    affiliation.
Physicians Committee for Responsible Medicine, 5100 Wisconsin Ave., NW,
    Suite 404, Washington, DC 20016; 202-686-2210. Promotes nutrition,
    preventive medicine, ethical research practices, and compassionate med-
    ical policy. Publishes *Good Medicine*, a quarterly journal.
Physicians for Global Survival, 170 A Rue Booth St., Ottawa, Ontario K1R
    7W1, Canada; 613-233-1982. The Canadian equivalent to Physicians for
    Social Responsibility.
Physicians for Social Responsibility, 1101 14th St., NW, Suite 700, Washington,
    DC; 202-898-0150. The organization that has been leading the effort to
    educate the public about the medical consequences of nuclear war and
    environmental deterioration.

Alternative Approaches to Cancer: Organizations

Center for Advancement in Cancer Education; P.O. Box 48, Wynnewood, PA
    19096-0048; 610-642-4810.
People Against Cancer; P.O. Box 10, Otho, IA 50569; 515-972-4444.

Alternative Approaches to Cancer: Services for Patients

Patrick McGrady's *CanHelp*; 206-437-2291.
Ralph Moss's *Healing Choices*; contact Anne Beattie: 718-636-4433.

Alternative Approaches to Cancer: Books

*Breast Cancer: What You Should Know (But May Not Be Told) About Preven-
    tion, Diagnosis, and Treatment*, Steve Austin, N.D., and Cathy Hitchcock,
    M.S.W. (Rocklin, CA: Prima Publishing, 1994).

Cancer Therapy: The Independent Consumer's Guide to Non-Toxic Treatment and Prevention, Ralph Moss, Ph.D. (Brooklyn, NY: Equinox Press, 1992).

Choices in Healing: Integrating the Best of Conventional and Complementary Approaches to Cancer, Michael Lerner (Cambridge, MA: MIT Press, 1994).

Options: The Alternative Cancer Therapy Book, Richard Walters (Garden City Park, NY: Avery, 1993).

Patient No More: The Politics of Breast Cancer, Sharon Batt (Charlottetown, PEI, Canada: Gynergy, 1994).

Questioning Chemotherapy, Ralph Moss, Ph.D. (Brooklyn, NY: Equinox Press, 1995).

Save Yourself From Breast Cancer: Life Choices That Can Help You Reduce the Odds, Robert Kradjian, M.D. (New York: Berkley Books, 1994).

The Cancer Industry: The Classic Expose of the Cancer Establishment, Ralph Moss, Ph.D. (New York: Paragon House, 1989).

The Cancer Prevention Diet: Michio Kushi's Blueprint for the Relief and Prevention of Disease, Michio Kushi (New York: St. Martin's Press, 1993).

The Essence of Essiac, Sheila Snow, Box 396, Port Carling, Ontario POBIJO Canada.

Specific Alternative Cancer Approaches Mentioned in *Reclaiming Our Health*

Nicholas Gonzalez, M.D.: 36 E 36th St, #204, New York, NY 10016; 212-213-3337.

Essiac: Resperin Corporation; 613-820-9311. Elaine Alexander, 6690 Oak St., Vancouver, BC V6P 3Z2, Canada; 604-261-1270.

Hoxsey: BioMedical Center, P.O. Box 727, 3170 General Ferreira, Colonia Juarez, Tijuana, Mexico 22000; 011-52-66-84-9011.

Gerson: Gerson Institute, P.O. Box 430, Bonita, CA 91908; 619-585-7600.

Macrobiotics: Kushi Institute of the Berkshires, P.O. Box 7, Becket, MA 01223; 413-623-5742.

Stanislaw Burzynski, M.D.: 12000 Richmond, Suite 260, Houston, TX 77082; 281-531-6464. (Burzynski Legal Defense Fund: P.O. Box 1770, Pacific Palisades, CA 90272).

Georg Springer, M.D.: Heather M. Bligh Cancer Research Laboratories, 3333 Green Bay Road, North Chicago, IL 60064; 847-578-3435.

Keith Block, M.D.: Block Medical Center, 1800 Sherman Ave., Suite 515, Evanston, IL 60201; 847-492-3040.

Glenn Warner, M.D.: Northwest Oncology Associates, Lincoln Center, 515 116th Ave., N.E., #220, Bellevue, WA 98004; 206-292-2277.

Alternative Approaches to HIV/AIDS

Jon D. Kaiser, M.D., The Wellness Center, 1635 Divisadero, Suite 625, San Francisco, CA 94114; 415-436-0100.

Joan Priestley, M.D., The Omni Medical Center, 615 E. 82nd, Suite 300, Anchorage, AL 59518; 907-344-7775.

AIDS Alternative Health Project, 4753 N. Broadway, Chicago, IL 60640; 312-561-2800.

Bastyr University AIDS Research Center, 144 N.E. 54th St., Seattle, WA 98105; 800-475-0135.

Consumer Advocacy and Health Freedom

Alternative Therapies in Health and Medicine, 101 Columbia, Aliso Viejo, CA 92656; 800-899-1712. A bimonthly journal edited by Larry Dossey, M.D. Provides information on the practical use of alternative therapies in preventing and treating disease, and promoting health.

Citizens for Alternative Health Care, P.O. Box 25312, Seattle, WA 98125-2212; 206-526-8091. Publishes *Progressive Health Choices*, a quarterly focusing on alternative medicine issues in the Pacific Northwest.

Citizens for Health, P.O. Box 2260, Boulder, CO 80306. One of the foremost citizen advocacy groups for health freedom.

People's Medical Society, 462 Walnut St., Allentown, PA 18102; 610-770-1670. A health-care consumer advocacy group.

Public Citizen Health Research Group, 1600 20th St., NW, Washington, DC 20009. Publishes a monthly *HealthLetter*, focusing on political and economic health-care realities. Can provide the cesarean section rate for specific hospitals.

Healing Our Planet

Choices for Our Future: A Generation Rising for Life on Earth, Ocean Robbins and Sol Solomon (Summertown, TN: The Book Publishing Co., 1994). An outstanding guide to taking positive action, geared for young people of all ages.

Food and Water, RR1, Box 68-D, Walden, VT 05873; 802-563-3300 or 800-EAT-SAFE. A nonprofit, consumer-advocacy organization working for safe food and a clean environment.

WorldWatch, 1776 Massachusetts Ave., NW, Washington, DC 20036; 202-452-1999. A monthly journal that tracks key indicators of the earth's well-being. Does not shy away from the immensity of the problems, yet consistently offers practical solutions.

Useful Guides for Patients Who May Need Conventional Medical Care

Confessions of a Medical Heretic, Robert S. Mendelsohn, M.D. (New York: Warner Books, 1979).

Dr. Dean Ornish's Program for Reversing Heart Disease, Dean Ornish, M.D. (New York: Ballantine Books, 1990).

Examining Your Doctor: A Patient's Guide to Avoiding Harmful Medical Care, Timothy McCall, M.D. (New York: Birch Lane Press, 1995).

Good Operations, Bad Operations: The People's Medical Society Guide to Surgery, Charles Inlander (New York: Viking, 1993).

How to Live Between Office Visits, Bernie Siegel, M.D. (New York: Harper-Collins, 1993).

How to Raise a Healthy Child in Spite of Your Doctor, Robert S. Mendelsohn, M.D. (Chicago: Contemporary Books, 1984).

Plastic Surgery Hopscotch: A Resource Guide for Those Considering Cosmetic Surgery, John McCabe (Santa Monica, CA: Carmania Books, 1995).

Surgery Electives: What to Know Before the Surgeon Operates, John McCabe (Santa Monica, CA: Carmania Books, 1996).

Take This Book to the Hospital With You: A Consumer's Guide to Surviving Your Hospital Stay, Charles Inlander and Ed Weiner (Emmaus, PA: Rodale Press, 1993).

Worst Pills, Best Pills II: The Older Adult's Guide to Avoiding Drug-Induced Death or Illness, Sidney Wolfe, M.D. (Washington, DC: Public Citizen Health Research Group, 1993).

Notes

Chapter 1: Reclaiming Our Health

1. Nicholas Kristof, "China Sets Example in Health Care," New York Times, *Ann Arbor News*, April 14, 1991, A-6. Jane Lii, "China Booms, the World Holds Its Breath," *New York Times Magazine*, Feb. 18, 1996, p. 27.
2. Anne Moffat, "China: A Living Lab for Epidemiology," *Science*, May 4, 1990, pp. 553–55.
3. Cinda Chima, quoted in "Malnourishment in U.S. Hospitals—Undiagnosed, Untreated," *Cleveland Plain Dealer*, Feb. 22, 1994.
4. John McDougall, *The McDougall Plan* (Clinton, NJ: New Win Publishers, 1983), p. 7.
5. Philip Kapleau, *To Cherish All Life* (San Francisco: Harper and Row, 1981), p. 59.
6. Bernie Siegel, *A Hope and a Prayer* (Santa Fe: Realidad Productions, 1986).
7. Ibid.
8. M. Roemer and J. Schwartz, "Doctor Slowdown: Effects on the Population of Los Angeles County," *Social Science and Medicine*, Dec. 1979, vol. 13C, pp. 214–17. T. Preston, *The Clay Pedestal* (Seattle: Madrona, 1981), pp. 134–35.
9. American Medical Association, *Winter Catalog 1996*, p. 37.
10. Lucy Moll, "Medical Care: Where's the Choice?," *Vegetarian Times*, Dec. 1988, pp. 44–52.
11. J. Harpignies, "The Greening of Medicine," *Lapis*; New York Open Center, Summer 1995.
12. Sandra Bertman, *Facing Death* (Taylor and Francis, 1991), p. 4.
13. Ibid. See also Bernard Lo, "Improving Care Near the End of Life: Why Is It So Hard?," editorial, *Journal of the American Medical Association*, 274(20), Nov. 22/29, 1995, pp.1634–46. Alfred Connors et al., "A Controlled Trial to Improve Care for Seriously Ill Hospitalized Patients," *Journal of the American Medical Association*, 274(20), Nov. 22/29, 1995, pp. 1591–98.

Chapter 2: The Goddess in Stirrups

1. Cited in Jessica Mitford, *The American Way of Birth* (New York: Plume, 1993), pp. 29–33.
2. Ibid.
3. "The State of the World's Children, 1996," UNICEF.
4. Ibid.
5. The Alan Guttmacher Institute, "Facts in Brief," March 15, 1993.
6. Ibid.
7. T. K. Eskes, "Home Deliveries in the Netherlands: Perinatal Mortality and Morbidity," *International Journal of Gynaecology and Obstetrics*, 1992, 38(3), pp. 161–69. Pieter Treffers et al., "Regional Perinatal Mortality and Regional Hospitalization at Delivery in the Netherlands," *British Journal of Obstetrics and Gynaecology*, 1986, 93(7), pp. 690–93. Pieter Treffers et al., "Letter From Amsterdam: Home Births and Minimal Medical Interventions," *Journal of the American Medical Association*, 264:17, Nov. 7, 1990. Theresa Malone, "American and Dutch Women . . ." *American College of Obstetricians and Gynecologists News Release*, May 24, 1988. S. Scherjon, "A Comparison Between the Organization of Obstetrics in Denmark and the Netherlands," *British Journal of Obstetrics and Gynaecology*, 1986, 93, pp. 684–89. S. M. Damstra-Wijmenga, "Home Confinement: The Positive Results in Holland," *Journal of the Royal College of General Practitioners*, 1984, 34(265), pp. 425–30.
8. Nancy W. Cohen and Lois J. Estner, *Silent Knife: Cesarean Prevention and Vaginal Birth After Cesarean* (New York: Bergin and Garvey, 1983), p. 3.
9. Letters from *The Ladies Home Journal* cited in Mitford, as per note 1, pp. 60–62.
10. As per note 3.

11. Henci Goer, *Obstetric Myths Versus Research Realities: A Guide to the Medical Literature* (Westport, CT: Bergin and Garvey, 1995), p. 321.
12. J. P. Rooks et al., "Outcomes of Care in Birth Centers: The National Birth Center Study," *New England Journal of Medicine*, Dec. 28, 1989, 321(26), pp. 1804–11.
13. Kittie Ernst, cited in Diana Korte and Roberta Scaer, *A Good Birth, A Safe Birth: Choosing and Having the Childbirth Experience You Want* (Cambridge, MA: Harvard Common Press, 1992), p. 46.
14. A. Scupholme and A. S. Kamons, "Are Outcomes Compromised When Mothers Are Assigned to Birth Centers for Care?," *Journal of Nurse Midwifery*, 1987, 32(4), pp. 211–15. A. Scupholme et al., "A Birth Center Affiliated With the Tertiary Care Center: Comparison of Outcome," *Obstetrics and Gynecology*, 1986, 67(4), pp. 598–603.
15. Examples cited in J. Mitford, as per note 1, pp. 72–73.
16. Christiane Northrup, *Women's Bodies, Women's Wisdom: Creating Physical and Emotional Health and Healing* (New York: Bantam, 1994), p. 391.
17. Suzanne Arms, *Immaculate Deception II: A Fresh Look at Childbirth* (Berkeley, CA: Celestial Arts, 1994), pp. 164–65.
18. Cited in D. Korte, as per note 13, p. 17.
19. Henci Goer, *Obstetric Myths Versus Research Realities: A Guide to the Medical Literature* (Westport, CT: Bergin and Garvey, 1995).
20. Marjorie Tew, "Do Obstetric Intranatal Interventions Make Birth Safer?," *British Journal of Obstetrics and Gynaecology*, July 1986, 93(7), pp. 684–89. Marjorie Tew, *Safer Childbirth? A Critical History of Maternity Care* (London: Chapman and Hall, 1988). Marjorie Tew, "Place of Birth and Perinatal Mortality," *Journal of the Royal College of General Practitioners*, August 1985, 35(277), pp. 390–94.
21. Barry Levy et al., "Reducing Neonatal Mortality Rate With Nurse-Midwives," *American Journal of Obstetrics and Gynecology*, 109, Jan. 1971.
22. D. Korte, as per note 13, p. 57.
23. Ibid.
24. M. Ward Hinds et al., "Neonatal Outcome in Planned vs. Unplanned Out-of-Hospital Births in Kentucky," *Journal of the American Medical Association* 253:11, Mar. 15, 1985, pp. 1578–82. Wayne Schramm et al., "Neonatality in Missouri Home Births, 1978–1984," *American Journal of Public Health*, 1987, 77(8), pp. 930–35. Deborah Sullivan et al., "Four Years' Experience by Licensed Midwives in Arizona," *American Journal of Public Health*, June 1983, 73(6), pp. 641–45. Claude Burnett et al., "Home Delivery and Neonatal Mortality in North Carolina," *Journal of the American Medical Association*, 244:24, Dec. 19, 1980, pp. 2741–45.
25. Ibid.
26. Chamberlain et al. in Sheila Kitzinger, *Homebirth* (New York: Dorling Kindersley, 1991).
27. P. E. Treffers et al., "Regional Perinatal Mortality and Regional Hospitalization at Delivery in the Netherlands," *British Journal of Obstetrics and Gynaecology*, 1986, 93(7).
28. D. Korte, as per note 13, p. 58.
29. Ibid.
30. "Mothering Perinatal Healthcare Statistics and Sources," *Mothering*, Fall 1993.
31. D. Korte, as per note 13, p. 58. D. B. Haire et al., "Maternity Care and Outcomes in a High-Risk Service: The North Central Bronx Hospital Experience," *Birth*, 1991, 18(1), pp. 33–37. See also J. Mitford, as per note 1, pp. 214–15.
32. J. Faison et al., "The Childbearing Center: An Alternative Birth Setting," *Obstetrics and Gynecology*, 1979, 54(4), pp. 527–32. C. Reinke, "Outcomes of the First 527 Births at the Birthplace in Seattle," *Birth*, 1982, 9(4), pp. 231–38. E. Zabrek et al., "Nurse-Midwifery Prototypes: The Alternative Birth Center in Jacksonville, Florida," *Journal of Nurse Midwifery*, 1983, 28(4), pp. 31–36. P. Eakins et al., "Obstetrical Outcomes at the Birth Place in Menlo Park: The First Seven Years," *Birth*, 1989, 16(3), pp. 123–29. A. Scupholme, as per note 14. A. B. Bennetts et al., "The Freestanding Birth Center," *Lancet*, 1:8268, Feb. 13, 1982, pp. 378–80. P. Eakins, "Freestanding Birth Centers in California: Program and Medical Outcome," *Journal of Reproductive Medicine* 1989, 34(12), pp. 960–70. J. P. Rooks et al., "Outcomes of Care in Birth Centers: The National Birth Center Study," *New England Journal of Medicine*, Dec. 28, 1989, 321(26), pp. 1804–11. G. Baruffi et al., "A Study of Pregnancy Outcomes in a Maternity Center and a Tertiary Care Hospital," *American Journal of Public Health*, 1984, 74(9), pp. 973–78. E. Feldman et al., "Outcomes and Procedures in Low Risk Birth: A Comparison of Hospital and Birth Center Settings," *Birth*, Mar. 1987, 14(1), pp. 18–24. Eunice Ernst, "Outcomes of 20,000 Women Who Sought Freestanding Birth Center Care: A National Collaborative Study," Eighth Birth Conference, San Francisco, CA, Mar. 1989.
33. R. Goodlin, "Low-Risk Obstetric Care for Low-Risk Mothers," *Lancet*, 1:8176, May 10, 1980.

34. Ibid.
35. Ibid.
36. Michelle Winkler, "Between the Lines," *The Doula*, Spring 1994, p. 2.
37. Suzanne Arms, as per note 17, p. 155.
38. D. Korte, as per note 13, p. 51. Mark Durand, "The Safety of Home Birth: The Farm Study," *American Journal of Public Health*, 1992, 82(3), pp. 450–53.
39. Joyce Vissell was kind enough to write this account specifically for *Reclaiming Our Health*.
40. Cited in George Annas, *Judging Medicine* (Clifton, NJ: Human Press, 1988), p. 117.
41. Lewis Mehl et al., "Outcomes of Elective Home Births: A Series of 1,146 Cases," *Journal of Reproductive Medicine*, 1977, 19(5), pp. 281–90. See also T. K. Eskes, as per note 7. R. Campbell et al., "Place of Delivery: A Review," *British Journal of Obstetrics and Gynaecology*, 1986, 93(7), pp. 675–83. R. Campbell et al., "Home Births in England and Wales: Perinatal Mortality According to Intended Place of Delivery," *British Medical Journal*, 1984, 289(6447), pp. 721–24. Pieter Treffers et al., as per note 7. J. F. Murphy et al., "Planned and Unplanned Deliveries at Home," *British Medical Journal*, 1984, 288(6428), pp. 1429–32. Marjorie Tew, as per note 20. J. M. Shearer, "Five Year Prospective Study of Risk of . . . Home Birth," *British Medical Journal*, 1985, 291(6507), pp. 1478–80. C. Ford et al., "Outcome of Planned Home Births in an Inner City Practice," *British Medical Journal*, 1991, 303(6816), pp. 1517–19. K.A. Howe, "Home Births in Southwest Australia," *Australian Medical Journal*, 1988, 149(6), pp. 296–302. M. Crotty, "Planned Home Births in South Australia," *Australian Medical Journal*, 1990, 153, pp. 664–71. H. Woodcock, "Planned Homebirths in Western Australia 1981–1987: A Descriptive Study," *Australian Medical Journal* 1990, 153, pp. 672–78. H. Tyson, "Outcomes of 1,001 Midwife-Attended Home Births in Toronto, 1983–1988," *Birth*, 1991, 18(1), pp. 14–19. M. Koehler et al., "Outcomes of a Rural Sonoma County Home Birth Practice, 1976–1982," *Birth*, 1984, 11(3), pp. 165–69. R. Anderson et al., "A Descriptive Analysis of Home Births Attended by Certified Nurse Midwives," *Journal of Nurse Midwifery*, 1991, 36(2), pp. 95–103. Mark Durand, as per note 38. See also note 24.
42. "Midwifery," *Los Angeles Times*, April 28, 1992, p. E1.
43. "Health Department Data Shows Danger of Home Births," press release from the American College of Obstetricians and Gynecologists, Jan. 4, 1978. This study was used during the 1991 Florida legislative session to "prove" the dangers of home birth, in the attempt to defeat a bill that would allow training for traditional midwives in the state. See Suzanne Suarez, "Midwifery Is Not the Practice of Medicine," *Yale Journal of Law and Feminism*, Spring 1993, 5(2), p. 315, note 277.
44. Murray Enkin et al., *Effective Care in Pregnancy and Childbirth* (England: Oxford University Press, 1989).
45. Henci Goer, "Guide Provides Information on Obstetric Management," *Genesis*, May–June 1991, quoted in D. Korte, as per note 13, p. 103.
46. "The Art of Midwivery," interview with Raven Lang, *The Doula*, 1986.

Chapter 3: Birth, Hospitals, and the Human Spirit

1. Diana Korte and Roberta Scaer, *A Good Birth, A Safe Birth: Choosing and Having the Childbirth Experience You Want* (Cambridge, MA: Harvard Common Press, 1992), p. 94.
2. J. R. Wilson et al., *Obstetrics and Gynecology*, 4th ed. (St. Louis: C. V. Mosby Co., 1971); cited in Claudia Dreifus, ed., *Seizing Our Bodies: The Politics of Women's Health* (New York: Vintage Books, 1977), pp. 213–14.
3. Marcel Heiman, "Psychiatric Complications: A Psychoanalytic View of Pregnancy," in Joseph Rovinsky and Alan Guttmacher, eds., *Medical, Surgical, and Gynecological Complications of Pregnancy*, 2nd ed. (Baltimore: Williams and Wilkins Co., 1965), p. 476.
4. Stuart Asch, "Psychiatric Complications: Mental and Emotional Problems," in Rovinsky and Guttmacher, as per note 3, pp. 461–64.
5. Ernest Friedman, letter, *Journal of the American Medical Association*, 1991, 266(21), p. 2984.
6. J. Whitridge Williams, *Williams Obstetrics*, 18th ed. (East Norwalk, CT: Appleton and Lang, 1989); cited in Jessica Mitford, *The American Way of Birth* (New York: Plume, 1993), p. 95.
7. Cited in *The Doula*, Summer 1992, p. 9.
8. C. L. Haq, "Vaginal Birth After Cesarean Delivery," *American Family Physician*, 1988, 37(6), pp. 167–71. M. G. Rosen et al., "Vaginal Birth After Cesarean: A Meta-Analysis of Morbidity and Mortality," *Obstetrics and Gynecology*, 1991, 77(3), pp. 465–70. L. J. Roberts, "Elective Section After Two Sections: Where's the Evidence?," *British Journal of Obstetrics and Gynaecology*, 1991, 98(12), pp. 1199–1202. K. M. Pruett et al., "Unknown Uterine Scar and Trial of Labor," *American Journal of Obstetrics and Gynecology*, 1988, 159(4), pp. 807–10. "Number of Cesarean Deliveries Can Be Reduced," Oct. 5, 1981, U.S. Dept. of Health and Human Services, *Research Resource Reporter*.

9. J. R. Evrard et al., "Cesarean Section and Maternal Mortality in Rhode Island," *Obstetrics and Gynecology*, Nov. 1977, 50(5), pp. 594–47. National Institutes of Child Health and Human Development, *Draft Report of the Task Force on Cesarean Childbirth*, NIH, Sept. 1980.
10. Susan Doering, "Unnecessary Cesareans," *Compulsory Hospitalization*, 48(2), pp. 145–52.
11. M. E. Avery, "Does Delivery by Section Matter to the Infant?," *New England Journal of Medicine*, 1971 (285), p. 917.
12. J. P. Phelan et al., "Vaginal Birth After Cesarean," *American Journal of Obstetrics and Gynecology*, Dec. 1987, pp. 1510–15. See also E. P. Kirk, "Vaginal Birth After Cesarean or Repeat Cesarean Section: Medical Risks or Social Realities," *American Journal of Obstetrics and Gynecology*, 1990, 162(6), pp. 1398-1405.
13. Myron Wegman, "Annual Summary of Vital Statistics," *Pediatrics*, 94(6), pp. 792–803, and previous annual summaries.
14. "Cesarean Birth Rate Goal for 2000: 50%," *Birth Gazette*, Summer 1995, 11(3), p. 34.
15. Marsden Wagner, "An Epidemic of Unnecessary Cesareans," *Mothering*, Fall 1993, p. 72.
16. Lynn Silver and Sidney Wolfe, "Unnecessary Sections: How to Cure a National Epidemic," Public Citizen Health Research Group, Washington, DC; quoted in D. Korte, as per note 1, p. 135.
17. Marsden Wagner, as per note 15, p. 71.
18. Mortimer Rosen, *The Cesarean Myth* (New York: Viking, 1989), p. 21.
19. Ibid.
20. Nancy Cohen and Lois Estner, *Silent Knife: Cesarean Prevention and Vaginal Birth After Cesarean* (Westport, CT: Bergin and Garvey, 1983), p. 37.
21. Nancy Cohen, *Open Season: Survival Guide for Natural Childbirth and VBAC in the 90s* (Westport, CT: Bergin and Garvey, 1991), p. 25.
22. Kathleen Kendall-Tackett, "Coming to Terms With a Negative Birth Experience," *The Doula*, Fall 1994, p. 10.
23. Jane Brody, "Postpartum Depression: Shedding Light on the Blues," *New York Times*, Oct. 25, 1994
24. Diana Korte, as per note 1, p. 183.
25. Melina Sacks, "Baby-Bonding," *San Jose Mercury News*, Jan. 2, 1996, p. E-1.
26. "Food for Labor: NPO or YES?" *Mothering*, no. 73, Winter 1994, p. 26.
27. Diana Korte, as per note 1, p. 144.
28. *Maternal Health News*, 14(2); cited in *Mothering*, no. 62, Winter 1992, p. 24.
29. Louis Saldana, "Management of Pregnancy After Cesarean Section," *American Journal of Obstetrics and Gynecology*, 1979 (135), p. 555.
30. M. Granat, "Oxytocin Contraindicated in Presence of Uterine Scar," *Lancet*, 1976 (25), p. 1411.
31. R. Caldeyro-Barcia et al., "Effects of Rupture of Membranes on Fetal Heart Rate Pattern," *International Journal of Gynecology and Obstetrics*, 1972 (19), p. 169. R. Caldeyro-Barcia, "Some Consequences of Obstetrical Interferences," *Birth and Family Journal*, 1977, 2(34), p. 73.
32. M. G. Rosen et al., "The Paradox of Electronic Fetal Monitoring: More Data May Not Enable Us to Predict or Prevent Infant Neurological Morbidity," *American Journal of Obstetrics and Gynecology*, Mar. 1993. K. Shy et al., "Evaluating a New Technology: The Effectiveness of Electronic Fetal Monitoring," *Annual Review of Public Health*, 1987(8), pp. 165–90. A. Prentice et al., "Fetal Heart Rate Monitoring During Labor: Too Frequent Intervention, Too Little Benefit?," *Lancet*, 1987 (2), pp. 1375–77. H. F. Sandmire, "Whither Electronic Fetal Monitoring?" *Obstetrics and Gynecology*, 1990, 76(6), pp. 1130–34. R. Freeman, "Intrapartum Fetal Monitoring: A Disappointing Story," *New England Journal of Medicine*, 1990, 322(9), pp. 624–26. J. Lumley, "The Irresistible Rise of Electronic Fetal Monitoring," *Birth*, 1982, 9(3), pp. 150–52.
33. A. D. Haverkamp et al., "The Evaluation of Continuous Heart Rate Monitoring in High Risk Pregnancy," *American Journal of Obstetrics and Gynecology*, 1976 (125), p. 310. K. Levino et al., "A Prospective Comparison of Selective and Universal Electronic Fetal Monitoring in 34,995 Pregnancies," *New England Journal of Medicine*, 315(10), 1986. E. Friedman, "The Obstetrician's Dilemma: How Much Fetal Monitoring and Cesarean Section Is Enough?," *New England Journal of Medicine*, 315(10), 1986.
34. Cited in N. Cohen, as per note 20, p. 181.
35. "Is Fetal Heart Rate Monitoring Worthwhile?," paper presented to the American Association for the Advancement of Science, Toronto, Canada, Jan. 1981; cited in N. Cohen, as per note 21, p. 181. A. Prentice, as per note 32.
36. Cited in N. Cohen, as per note 20, p. 182.
37. Ibid.
38. Cited in Diana Korte, as per note 1, p. 150.

39. J. Murphy et al., "The Relation of Electronic Fetal Monitoring Patterns to Infant Outcomes," *American Journal of Epidemiology*, 1991 (114), p. 1539.
40. Diana Korte, as per note 1, p. 124.
41. Christiane Northrup, *Women's Bodies, Women's Wisdom: Creating Physical and Emotional Health and Healing* (New York: Bantam, 1994), p. 393.
42. N. Cohen, as per note 20, p. 193.
43. Argentine Episiotomy Trial Collaborative Group, "Routine vs. Selective Episiotomy: A Randomised Controlled Trial," *Lancet*, 1993 (342), pp. 1517–18.
44. P. Shiono et al., "Midline Episiotomies: More Harm Than Good," *American Journal of Obstetrics and Gynecology*, 1991, 77(5), pp. 765–70.
45. Sheila Kitzinger, *Some Women's Experiences of Episiotomy* (London: National Childbirth Trust); cited in N. Cohen, as per note 21, p. 194. J. Thorp et al., "Episiotomy: Can Its Routine Use Be Defended?," *American Journal of Obstetrics and Gynecology*, 1989, 160(5).
46. Quoted in N. Cohen, as per note 20, p. 209.
47. Ellen Switzer and Joan Kline, "Pregnancy and Childbirth 1982: Options," *Family Circle Magazine*, Mar. 16, 1982.
48. Marshall Klaus et al., "The Dublin Experience," *Mothering*, Fall 1994, pp. 68–75.
49. John Kennell et al., "Continuous Emotional Support During Labor in a U.S. Hospital," *Journal of the American Medical Association*, May 1, 1991, 265(17).
50. Diana Korte, as per note 1, p. 218.
51. Ibid.
52. Ibid.
53. Michel Odent, "Birth Under Water," *Lancet*, Dec. 24/31, 1983.
54. Quoted in *The Doula*, Summer 1994, p. 37.

Chapter 4: A Modern-Day Witch-Hunt

1. Bev Eaton, "Midwives Make a Comeback: The Search for the Personal Touch," *Hartford Courant*, Mar. 1988, Section E, p. 1; cited in N. Cohen, *Open Season: A Survival Guide for Natural Childbirth and VBAC in the 90s* (Westport, CT: Bergin and Harvey, 1991), p. 166.
2. N. Cohen, as per note 1, p. 166.
3. Suzanne Arms, *Immaculate Deception II: A Fresh Look at Childbirth* (Berkeley, CA: Celestial Arts, 1994), p. 156.
4. Jessica Mitford, *The American Way of Birth* (New York: Plume, 1993), p. 232.
5. Quoted in J. Mitford, as per note 4, p. 234.
6. J. Mitford, as per note 4, p. 273.
7. Monica Sjoo and Barbara Mor, *The Great Cosmic Mother: Rediscovering the Religion of the Earth* (San Francisco: HarperCollins, 1987), p. 298.
8. Montague Summers, trans., *Malleus Maleficarum* (London: Fortune Press, 1948), quoted in Jessica Mitford, as per note 4, p. 20.
9. M. Sjoo and B. Mor, as per note 7, p. 298.
10. Margot Edwards and Mary Waldorf, *Reclaiming Birth: History and Heroines of American Childbirth Reform* (Trumansburg, NY: Crossing Press, 1984), p. 147.
11. J. Mitford, as per note 4, p. 20.
12. M. Sjoo and B. Mor, as per note 7, p. 302.
13. J. Mitford, as per note 4, p. 21.
14. M. Sjoo and B. Mor, as per note 7, p. 303.
15. Ibid., p. 302.
16. Barbara Ehrenreich and Deirdre English, *Witches, Midwives and Nurses: A History of Women Healers* (New York: The Feminist Press, 1973), p. 7.
17. Ibid.
18. M. Sjoo and B. Mor, as per note 7, p. 309.
19. Thomas Szasz, *The Manufacture of Madness* (New York: Harper, 1970), pp. 82–94. B. Ehrenreich, as per note 16, p. 12.
20. Ibid., p. 12.
21. N. Cohen, as per note 1, p. 169.
22. B. Ehrenreich, as per note 16, p. 18.
23. Ibid., p. 19.
24. M. Sjoo and B. Mor, as per note 7, p. 305.
25. B. Ehrenreich, as per note 16, p. 13.

26. M. Sjoo and B. Mor, as per note 7, p. 306.
27. J. Mitford, as per note 4, p. 23.
28. Robertson's remark was widely quoted in the national press. It appeared in a column by Molly Ivins in the *San Francisco Chronicle*, among many other places.
29. M. Edwards, as per note 10, p. 148.
30. Ibid., p. 149.
31. B. Ehrenreich, as per note 16, p. 93.
32. Ibid., pp. 95–96.
33. M. Edwards, as per note 10, p. 153.
34. Ibid., p. 154.
35. Ibid.
36. J. Mitford, as per note 4, p. 228.
37. *Santa Cruz Times*, March 14, 1974.
38. "Midwives Busted in Santa Cruz," *Playgirl*, July 1974, p. 5.
39. M. Edwards, as per note 10, p. 167.
40. "Woman Arrested in Baby Death," *San Luis Obispo Telegram-Tribune*, July 7, 1978, p. A-1.
41. M. Edwards, as per note 10, p. 167.
42. "Child Death," *San Luis Obispo Telegram-Tribune*, July 8, 1978.
43. "Midwife Faces Murder Charge in Home Birth Tragedy," *San Francisco Examiner-Chronicle*, July 9, 1978, p. A-4.
44. M. Edwards, as per note 10, p. 168.
45. "Midwife Freed in Infant Death: Judge Blasts Doctors," Associated Press, San Luis Obispo.
46. M. Edwards, as per note 10, p. 168.
47. Sylvia Reichmann, *Transitions* (Marble Hill, MO: NAPSAC International, 1988), pp. 121–22.
48. M. Edwards, as per note 10, p. 169.
49. Ibid., p. 170.
50. Ibid., pp. 170–71. Associated Press, May 3, 1978.
51. M. Edwards, as per note 10, p. 172.
52. Scott Thurm, "Why Medical Oversight System Is Still Stuck," *San Jose Mercury News*, Feb. 5, 1995.
53. Robert Fellmeth, *Physician Discipline in California: A Code Blue Emergency; An Initial Report on the Physician Discipline System of the Board of Medical Quality Assurance*, Center for Public Interest Law, University of San Diego School of Law, April 5, 1989.
54. Ibid., p. 95.
55. Ibid., p. 96.
56. J. Mitford, as per note 4, p. 224.
57. Gabe Fuentes, "Klvana Gets 53 Years to Life," *Los Angeles Times*, Feb. 6, 1990.
58. Gabe Fuentes and Stephanie Chavez, "Obstetrician Convicted of Murdering 8 Babies, Fetuses," *Los Angeles Times*, Dec. 19, 1989.
59. Ibid.
60. Ibid.
61. J. Mitford, as per note 4, p. 226.
62. G. Fuentes, as per note 58.
63. G. Fuentes, as per note 57.
64. "State Storms Into Midwife's Home," *Sacramento Union*, April 10, 1990, p. B-1. J. Mitford, as per note 4, p. 229.
65. Ibid., p. 230.
66. Diana Korte, "Midwives on Trial," *Mothering*, no. 76, Fall 1995, p. 56.
67. Tupper Hall, "Regulatory Boards Mired in Red Tape," *San Francisco Examiner*, Feb. 16, 1992, p. A-1.
68. Scott Thurm, "Why Medical Oversight System Is Still Stuck," *San Jose Mercury News*, Feb. 5, 1995.
69. Ibid., p. A-18.
70. N. Cohen, as per note 1, p. 170.
71. Ibid.
72. "Midwives Seek to Give Pregnant Women More Choices," *Associated Press*, Mar. 7, 1994; cited in *Birth Gazette*, Summer 1994, p. 22.
73. Suzanne Suarez, "Midwifery Is Not the Practice of Medicine," *Yale Journal of Law and Feminism*, Spring 1993, 5(2), p. 322.
74. *Birth Gazette*, Spring 1994, vol. 10, no. 2, p. 2.
75. Ibid., p. 15.
76. Ibid., p. 2.

77. Ibid., pp. 11–12.
78. M. Edwards, as per note 10, p. 177.
79. Ibid., p. 181.
80. S. Reichmann, as per note 47, p. 46.
81. Sarah Phelan, "Labor of Love," unpublished.
82. Quoted in N. Cohen, as per note 1, p. 178.
83. S. Reichmann, as per note 47, back cover.
84. Hannah Lapp, "The Home Birth Controversy," *The Freeman*, June 1992, p. 240.
85. Ibid.
86. "Florida Calls for Use of Midwives," *Santa Cruz Sentinel*, Jan. 11, 1994.
87. S. Suarez, as per note 73, p. 321.
88. D. Korte, as per note 66, pp. 58–59.
89. J. L. English, "Fettered but Not Silenced," *Midwifery Today*, issue 8, 1988, p. 28.
90. J. Mitford, as per note 4, pp. 14–17.
91. J. L. English, as per note 89, p. 28.
92. J. Mitford, as per note 4, p. 16.
93. J. L. English, as per note 89, p. 28.
94. Ibid., p. 29.
95. Ibid.
96. J. Mitford, as per note 4, p. 17.

Chapter 5: Awakening From Patriarchal Medicine

1. Barbara Ehrenreich and Deirdre English, *For Her Own Good: 150 Years of the Experts' Advice to Women* (Garden City, NY: Anchor Doubleday, 1978), p. 123.
2. John S. Haller and M. Robin, *The Physician and Sexuality in Victorian America* (Urbana: University of Illinois Press, 1974), p. 103.
3. Edward Clarke, *Sex in Education* (Boston: Houghton Mifflin, 1873).
4. G. J. Barker-Benfield, "The Spermatic Economy: A Nineteenth Century View of Sexuality," *Feminist Studies*, Summer 1972, pp. 45–74. Leslie Laurence and Beth Weinhouse, *Outrageous Practices: The Alarming Truth About How Medicine Mistreats Women* (New York: Fawcett Columbine, 1994), p. 124.
5. B. Ehrenreich, as per note 1, p. 124.
6. G. J. Barker-Benfield, *The Horrors of the Half-Known Life: Male Attitudes Toward Women and Sexuality in Nineteenth Century America* (New York: Harper and Row, 1976), p. 122.
7. Samuel Haber, "The Professions and Higher Education in America: A Historical View," in Margaret Gordon, ed., *Higher Education and the Labor Market* (New York: McGraw-Hill, 1974), p. 264.
8. Anna Robeson Burr, *Weir Mitchell: His Life and Letters* (New York: Duffield and Co., 1929).
9. Charlotte Perkins Gilman, *The Living of Charlotte Perkins Gilman: An Autobiography* (New York: Harper Colophon Books, 1975), p. 96.
10. Ibid.
11. Charlotte Perkins Gilman, *Herland* (New York: Pantheon Books, 1979).
12. Carroll Smith-Rosenberg, "The Hysterical Woman: Sex Roles in Nineteenth Century America," *Social Research*, Winter 1972, pp. 652–78. Carroll Smith-Rosenberg, *Disorderly Conduct: Visions of Gender in Victorian America* (New York: Alfred Knopf, 1985). B. Ehrenreich, as per note 1, p. 139.
13. Diana Scully and Pauline Bart, "A Funny Thing Happened on the Way to the Orifice: Women in Gynecology Textbooks," *American Journal of Sociology*, 78(4), 1973, p. 1045. L. Laurence, as per note 4, p. 330.
14. B. Ehrenreich, as per note 1, p. 34.
15. Ibid., pp. 33–68.
16. Ibid., p. 109.
17. Ibid., p. 43.
18. Dolores Burns, ed., *The Greatest Health Discovery: Natural Hygiene, and Its Evolution Past, Present, and Future* (Chicago: Natural Hygiene Press, 1972), p. 30; cited in B. Ehrenreich, as per note 1, p. 44.
19. Richard Walters, *Options* (Garden City Park, NY: Avery Publishing, 1993), p. 288.
20. "Report on Criminal Abortion," *Transactions of the American Medical Association*, 1859, p. 75.
21. Howard Wolinsky and Tom Brune, *The Serpent on the Staff: The Unhealthy Politics of the American Medical Association* (New York: Tarcher/Putnam, 1994), pp. 174–79.
22. Betsy Hartmann, *Reproductive Rights and Wrongs* (Boston: South End Press, 1994), p. 259.
23. Horatio Storer, "The Criminality and Physical Evils of Forced Abortion," *Transactions of the American Medical Association*, 1865.

24. James Mohr, *Abortion in America: The Origins and Evolution of National Policy, 1800–1900* (New York: Oxford University Press, 1978).
25. Ibid., pp. 147–48.
26. Report of the Committee on Criminal Abortions, *Transactions of the American Medical Association*, 1871, pp. 246, 251.
27. James Reed, "Doctors, Birth Control, and Social Values: 1830–1970," in M. Vogel and C. Rosenberg, eds., *The Therapeutic Revolution* (University of Pennsylvania Press, 1979), pp. 109–33.
28. "Induced Termination of Pregnancy Before and After Roe v. Wade: Trends in the Mortality and Morbidity of Women," American Medical Association Council on Scientific Affairs, Report H.
29. Jodi Jacobson, "Abortion in a New Light," *WorldWatch*, Mar.–Apr. 1990, p. 33.
30. Ibid.
31. Ibid. Jodi Jacobson, *Planning the Global Family*, WorldWatch Paper 80, 1987.
32. Jodi Jacobson, "Out From Behind the Contraceptive Iron Curtain," *WorldWatch*, Sept.–Oct. 1990, pp. 29–34.
33. Ibid.
34. Ibid., p. 33.
35. "Adolescent Pregnancy Rates in the U.S.: Contemporary," *Ob-Gyn*, Feb. 1994.
36. American Medical Association Policy Statement I, 1994; Policy: Teenage Pregnancy; No. 75.999. Obtained from AMA, Oct. 3, 1995.
37. B. Ehrenreich, as per note 1, pp. 114–15.
38. L. Laurence, as per note 4, p. 21.
39. J. Reed, as per note 27.
40. L. Laurence, as per note 4, p. 21.
41. *Developing New Contraceptives: Obstacles and Opportunities*, National Research Council Institute of Medicine, National Academy Press, Washington, 1990, p. 39.
42. Elmer De-Witt, *Time*, Feb. 26, 1990, p. 44.
43. B. Ehrenreich, as per note 1, p. 63.
44. Shryock, *Medicine in America: Historical Essays*, p. 84; cited in B. Ehrenreich, as per note 1, p. 65.
45. Thomas Woody, *A History of Women's Education in the United States, Vol. II* (New York: Octagon Books, 1974), p. 346.
46. L. Laurence, as per note 4, p. 40.
47. Ibid., p. 42.
48. Ibid.
49. Neil Baum, "How to Market Your Medical Practice to Women," *American Medical News*, July 5, 1993, p. 25.
50. L. Laurence, as per note 4, p. 30. Personal communication with one of Dr. Burt's nurses.
51. Ibid., p. 315.
52. John M. Smith, *Women and Doctors* (New York: Atlantic Monthly Press, 1992), p. 89.

Chapter 6: Cycles, Fertility, and Personal Power

1. Christiane Northrup, *Women's Bodies, Women's Wisdom: Creating Physical and Emotional Health and Healing* (New York: Bantam, 1994), p. 105.
2. Laurie Garrett, *The Coming Plague: Newly Emerging Diseases in a World Out of Balance* (New York: Penguin, 1994), p. 668, note 5.
3. D. E. Marlowe et al., "Measurement of Tampon Absorbency," Bureau of Medical Devices, U.S. Food and Drug Administration, Rockville, MD, 1981.
4. L. Garrett, as per note 2, pp. 390–410.
5. Ibid.
6. C. Northrup, as per note 1, pp. 97–98.
7. Ibid., pp. 99–100. W. Menaker, "Lunar Periodicity in Human Reproduction," *American Journal of Obstetrics and Gynecology*, 77(4), 1959, pp. 905–14.
8. C. Northrup, as per note 1, pp. 98–100.
9. E. Hartman, "Dreaming Sleep and the Menstrual Cycle," *Journal of Nervous and Mental Disease*, 143, 1966, pp. 406–16. E. Swanson and D. Foulkes, "Dream Content and the Menstrual Cycle," *Journal of Nervous and Mental Disease*, 145, 1968, pp. 358–63.
10. C. Northrup, as per note 1, p. 101.
11. J. Wurtman et al., "Effect of Nutrient Intake on Premenstrual Depression," *American Journal of Obstetrics and Gynecology*, 1989, 16(5), pp. 1228–34.
12. D. Jones, "Influence of Dietary Fat on Self-reported Premenstrual Symptoms," *Physiology and Behavior*, 1987, 40(4), pp. 483–87.

13. B. Goldin et al., "Estrogen Excretion Patterns and Plasma Levels in Vegetarian and Omnivorous Women," *New England Journal of Medicine*, vol. 307, 1982, pp. 1542–47. B. Goldin et al., "Effect of Diet on Excretion of Estrogens in Pre- and Post-Menopausal Women," *Cancer Research*, vol. 41, 1981, pp. 3771–73.
14. G. Gogi et al., "Effect of Nutritional . . . on Symptoms of Premenstrual Tension," *Journal of Reproductive Medicine*, vol. 83, 1982, pp. 527–31.
15. Stanley West, *The Hysterectomy Hoax* (New York: Doubleday, 1994), p. 140.
16. J. Prior et al., "Conditioning Exercise Decreases Premenstrual Symptoms: A Prospective Controlled Six-Month Trial," *Fertility and Sterility*, vol. 47, 1987, pp. 402–9.
17. I. Goodale et al., "Alleviation of Premenstrual Syndrome Symptoms With the Relaxation Response," *Obstetrics and Gynecology*, Apr. 1990, pp. 649–89.
18. B. Parry et al., "Morning vs. Evening Bright Light Treatment of Late Luteal Phase Dysphoric Disorder," *American Journal of Psychiatry*, vol. 147, 1991, p. 9.
19. T. Oleson et al., "Randomized Controlled Study of Premenstrual Symptoms Treated With Ear, Hand, and Foot Reflexology," *Obstetrics and Gynecology*, 1993, vol. 82, pp. 906–11.
20. John Lee, *Natural Progesterone: The Multiple Roles of a Remarkable Hormone* (Sebastopol, CA: BLL Publishing, 1993).
21. Ibid., p. 52.
22. Ibid.
23. C. Northrup, as per note 1, pp. 109–13.
24. R. Michael et al., "Human Vaginal Secretion and Volatile Fatty Acid Content," *Science*, vol. 186, 1974, pp. 1217–19.
25. M. Mintz, *At Any Cost: Corporate Greed, Women, and the Dalkon Shield* (New York: Pantheon, 1985), p. 3.
26. "Piercing the Dalkon Shield," *National Law Journal*, June 16, 1980, p. 13.
27. M. Mintz, as per note 25, p. 264.
28. Jane Zones, National Organization of Women, quoted in "Dow Corning Goes Bankrupt," *San Jose Mercury News*, May 16, 1995, p. A-1.
29. John M. Smith, *Women and Doctors* (New York: Atlantic Monthly Press, 1992), p. 83.
30. Ibid., p. 84.
31. Ibid.
32. Leslie Laurence and Beth Weinhouse, *Outrageous Practices: The Alarming Truth About How Medicine Mistreats Women* (New York: Fawcett Columbine, 1994), p. 195.
33. Sharon Batt, *Patient No More: The Politics of Breast Cancer* (Charlottetown, P.E.I., Canada: Gynergy, 1994), pp. 123–24.
34. Harris Lippman, "On Oral Contraceptives," *New England Journal of Medicine*, July 30, 1992, p. 322. Harris Lippman, "On Risk Factors That Could Be Modified," *New England Journal of Medicine*, Aug. 13, 1992, p. 478.
35. C. Northrup, as per note 1, pp. 336–37. T. Hilgers et al., "Natural Family Planning . . ." *Obstetrics and Gynecology*, 1981, 58(3), pp. 345–50.
36. Margaret Nofziger, *A Cooperative Method of Natural Birth Control*, 4th ed. (Summertown, TN: The Book Publishing Company, 1993).

Chapter 7: When in Doubt, Take It Out

1. Celso Ramon Garcia et al., "Preservation of the Ovary: A Reevaluation," *Fertility and Sterility*, 42(4), Oct. 1984, pp. 510–14. John Smith, *Women and Doctors* (New York: Atlantic Monthly Press, 1992), p. 14. Christiane Northrup, *Women's Bodies, Women's Wisdom* (New York: Bantam, 1994), p. 152.
2. Stanley West, *The Hysterectomy Hoax* (New York: Doubleday, 1994), p. 1.
3. Ibid., p. 23.
4. Ibid.
5. C. Northrup, as per note 1, p. 151.
6. S. West, as per note 2, p. 15.
7. Ibid., p. 20.
8. C. Northrup, as per note 1, p. 154.
9. Patrick Jenkins, "NOW Told of Unnecessary Surgery for Women," *Princeton Star Ledger*, Oct. 30, 1994, Sec. 1, p. 20.
10. S. West, as per note 2, pp. 28–29.
11. Ibid., p. 42.
12. Ibid., p. 34.

13. Ibid., p. 20.
14. K. McNatty et al., "The Production of Progesterone, Androgens, and Estrogens . . ." *Journal of Clinical Endocrinology and Metabolism,* vol. 49, 1979, p. 687.
15. C. Garcia, as per note 1.
16. S. West, as per note 2, p. 174.
17. C. Northrup, as per note 1, p. 172.
18. Ibid., p. 185.
19. Ibid.
20. Ibid., p. 166.
21. Ibid., pp. 167–68.
22. Ibid., p. 168.
23. Lynn Payer, *Medicine and Culture* (New York: Penguin, 1988), p. 130.
24. C. Northrup, as per note 1, pp. 561–62.
25. *Understanding Hysterectomy,* American College of Obstetricians and Gynecologists, 1987; quoted in "Sexual Response After Hysterectomy," *HealthFacts,* Center for Medical Consumers, New York, vol. 15, no. 139, 1990, p. 1.
26. Naomi Stokes, *The Castrated Woman* (New York: Franklin Watts, 1986), p. 39.
27. Harry Huneycutt et al., *All About Hysterectomy* (New York: Dial Press, 1977); cited in N. Stokes, as per note 26.
28. W. Gifford-Jones, *On Being a Woman* (New York: Macmillan, 1969).
29. W. Gifford-Jones, *What Every Woman Should Know About Hysterectomy* (New York: Funk and Wagnall, 1977); cited in N. Stokes, as per note 26.
30. N. Stokes, as per note 26, p. 64. See also S. West, as per note 2, pp. 31–32, 47–51.
31. S. West, as per note 2, p. 48.
32. N. Stokes, as per note 26, p. 78.
33. Ibid., p. 79.
34. Ibid., pp. 64–65.
35. Ibid., p. 59.
36. Ibid., p. 4.
37. In 1995, the American College of Obstetricians and Gynecologists published an updated version of *Understanding Hysterectomy,* in which it states: "Some women may notice a change in their sexual response after a hysterectomy. . . . Some women have a heightened response, however."

Chapter 8: Menopause Naturally

1. Leslie Laurence and Beth Weinhouse, *Outrageous Practices* (New York: Fawcett Columbine, 1994), p. 234.
2. Christiane Northrup, *Women's Bodies, Women's Wisdom* (New York: Bantam, 1994), p. 431.
3. Tamara Slayton, *Reclaiming the Menstrual Matrix: Evolving Feminine Wisdom: A Workbook* (Petaluma, CA: Menstrual Health Foundation, 1990), p. 41.
4. Carolyn DeMarco, *Take Charge of Your Body: Women's Health Advisor* (Winlaw, B.C., Canada: Well Women Press, 1994), p. 209.
5. David Reuben, *Everything You Always Wanted to Know About Sex but Were Afraid to Ask* (New York: David McKay Co., 1969), p. 293.
6. Russell Mokhiber, "DES," in *Corporate Crime and Violence: Big Business Power and the Abuse of the Public Trust* (San Francisco: Sierra Club Books, 1988), p. 173.
7. Susan Bell, "The Synthetic Compound Diethylstilbestrol (DES) 1938–1941: The Social Construction of a Medical Treatment," Brandeis University Dissertation, 1980, p. 28.
8. Helen Haberman, "Help for Women Over 40," *Hygeia,* Nov. 1941, pp. 898–99; this article was also condensed in the *Reader's Digest,* Nov. 1941, pp. 67–68. Diana Dutton, *Worse Than the Disease: Pitfalls of Medical Progress* (New York: Cambridge University Press, 1988), p. 46.
9. William Laurence, "Time Is Reversed by New Extract," *New York Times,* May 14, 1939, p. 39. See also W. Laurence, "New Method Used in Rejuvenation," *New York Times,* Aug. 24, 1939, p. 13, and W. Laurence, "New Remedy Used in Ills of Women," *New York Times,* Oct. 21, 1939, p. 13.
10. D. Dutton, as per note 8, p. 31.
11. Evan Wylie, "Why You Won't Lose Your Baby," *Good Housekeeping,* Mar. 1960, pp. 82–83, 118–19.
12. Robert Meyers, *DES: The Bitter Pill* (New York: Seaview/Putnam, 1983), p. 143.
13. D. Dutton, as per note 8, p. 87.
14. F. McCrea, "The Politics of Menopause: The 'Discovery' of a Deficiency Disease," *Social Problems* 31, 1983, pp. 111–23. Gail Vines, *Raging Hormones: Do They Rule Our Lives?* (Berkeley, CA: Univer-

sity of California Press, 1993), p. 125. Nancy Sommers and James Ridgeway, "Can a Woman Be Feminine Forever?," *The New Republic*, Mar. 19, 1966, pp. 15–16.

15. Robert Wilson, *Feminine Forever* (New York: David McKay, 1966).
16. B. Stadel and N. Weiss, "Characteristics of Menopausal Women . . ." *Journal of Epidemiology*, vol. 102, 1975, p. 215.
17. Donald Smith et al., "Association of Exogenous Estrogen and Endometrial Carcinoma," *New England Journal of Medicine*, 293(23), 1975, p. 1164. Harry Ziel and William Finkle, "Increased Risk of Endometrial Carcinoma Among Users of Conjugated Estrogens," *New England Journal of Medicine*, 293(23), 1975, p. 1167. Noel Weiss et al., "Increasing Incidence of Endometrial Cancer in the United States," *New England Journal of Medicine*, 294(23), 1976, p. 1259. Thomas Mack et al., "Estrogens and Endometrial Cancer . . ." *New England Journal of Medicine*, 294(23), 1976, p. 1262.
18. C. DeMarco, as per note 4, p. 214.
19. C. Northrup, as per note 2, p. 434.
20. Karen Stabiner, "In the Menopause Market: A Gold Mine of Ads," *New York Times*, Apr. 4, 1994, p. D6.
21. L. Laurence, as per note 1, p. 228.
22. Cynthia Pearson, "Women at Midlife: Consumers of Second-Rate Health Care?," testimony before the Subcommittee on Housing and Consumer Interests, Select Committee on Aging, House of Representatives, Washington, May 30, 1991.
23. "Estrogen: Every Woman's Dilemma," *Time*, June 26, 1995.
24. Personal communication with author, Jan. 1996.
25. C. Northrup, as per note 2, pp. 464–65.
26. "Women's Information About Menopause Is Limited," North American Menopause Society, Sept. 4, 1993.
27. "Estrogen: Every Woman's Dilemma," *Time*, June 26, 1995, pp. 46–53.
28. Susan Weed, *Menopausal Years: The Wise Woman Way* (Woodstock, NY: Ash Tree Publishing, 1992), p. 55.
29. Y. Beyene, *From Menarche to Menopause: Reproductive Lives of Peasant Women in Two Cultures* (Albany: State University of New York Press, 1989). "Menopause," *Newsweek*, May 25, 1992, pp. 39–44.
30. C. DeMarco, as per note 4, p. 220.
31. Robert Freedman and Suzanne Woodward, "Behavioral Treatment of Menopausal Hot Flashes," *American Journal of Obstetrics and Gynecology*, 167(2), 1992, pp. 436–39.
32. Susan Lark, *The Estrogen Decision* (Los Altos, CA: Westchester Publishing, 1994). Sadja Greenwood, *Menopause, Naturally* (CA: Volcano Press, 1992). C. DeMarco, as per note 4. S. Weed, as per note 28.
33. Tori Hudson et al.,"A Pilot Study Using Botanical Medicines in the Treatment of Menopause Symptoms," *Townsend Letter for Doctors*, Dec. 1994, p. 1372.
34. Editorial, *New England Journal of Medicine*, Aug. 27, 1992; cited in C. DeMarco, as per note 4, p. 230.
35. John Robbins, *Diet for a New America* (Walpole, NH: Stillpoint, 1987), pp. 186–96.
36. *American Journal of Clinical Nutrition*, March 1983.
37. T. Remer et al., "Estimation of the Renal Net Acid Excretion by Adults Consuming Diets Containing Variable Amounts of Protein," *American Journal of Clinical Nutrition*, 59, 1994, pp. 1356–61.
38. J. Robbins, as per note 35.
39. C. DeMarco, as per note 4, p. 226.
40. B. Nordin et al., "The Nature and Significance of the Relationship Between Urinary Sodium and Urinary Calcium in Women," *Journal of Nutrition*, 123, 1993, pp. 1615–22. J. Hopper et al., "The Bone Density of Female Twins Discordant for Tobacco Use," *New England Journal of Medicine*, 330, 1994, pp. 387–92.
41. J. Lee, "Osteoporosis Reversal With Transdermal Progesterone," *Lancet*, 336, 1990, p. 1327.
42. J. Lee, "Osteoporosis Reversal: The Role of Progesterone," *Clinical Nutritional Review*, 10, 1990, pp. 384–91. J. Lee, "Is Natural Progesterone the Missing Link in Osteoporosis Prevention and Treatment?," *Medical Hypotheses*, 35, 1991, pp. 316–18. J. Prior, "Progesterone as a Bone-Trophic Hormone," *Endocrine Review*, 11, 1990, pp. 386–98. J. Prior et al., "Progesterone and the Prevention of Osteoporosis," *Canadian Journal of Obstetrics and Gynecology*, 3, 1991, p. 178.
43. Dean Ornish, *Dr. Dean Ornish's Program for Reversing Heart Disease* (New York: Random House, 1990).
44. Lila Nachtigall, *Estrogen: The Facts Can Change Your Life* (New York: HarperCollins); cited in "Estrogen: Every Woman's Dilemma," *Time*, June 26, 1995, p. 50.
45. Germaine Greer, *The Change: Women, Aging and the Menopause* (New York: Fawcett Columbine, 1991), p. 10.
46. Quoted in Helen Nearing, *Light on Aging and Dying* (Gardiner, ME: Tilbury House, 1995), p. 30.

47. J. Meyers, et al., "Six-Month Prevalence of Psychiatric Disorder in Three Communities," *Archives of General Psychiatry*, 41, 1984, p. 959.
48. G. Greer, as per note 45.
49. C. Northrup, as per note 2, p. 460.
50. G. Greer, as per note 45, p. 118.
51. G. Colditz et al., "The Use of Estrogens and Progestins and the Risk of Breast Cancer in Postmenopausal Women," *New England Journal of Medicine*, 332, June 1995, pp. 1589–93.
52. Ibid.
53. S. Greenwood, as per note 32, p. 114.
54. People for the Ethical Treatment of Animals, P.O. Box 42516, Washington, DC, 20015.
55. Paula Moore, "On Your Mind," *Natural Health*, Sept.–Oct. 1995.
56. G. Greer, as per note 45, p. 24.
57. Audre Lorde, *The Cancer Journals* (San Francisco: Aunt Lute Books, 1980), p. 63.
58. Quoted in "Estrogen: Every Woman's Dilemma," *Time*, June 26, 1995.
59. S. Greenwood, as per note 32, p. 203.
60. T. Slayton, as per note 3, p. 41.
61. G. Greer, as per note 45, p. 49.
62. Quoted in H. Nearing, as per note 46, p. 11.
63. Marianne Williamson, *A Woman's Worth* (New York: Ballantine, 1993), p. 12.

Chapter 9: Hugs, Not Drugs
1. "Ritalin Maker Opens Drive to End Abuse," Associated Press, *New York Times*, Mar. 28, 1996, p. A-13.
2. J. Swanson et al., "Treatment of ADHD: Beyond Medication," *Beyond Behavior*, 4(1), 1992, pp. 13–22. Diane McGuinness, "Attention Deficit Disorder: The Emperor's New Clothes . . ." in S. Fisher et al., eds., *The Limits of Biological Treatments for Psychological Distress* (New York: Erlbaum, 1989), pp. 151–88. Gerald Coles, *The Learning Mystique: A Critical Look at 'Learning Disabilities'* (New York: Pantheon, 1987). Peter Breggin, *The War Against Children* (New York: St. Martin's Press, 1994), p. 98.
3. Alfie Kohn, "Suffer the Restless Children," *Atlantic Monthly*, Nov. 1989, p. 98.
4. Patrice Fitch, "In Amanda's Room," *Mothering*, Winter 1995, p. 66.
5. A. Kohn, as per note 3, p. 100. P. Breggin, as per note 2, p. 84.
6. R. Brown et al., "Effects of Methylphenidate on Cardiovascular Responses in Attention Deficit Hyperactivity Disordered Adolescents," *Journal of Adolescent Health Care*, 10, 1989, pp. 179–83. Laurence Greenhill et al., "Prolactin: Growth Hormone and Growth Responses in Boys With Attention Deficit Disorder and Hyperactivity Treated With Methylphenidate," *Journal of the American Academy of Child Psychiatry*, 23, 1984, pp. 58–67. Kevin Kelly et al., "Attention Deficit Disorder and Methylphenidate . . ." *International Journal of Clinical Psychopharmacology*, 3, 1988, pp. 167–81. Rachel Klein et al., "Methylphenidate and Growth in Hyperactive Children," *Archives of General Psychiatry*, 45, 1988, pp. 1127–30. Richard Scarnati, "An Outline of Hazardous Side Effects of Ritalin (Methylphenidate)," *International Journal of Addictions*, 21, 1986, pp. 837–41. John Talbott et al., *Textbook of Psychiatry* (Washington, DC: American Psychiatric Press, 1988), pp. 990–93. M. Dulcan, "Comprehensive Treatment of Children and Adolescents With Attention Deficit Disorders: The State of the Art," *Clinical Psychology Review*, 1986, pp. 539–70.
7. FDA-approved information from Ciba-Geigy, *Physicians' Desk Reference*, 1993. P. Breggin, as per note 2, p. 84.
8. Fred Baughman, "Correspondence," *Journal of the American Medical Association*, 269, May 12, 1993, p. 2369.
9. William Crook, Letter, *Mothering*, Fall 1991, p. 18.
10. Peter Breggin, *Toxic Psychiatry* (New York: St. Martin's Press, 1991), p. 311.
11. Editorial, "Hyperactivity in Childhood," *New England Journal of Medicine*, 323, Nov. 15, 1990, pp. 1413–15. Diane McGuinness, "Stimulants and Children," *Mothering*, Summer 1991, p. 111.
12. Antonia Black, "The Drugging of America's Children," *Redbook*, Dec. 1994, p. 44.
13. "The Risks of Ritalin," *Mothering*, Spring 1989, pp. 81–82. *Brain/Mind Bulletin*, Dec. 1988, p. 4. D. Wollner, Letter, *Mothering*, Winter 1992, p. 14.
14. Daniel Safer et al., "A Survey of Medication Treatment for Hyperactive/Inattentive Children," *Journal of the American Medical Association*, Oct. 15, 1988, pp. 2256–58. Daniel Safer et al., "Effect of a Media Blitz and a Threatened Lawsuit on Stimulant Treatment," *Journal of the American Medical Association*, Aug. 26, 1992, pp. 1004–7.
15. A. Black, as per note 12.

16. As per note 1. See also "U.C. Professor Critical of Ritalin Dependency," *San Jose Mercury News*, Mar. 3, 1996, p. 5-B.
17. A. Kohn, as per note 3, p. 96.
18. Ibid., p. 93.
19. P. Breggin, as per note 2, p. 77.
20. P. Breggin, as per note 2, p. 313.
21. Ibid., p. 272.
22. John Gatto, "Our Children Are Dying in Our Schools," *New Age Journal*, Sept.–Oct. 1990, p. 62.
23. Colleen Bollen, "When Children Take Action," *Mothering*, Spring 1994, pp. 89–91.
24. Riak Jordan, *Plain Talk About Spanking*, Parents and Teachers Against Violence, Danville, CA, p. 5. Irwin Hyman, *Reading, Writing and the Hickory Stick* (Lexington, MA: Lexington Books, 1990).
25. "Attitude of Primary Care Physicians Toward Corporal Punishment," *Journal of the American Medical Association*, 267, June 17, 1992.
26. Stephen Ceci et al., "Hyperactivity and Incidental Memory: Evidence for Attentional Diffusion," *Child Development* 55(6), Dec. 1984, pp. 2192–2203.
27. Jules Henry, "A Cross-Cultural Outline of Education," *Current Anthropology* 1, 4, 1960, p. 268.
28. Thomas Armstrong, "Hyperactivity: Whose Problem?," *Mothering*, Summer 1991, pp. 103–7.
29. Robert Conot, *A Streak of Luck* (New York: Seaview Books, 1979), p. 9.
30. R. Jacob et al., "Formal and Informal Classroom Settings: Effects on Hyperactivity," *Journal of Abnormal Child Psychology*, 6, 1978, pp. 47–59.
31. Personal communication with author.
32. Eric Chivia et al., eds., *Critical Condition: Human Health and the Environment* (Cambridge, MA: MIT Press, 1994).
33. Herbert Needleman et al., "Bone Lead Levels and Delinquent Behavior," *Journal of the American Medical Association*, 275(5), Feb. 7, 1996, pp. 363–69. "Study Links Lead Exposure to Inner-City Crime," Los Angeles Times, *San Jose Mercury News*, Feb. 7, 1996, 4A.
34. Ben Feingold, *Why Your Child Is Hyperactive* (New York: Random House, 1975).
35. K. Conners et al., "Food Additives and Hyperkinesis," *Pediatrics*, 58, 1976, p. 154. J. Harley et al., "Hyperkinesis and Food Additives: Testing the Feingold Hypothesis," *Pediatrics*, 61, 1978, p. 818. J. Harley et al., "Synthetic Food Colors and Hyperactivity in Children," *Pediatrics*, 62, 1978, p. 975. B. Weiss et al., "Behavioral Responses to Artificial Food Colors," *Science*, 207, 1980, p. 1487.
36. J. Swanson et al., "Food Dyes Impair Performance of Hyperactive Children . . ." *Science*, 207, 1980, p. 1485.
37. Autism Research Institute (formerly Child Behavior Research Institute), San Diego, June 1992.
38. J. Swanson, as per note 36.
39. J. Egger et al., "Controlled Trial of Oligoantigenic Treatment in the Hyperkinetic Syndrome," *Lancet*, 1985, p. 540.
40. Feingold Association of the United States, Alexandria, VA.
41. Stephen Schoenthaler, "Institutional Nutritional Policies and Criminal Behavior," *Nutrition Today*, 20(3), 1985, p. 16.
42. Stephen Schoenthaler, "Diet and Crime: An Empirical Examination of the Value of Nutrition in the Control and Treatment of Incarcerated Juvenile Offenders," *International Journal of Biosocial Research*, 4(1), 1983, pp. 25–39. Stephen Schoenthaler, "Types of Offenses Which Can Be Reduced in an Institutional Setting Using Nutritional Intervention: A Preliminary Empirical Evaluation," *International Journal of Biosocial Research*, 4(2), 1983, pp. 74–84.
43. Stephen Schoenthaler, "The Los Angeles Probation Department Diet Behavior Program: An Empirical Evaluation of Six Institutions," *International Journal of Biosocial Research*, 5(2), 1983, pp. 88–98. Stephen Schoenthaler, "The Northern California Diet-Behavior Program: An Empirical Examination of 3,000 Incarcerated Juveniles in Stanislaus County Juvenile Hall," *International Journal of Biosocial Research*, 5(2), 1983, pp. 99–106.
44. Stephen Schoenthaler, "The Alabama Diet-Behavior Program: An Empirical Evaluation at the Coosa Valley Regional Detention Center," *International Journal of Biosocial Research*, 5(2), 1983, pp. 79–87. Stephen Schoenthaler, "Diet and Behavior," *Nutrition Today*, 20(6), 1985, p. 34. Stephen Schoenthaler, "Diet and Delinquency: Empirical Testing of Eight Theories," Proceedings of the American College of Nutrition, International Conference on Nutrients and Brain Function, Feb. 19–20, 1986.
45. Cited by Autism Research Institute (formerly Child Behavior Research Institute), San Diego, June 1992.
46. Jane Hersey, Letter, *Mothering*, Winter 1992, p. 14.
47. Stephen Schoenthaler et al., "The Impact of a Low Food Additive and Sucrose Diet on Academic

Performance in 803 New York City Public Schools," *International Journal of Biosocial Research*, 8(2), 1986, pp. 185–95. See also Alex Schauss et al., *Eating for A's* (New York: Pocket Books, 1991).

48. Ibid.

49. Ibid.

50. Doris Rapp, *Is This Your Child?* (New York: William Morrow, 1991), pp. 355–59.

51. LynNell Hancock, "Mother's Little Helper," *Newsweek*, Mar. 18, 1996, p. 52. "U.C. Professor Critical of Ritalin Dependency," *San Jose Mercury News*, Mar. 31, 1996, pp. 5-B.

52. *Journal of the American Dietetic Association*, Sept. 1994, p. 975.

53. Ibid.

54. Amy O'Connor, "In The News," *Vegetarian Times*, Oct. 1995, p. 20.

55. "Medication for Children With an Attention Deficit Disorder (RE 7103)," *American Academy of Pediatrics*, Committee on Children With Disabilities, Committee on Drugs, *Pediatrics*, 80(5), Nov. 1987.

Chapter 10: Medical Monopoly: The Game Nobody Wins

1. Howard Wolinsky and Tom Brune, *The Serpent on the Staff: The Unhealthy Politics of the American Medical Association* (New York: Tarcher/Putnam, 1994), p. xvi.

2. Ibid., p. 3.

3. Ibid., p. 68.

4. Ibid., p. 84.

5. Ibid., p. 88.

6. Dana Ullman, "Article on Homeopathy History . . ." *Alternative Therapies*, Sept. 1995, p. 13. Dana Ullman, *Discovering Homeopathy* (Berkeley, CA: North Atlantic Books, 1988), p. 40.

7. Paul Starr, *The Social Transformation of American Medicine* (New York: Basic Books, 1982), p. 98.

8. Ibid.

9. "Manga Report: Executive Summary," *Townsend Letter for Doctors*, July 1994, p. 814.

10. Cited in Anthony Cichoke, "Does Chiropractic Work?," *Townsend Letter for Doctors*, June 1995, p. 28.

11. B. Koes et al., "Randomized Clinical Trial of Manipulative Therapy . . ." *British Medical Journal*, 304, Mar. 7, 1992, pp. 601–5.

12. P. Ebrall, "Mechanical Low-Back Pain: A Comparison of Medical and Chiropractic Management . . ." *Chiropractic Journal of Australia*, 22(2), June 1992, pp. 47–53.

13. H. Wolinsky, as per note 1, p. 126.

14. Robert B. Throckmorton, legal counsel Iowa Medical Society, "The Menace of Chiropractic," remarks given to the North Central Medical Conference, Minneapolis, MN, Nov. 11, 1962; *plaintiff's exhibit 172, Wilk et al. vs. AMA et al.*

15. Ibid.

16. H. Wolinsky, as per note 1, p. 128.

17. Ibid.

18. H. Doyl Taylor, deposition for *Wilk et al. vs. AMA et al.*, Apr. 28, 1987, Phoenix. AZ.

19. Ibid.

20. H. Wolinsky, as per note 1, pp. 128–29.

21. Ibid., p. 129. William Monaghan, deposition for *Wilk et al. vs. AMA et al.*, June 21, 1979, pp. 32–39.

22. Ralph Smith, *At Your Own Risk: The Case Against Chiropractic* (New York: Pocket Books, 1969), p. 26.

23. John Mennell, deposition for *Wilk et al. vs. AMA et al.*, p. 75.

24. Ibid.

25. Minutes from the "Chiropractic Workshop," Michigan State Medical Society, Lansing, May 10, 1973; exhibit 1283, *Wilk et al. vs. AMA et al.*

26. Personal communication with author.

27. Memo to the AMA Board of Trustees, Jan. 4, 1971; plaintiff's exhibit 464, *Wilk et al. vs. AMA et al.*

28. H. Wolinsky, as per note 1, pp. 132–33.

29. Chester Wilk, *Chiropractic Speaks Out: A Reply to Medical Propaganda, Bigotry, and Ignorance* (Park Ridge, IL: Wilk Publishing, 1973).

30. Ron Shaffer, "Scientologists Kept Files on 'Enemies,'" *Washington Post*, May 16, 1978, p. A1.

31. H. Wolinsky, as per note 1, p. 137.

32. Ibid.

33. Richard Lewis, "AMA Revamps Stand on Chiropractic," *American Medical News*, August 3/10, 1979, p. 1.

34. *Transcript of Proceedings, Wilk et al. vs. AMA et al.*, May 26, 1987, p. 1266.

35. "Assessing the Efficacy and Safety of Medical Technologies," *Office of Technology Assessment* (Washington, DC: U.S. Government Printing Office, 1978), p. 7.

36. *Transcript of Proceedings, Wilk et al. vs. AMA et al.*, May 26, 1987, p. 3132.
37. *Transcript of Proceedings, Wilk et al. vs. AMA et al.*, July 2, 1987, p. 3396.
38. Getzendanner, Memorandum Opinion and Order, p. 5.
39. Ibid., p. 48.
40. "Acute Low Back Pain in Adults: Clinical Practice Guidelines," *Agency for Health Care Policy and Research* (Washington, DC, 1994).
41. P. Joseph Lisa, *The Assault on Medical Freedom* (Norfolk, CT: Hampton Roads, 1994), pp. 13–17.
42. "Holistic Medicine," in *Alternative Health Methods* (Chicago: American Medical Association, 1993), p. 81.
43. American Medical Association, Winter Catalog 1996, p. 37.
44. Barbara Ehrenreich and Deirdre English, *Witches, Midwives and Nurses: A History of Women Healers* (New York: Feminist Press, 1973), p. 39.
45. Harold Speert, *Obstetrics and Gynecology in America: A History* (Baltimore, MD: Waverly Press, 1980), p. 142.
46. "Cheaper Primary Care: Nurses May Be the Answer," *Business Week*, April 12, 1993, p. 71. H. Sox, "Quality of Patient Care by Nurse Practitioners . . ." *Annals of Internal Medicine*, Sept. 1979, 91(3), p. 459.
47. Eric Patterson, "Nursing Our Medical System Back to Health," *Delicious*, June 1994, pp. 10–11.
48. Ibid.
49. Ibid.
50. H. Wolinsky, as per note 1, p. 143.
51. Personal communication with author.
52. "American Nurses Association Expresses Diasppointment at AMA Opposition to an Expanded Role for Nurses," American Nurses Association news release, Dec. 9, 1993.
53. Daniel Wirth, "The Effect of Non-Contact Therapeutic Touch on Healing Rate of Full Thickness Dermal Wounds," *Subtle Energies* 1(1), Winter 1990.
54. Daniel Wirth et al., "Full Thickness Dermal Wounds Treated With Non-Contact Therapeutic Touch," unpublished manuscript, 1991; cited in Michael Lerner, *Choices in Healing* (Cambridge, MA: MIT Press, 1994), p. 364.
55. Janet Quinn, "Therapeutic Touch as Energy Exchange: Testing a Theory," *Advances in Nursing Science* 6, 1984, pp. 42–49. Janet Quinn, "An Investigation of the Effects of Therapeutic Touch Done Without Physical Contact on Anxiety of Hospitalized Cardiovascular Patients," doctoral dissertation, New York University, 1982, University Microfilm #DA8226788. D. Krieger, "Theapeutic Touch: The Imprimatur of Nursing," *American Journal of Nursing*, 7, 1975, pp. 784–867. E. Keller, et al., "Effects of Therapeutic Touch on Tension Headache Pain," *Nursing Research*, 1986, pp. 101–4. T. Meehan, "An Abstract of the Effect of Therapeutic Touch on the Experience of Acute Pain in Post-Operative Patients," doctoral dissertation, New York University, 1985. P. Heidt, "An Investigation of the Effect of Therapeutic Touch on the Anxiety of Hospitalized Patients," doctoral dissertation, New York University, 1979.
56. Nancy Cohen, *Open Season: Survival Guide for Natural Childbirth and VBAC in the 90s* (Westport, CT: Bergin and Garvey, 1991), p. 99.
57. M. Lerner, as per note 54, p. 364.
58. Ibid.
59. Ibid.
60. Leon Jaroff, "A No-Touch Therapy," *Time*, Nov. 21, 1994, p. 88.
61. "Therapeutic Touch Under Withering Scrutiny," *National Council Against Health Fraud Newsletter*, Nov.–Dec. 1994.
62. Larry Dossey, *Healing Words* (San Francisco: Harper, 1993), p. 189.
63. M. Lerner, as per note 54, p. 365. M. Raucheisen, "Symptom Relief With the Use of Non-Invasive Techniques," *Oncology Nursing Forum*, 12 (2 Supplement), 1985, p. 94.

Chapter 11: Dedicated to the Health of America?

1. "Introduction," *Preventing Tobacco Use Among Young People: A Report of the Surgeon General*, U.S. Dept. of Health and Human Services, Centers for Disease Control and Prevention, Office on Smoking and Health, 1994.
2. U.S. Dept. of Commerce, *Statistical Abstract of the United States, 1993*, tables 126, 131, 135 (Washington, DC: U.S. Govt. Printing Office, 1993).
3. *The Health Consequences of Environmental Smoking: Report of the Surgeon General*, U.S. Dept. of Health and Human Services, Centers for Disease Control and Prevention, Office on Smoking and Health, 1986.

4. Geoffrey Cowley, "Poisons at Home and Work," *Newsweek*, June 29, 1992.
5. Michael Jacobson and Laurie Ann Mazur, *Marketing Madness* (Boulder, CO: Westview Press, 1995), p. 149.
6. Christiane Northrup, *Women's Bodies, Women's Wisdom: Creating Physical and Emotional Health and Healing* (New York: Bantam, 1994), p. 612.
7. B. Haglund et al., "Cigarette Smoking as a Risk Factor for Sudden Infant Death Syndrome," *American Journal of Public Health*, vol. 80, 1990, pp. 29–32.
8. Marjorie Williams, "Feminism's Unaddressed Issue: Health Risks to Women Who Smoke," *Washington Post*, Nov. 14, 1991, A1.
9. C. Northrup, as per note 6, p. 613.
10. *Preventing Tobacco Use*, as per note 1.
11. Ibid.
12. Kenneth Warner, *Selling Smoke: Cigarette Advertising and Public Health* (Washington, DC: American Public Health Association, 1986), p. 19.
13. Raymond Pearl, "Tobacco Smoking and Longevity," *Science*, Mar. 4, 1938.
14. Susan Wagner, *Cigarette Country: Tobacco in American History and Politics* (New York: Praeger, 1971), p. 69.
15. Russell Mokhiber, *Corporate Crime and Violence: Big Business Power and the Abuse of the Public Trust* (San Francisco: Sierra Club Books, 1989), p. 431.
16. Howard Wolinsky and Tom Brune, *The Serpent on the Staff: The Unhealthy Politics of the American Medical Association* (New York: Tarcher/Putnam, 1994), p. 145.
17. Ibid.
18. James Rorty, "The AMA and the Cigarette Business," *American Medicine Mobilizes* (New York: Norton, 1939). Michael Mulinos et al., "Irritating Properties of Cigarette Smoke as Influenced by Hygroscopic Agents," *New York State Journal of Medicine*, June 1, 1935, pp. 590–92.
19. H. Wolinsky, as per note 16, p. 146.
20. J. Rorty, as per note 18, p. 184. *Fortune*, Mar. 1938, p. 152.
21. "Deaths Following Elixir of Sulfaniliamide-Massengill," *Journal of the American Medical Association*, Oct. 30, 1937, pp. 1456–57.
22. Ernest Wynder et al., "Tobacco Smoking as a Possible Etiologic Factor in Bronchogenic Carcinoma," *Journal of the American Medical Association*, May 1950, pp. 329–38.
23. H. Wolinsky, as per note 16, p. 148.
24. "Cigarettes Under Fire: Blowing Away the PR Smoke Screen," *Media and Values*, Center for Media and Values, Los Angeles, Spring/Summer 1991, p. 16.
25. H. Wolinsky, as per note 16, p. 149.
26. M. Jacobson, as per note 5, p. 150.
27. "Cigarette Hucksterism and the AMA," *Journal of the American Medical Association*, April 3, 1954, p. 1180.
28. H. Wolinsky, as per note 16, p. 150.
29. M. Jacobson, as per note 5, p. 150.
30. Richard Harris, *A Sacred Trust* (New York: New American Library, 1966), p. 159.
31. R. Mokhiber, as per note 15, p. 434.
32. "AMA Position on Cigaret Smoking Outlined," *AMA News*, Apr. 13, 1964, p. 5.
33. "Smoking Study Funds Donated," and "Research Group Named," *AMA News*, Feb. 17, 1964, p. 1.
34. Joseph Hixon, "AMA at Last Finds Perils in Smoking," *Chicago Sun-Times*, June 25, 1964. Elizabeth Whelan, *A Smoking Gun: How the Tobacco Industry Gets Away With Murder* (Philadelphia: Stickley, 1984), p. 104.
35. Ibid.
36. H. Wolinsky, as per note 16, p. 152.
37. Ibid., p. 153.
38. Ibid.
39. "AMA View Decried in Tobacco Dispute," *New York Times*, Mar. 20, 1964, p. 23. "Lawmaker Assails Charges vs AMA on Tobacco," *Journal of the American Medical Association*, Apr. 6, 1954, pp. 15–16. "AMA Presents Cigarette Labeling View to FTC," ibid., pp. 29–31. "AMA Opposes Warning on Tobacco, Association Comes Under Sharp Criticism as It Takes Position Shared by Industry Against Mandatory Labeling of Cigarettes as Health Hazard," *Medical World News*, Apr. 10, 1964, pp. 51–53.
40. Drew Pearson and Jack Anderson, *The Case Against Congress: A Compelling Indictment of Corruption on Capitol Hill* (New York: Simon and Schuster, 1968), pp. 329–30.
41. H. Wolinsky, as per note 16, p. 158.

42. AMA-ERF Committee for Research on Tobacco and Health, *Tobacco and Health* (Chicago: American Medical Association, 1978).
43. *Smoking and Health: A Report of the Surgeon General*, U.S. Dept. of HEW, Centers for Disease Control and Prevention, Office on Smoking and Health, 1979, pp. i–v.
44. H. Wolinsky, as per note 16, p. 157.
45. Federal Trade Commission, "Staff Report of the Cigarette Advertising Investigation," Washington, DC, FTC, 1981.
46. James Sammons, letter to Dr. Stephen J. Dresnick, chairman AMA Resident Physicians Section, Oct. 11, 1979; cited in H. Wolinsky, as per note 16, p. 159.
47. "Residents Seek Bigger Vote," *American Medical News*, Aug. 1/9, 1980, p. 18. "Doctor's Dilemma," *Wall Street Journal*, Mar. 12, 1981, sec. 2, p. 29.
48. Wayne Stayskal, cartoon, *Chicago Tribune*, June 15, 1981, sec. 1, p. 27.
49. M. Jacobson, as per note 5, p. 159.
50. Howard Wolinsky, "AMA Burns Smoking Issue at Both Ends," *Chicago Sun-Times*, June 18, 1985, p. 3. Howard Wolinsky, "AMA's Chief Edgy About Tobacco Land," *Chicago Sun-Times*, June 19, 1985, p. 24.
51. Howard Wolinsky, "AMA's Mixed Smoke Signals," *Chicago Sun-Times*, June 19, 1985, p. 7. Howard Wolinsky, "AMA Boss Sells Tobacco Farm," *Chicago Sun-Times*, Oct. 25, 1985, p. 6.
52. H. Wolinsky, as per note 16, p. 165.
53. Ibid., p. 166.
54. Ibid., p. 167.
55. Ibid., p. 168.
56. *Washington Post*, Jan. 27, 1993, A-16.
57. H. Wolinsky, as per note 16, p. 171.
58. Jerry Bishop, "AMA Urges FDA Regulation of Tobacco," *New York Times*, July 14, 1995, p. B-3.
59. Joshua Sharfstein et al., "Campaign Contributions From the American Medical Political Action Committee to Members of Congress," *New England Journal of Medicine*, Jan. 6, 1994, p. 32.
60. "Philip Morris: Death, Disease, and Duplicity," *Multi-National Monitor*, Dec. 1994, p. 14.
61. George Milowe, "Help Stop the Tobacco Epidemic," *Townsend Letter for Doctors*, Aug.–Sept. 1994, p. 944.
62. Ibid.
63. J. Sharfstein, as per note 59.
64. "New Majority Agenda," *New York Times*, Nov. 11, 1994, p. A-26.
65. H. Wolinsky, as per note 16, p. 228.
66. "The AMA: It's Not Tobacco, It's Margarine," *Good Medicine*, Spring 1993, pp. 3–4.
67. Ibid.
68. Deborah Christie-Smith, "PCRM Campaigns to End Wasteful Tobacco Experiments," *Good Medicine*, Summer 1994, p. 7.
69. Jane Brody, "Health Toll for a Meat Diet Costs Billions," New York Times, *Santa Cruz Sentinel*, Nov. 22, 1995, p. C-4.

Chapter 12: Must We Kill to Cure?

1. "Effectiveness of Lumpectomy Reaffirmed for Localized Tumors," New York Times, *Santa Cruz Sentinel*, Nov. 16, 1994.
2. Lucien Israel, *Conquering Cancer* (New York: Random House, 1978), p. 95.
3. Cited in *The Cancer Chronicles*, Summer 1990, p. 1.
4. Sharon Batt, *Patient No More* (Charlottetown, PEI, Canada: Gynergy Books, 1994), p. 86.
5. Ralph Moss, *The Cancer Industry* (New York: Paragon House, 1991), p. 68.
6. Ibid., p. 65.
7. "Matters of State," *WorldWatch*, March–April 1995, p. 39.
8. John Laszlo, *Understanding Cancer* (New York: Harper and Row, 1987).
9. Richard Walters, *Options: The Alternative Cancer Book* (Garden City Park, NY: Avery, 1993), p. 13.
10. S. Batt, as per note 4, p. 81.
11. Leslie Freeman, ed., *Nuclear Witnesses: Insiders Speak Out* (New York: Norton, 1982), p. 27.
12. S. Batt, as per note 4, p. 82.
13. Constance Holden, "Low Level Radiation: A High Level Concern," *Science* Apr. 13, 1979, pp. 155–58. Jean Marx, "Low Level Radiation: Just How Bad Is It?" *Science*, Apr. 13, 1979, pp. 160–64.
14. John Gofman, *Preventing Breast Cancer* (San Francisco: Committee for Nuclear Responsibility, 1995), p. 303.

15. Ibid., p. 6.
16. Robert Harris and Jeremy Paxman, *A Higher Form of Killing: The Secret Story of Chemical and Biological Warfare* (New York: Hill and Wang, 1982), pp. 119–25.
17. S. Batt, as per note 4, p. 93.
18. J. Patterson, *The Dread Disease* (Cambridge, MA: Harvard University Press, 1987).
19. Ralph Moss, *Questioning Chemotherapy* (Brooklyn, NY: Equinox, 1995), p. 21.
20. J. Patterson, as per note 18, p. 146.
21. R Moss,. as per note 19, p. 20.
22. Ibid., p. 21.
23. Ibid., p. 22.
24. Ibid., p. 20.
25. John Cairns, "The Treatment of Diseases and the War Against Cancer," *Scientific American*, 253(5), Nov. 1985, pp. 51–59.
26. John Bailar and Elaine Smith, "Progress Against Cancer?," *New England Journal of Medicine*, 314, May 8, 1986, pp. 1226–33.
27. Abel Ulrich, *Chemotherapy of Advanced Epithelial Cancer* (Stuttgart: Hippokrates Verlag, 1990).
28. Tim Beardsley, "A War Not Won," *Scientific American*, Jan. 1994, p. 130.
29. R. Moss, as per note 19, p. 13.
30. Ibid., pp. 56–57, 66.
31. *Cecil's Textbook of Medicine*, 18th ed., 1988; cited in R. Moss, as per note 19, p. 57.
32. Albert Braverman, "Medical Oncology in the 1990s," *Lancet*, 337, 1991, pp. 901–2.
33. R. Moss, as per note 19, p. 40.
34. Ibid.
35. Ibid., p. 41.
36. M. Moore et al., "How Expert Physicians Would Wish to Be Treated if They Developed Genito-Urinary Cancer," *Proceedings of the American Society of Cancer Oncologists*, 1988.
37. R. Moss, as per note 19, p. 42.
38. Lester Grinspoon and James Bakalar, *Marijuana: The Forbidden Medicine* (New Haven, CT: Yale University Press, 1993), p. 25.
39. S. Loeb, *Chemotherapy Handbook* (Springhouse, PA: Springhouse Corp., 1994).
40. R. Moss, as per note 19, p. 68.
41. Christine Gorman, "The Disturbing Case of the Cure That Killed the Patient," *Time*, Apr. 3, 1995, p. 60.
42. Jon Marcus, "Boston Hospital Rocked by Fatal Drug Mistake," Associated Press, *Santa Cruz Sentinel*, Mar. 24, 1995, p. A-1.
43. K. Fields et al., "Maximum Tolerated Doses of Ifosfamide, Carboplatin, and Etoposide . . ." *Journal of Cancer Oncology*, 13, 1995, pp. 323–32.
44. Ibid.
45. V. DeVita et al., eds., *Cancer: Principles and Practice of Oncology* (Philadelphia: Lippincott, 1993).
46. Robert Kotlowitz, *New York Times Magazine*, Dec. 4, 1994.
47. F. DiMario et al., "Acute Mental Status Changes in Children With Systemic Cancer," *Pediatrics*, 85, 1990, pp. 353–60.
48. Personal communication with author.
49. J. Laszlo, as per note 8.
50. M. Kris et al., "Delayed Emesis Following Anti-Cancer Chemotherapy," *Support Care Cancer*, 2, 1994, pp. 297–300.
51. Lynn Payer, *Medicine and Culture* (New York: Holt, 1988), p. 31.
52. Jane Brody and Art Holleb, *You Can Fight Cancer and Win* (New York: Times Books, 1977).
53. *New York Times*, Oct. 8, 1976; cited in R. Moss, as per note 5, p. 27.
54. *New York Daily News*, Jan. 14, 1978; cited in R. Moss, as per note 5, p. 27.
55. S. Batt, as per note 4, pp. 27, 214.
56. Ibid., p. 218.
57. Audre Lorde, *The Cancer Journals* (San Francisco: Aunt Lute Books, 1980), p. 56.
58. Ibid.
59. S. Batt, as per note 4, pp. 27, 224.
60. Ibid., p. 225.
61. Ibid., p. 235.
62. Personal communication with author.
63. S. Batt, as per note 4, p. 226.

Chapter 13: Alternatives for Cancer

1. C. Frey et al., "Randomized Study of 5-FU and CCNU in Pancreatic Cancer," *Cancer*, 47, 1981, pp. 27–31.
2. "Michael Landon's Drama Moves the Nation," in R. Moss, ed., *The Cancer Chronicles*, Summer 1991, p. 1
3. Ibid., p. 8.
4. Robert Houston, *Misinformation From OTA on Unconventional Cancer Treatments: Invited Response for the U.S. Congress* (Otho, IA: Office of Technology Assessment, People Against Cancer, 1990), p. 10
5. Nicholas Gonzales, *One Man Alone: An Investigation of Nutrition, Cancer, and William Donald Kelley*, unpublished manuscript, 1987; cited in Richard Walters, *Options: The Alternative Cancer Book* (Garden City Park, NY: Avery, 1993), p. 212. "Portrait of a Healer: Nicholas Gonzales, M.D.," *The Cancer Chronicles*, Summer 1990, p. 10.
6. Ibid.
7. Harold Ladas, "Book Review," *Cancer Victors Journal*, Summer–Fall 1988, pp. 23–24.
8. Robert Maver, "Nutrition and Cancer: the Gonzales Study," *On the Risk*, 7(2), 1991; originally published in *Discoveries in Medicine* (Mutual Benefit Life).
9. Ralph Moss, *The Cancer Industry* (New York: Paragon House, 1991), p. 116.
10. "Physicians and Healers: Unwitting Partners in Health Care," *New England Journal of Medicine*, Jan. 2, 1992, p. 63.
11. Norman Paradis, "Making a Living Off the Dying," *New York Times*, Apr. 25, 1992, p. 23.
12. Michael Lerner, *Choices in Healing: Integrating the Best of Conventional and Complementary Approaches to Cancer* (Cambridge, MA: MIT Press, 1994), p. 34.
13. Ibid., p. 35.
14. Ibid., p. 36.
15. R. Walters, as per note 5, p. 125.
16. M. Lerner, as per note 12, p. 35.
17. Jurgen Schurhold, testimony before U.S. Senate Labor and Human Resources Committee Hearing on the Access to Medical Treatment Act (AMTA), July 22, 1994.
18. "Alternative Medicine Programs Growing in Israel," in Larry Dossey, ed., *Alternative Therapies*, July 1995, p. 27. James Carter, "Letter," in *Townsend Letter for Doctors*, Aug.–Sept. 1994, p. 913.
19. Lynn Payer, *Medicine and Culture* (New York: Holt, 1988), p. 66.
20. "Paris Doc Blasts War on Cancer," in R. Moss, as per note 2, July 1995, p. 7.
21. Dana Ullman, "The Mainstreaming of Alternative Medicine," *Healthcare Forum Journal*, Nov.–Dec., 1993, p. 26.
22. Emiko Ohnuki-Tierney, *Illness and Culture in Contemporary Japan: An Anthropological View* (New York: Cambridge University Press, 1984); cited in M. Lerner, as per note 12, p. 43.
23. Ibid.
24. American Cancer Society, Cancer Response System #8249, printed May 24, 1995. "Unconventional Methods of Treatment," *Cancer Facts*, National Cancer Institute, National Institutes of Health, Oct. 2, 1992.
25. Robert Paradowski, "About the Author," in Linus Pauling, *How to Live Longer and Feel Better* (New York: W. H. Freeman and Co., 1986), p. 307.
26. L. Pauling, as per note 25, p. 166.
27. Ibid.
28. Ewan Cameron and Linus Pauling, "Supplemental Ascorbate in the Supportive Treatment of Cancer: Prolongation of Survival Times in Terminal Human Cancer," *Proceedings of the National Academy of Sciences*, 73, 1976, pp. 3685–89.
29. L. Pauling, as per note 25, p. 171.
30. Evelleen Richards, "The Politics of Therapeutic Evaluation: The Vitamin C and Cancer Controversy," *Social Studies of Science*, SAGE, vol. 18, 1988, p. 665.
31. Ewan Cameron and Linus Pauling, *Cancer and Vitamin C* (Philadelphia: Camino Books, 1993), p. 130.
32. E. Creagan, et al., "Failure of High Dose Vitamin C Therapy to Benefit Patients With Advanced Cancer: A Controlled Trial," *New England Journal of Medicine*, 301, 1979, pp. 687–90. *Medical World News*, June 25, 1979; cited in E. Richards, as per note 30, p. 668.
33. R. Moss, as per note 9, p. 221.
34. E. Creagan and C. Moertel, "Vitamin C Therapy and Advanced Cancer," *New England Journal of Medicine*, 301, Dec. 20, 1979, p. 1399.
35. E. Cameron and L. Pauling, "Supplemental Ascorbate in the Supportive Treatment of Cancer:

Reevaluation of Prolongation of Survival Times in Terminal Human Cancer," *Proceedings of the National Academy of Sciences*, 75, 1978, pp. 4538–44. E. Cameron and L. Pauling , "Experimental Studies Designed to Evaluate the Management of Patients With Incurable Cancer," *Proceedings of the National Academy of Sciences*, 75, 1978, p. 6252. E. Cameron and L. Pauling, "Ascorbate and Cancer," *Proceedings of the American Philosophical Society*, 123, 1979, pp. 117–23.

36. F. Morishige and A. Murata, "Prolongation of Survival Times in Terminal Human Cancer by Administration of Supplemental Ascorbate," *Journal of the International Academy of Preventive Medicine*, 5, 1979, pp. 47–52.
37. Abram Hoffer and Linus Pauling, "Hardin Jones Biostatistical Analysis of Mortality Data for Cohorts of Cancer Patients . . ." *Journal of Orthomolecular Medicine*, 5, 1990, pp 143–54.
38. Charles Moertel, in "A Proposition: Megadoses of Vitamin C Are Valuable in the Treatment of Cancer. Affirmative: Linus Pauling. Negative: Charles Moertel," *Nutrition Review*, 44, 1986, p. 30.
39. E. Richards, as per note 30, p. 672.
40. E. Richards, "Vitamin C Suffers a Dose of Politics," *New Scientist*, Feb. 27, 1986.
41. R. Moss, as per note 9, p. 226.
42. Charles Moertel, "Current Concepts in Cancer Chemotherapy of Gastrointestinal Cancer," *New England Journal of Medicine*, 299, 1978, pp. 1049–52.
43. Ibid.
44. Frost and Sullivan Market Intelligence, cited in Ralph Moss, *Questioning Chemotherapy* (New York: Equinox Press, 1995), p. 75.
45. "Big Money in New Cancer Drugs," *The Cancer Chronicles*, Spring 1991, p. 5."Broder Steps Down at NCI: MSKCC Chief Heads Search Panel," *The Cancer Chronicles*, Feb. 1995, p. 2.
46. R. Moss, as per note 9, p. 83.
47. Ibid., p. 91.
48. R. Walters, as per note 5, p. 105.
49. Ibid.
50. Ibid., p. 109.
51. Ibid., p. 110.
52. Ibid.
53. Ibid., p. 112.
54. Ibid., p. 115.
55. Ken Ausebel, *Hoxsey: How Healing Becomes a Crime* (A Documentary), Realidad Productions, Santa Fe.
56. Benedict Fitzgerald, *The Fitzgerald Report: A Report to the Senate Interstate Commerce Committee on the Need for Investigation of Cancer Research Organizations*, Congressional Record, Aug. 3, 1953.
57. Harry Hoxsey, *You Don't Have to Die* (New York: Milestone Books, 1956), p. 59.
58. K. Ausebel, as per note 55.
59. Ibid.
60. Ibid.
61. American Cancer Society Cancer Response System #8308, printed May 24, 1995.
62. Ken Ausebel, "The Troubling Case of Harry Hoxsey," *New Age Journal*, July–Aug. 1988, p. 45.
63. R. Walters, as per note 5, p. 103.
64. Steve Austin and Cathy Hitchcock, *Breast Cancer* (Rocklin, CA: Prima Publishing, 1994), pp. 139–44.

Chapter 14: Heretics and Healing

1. Patricia Spain Ward, "History of Gerson Therapy," Contract Report for the U.S. Congress Office of Technology Assessment (OTA), revised June 1988, pp. 1–2, 8.
2. Ralph Moss, *Cancer Therapy* (New York: Equinox, 1992), pp. 187–88.
3. P. Ward, as per note 1, p. 12.
4. Ibid.
5. Mark McCarty, "Aldosterone and the Gerson Diet," *Medical Hypotheses*, 7, 1981, pp. 591–97.
6. Richard Walters, *Options: The Alternative Cancer Book* (Garden City Park, NY: Avery, 1993), p. 200.
7. A. Reed et al., "Mexico: Juices, Coffee Enemas, and Cancer," *Lancet*, Sept. 15, 1990, pp. 667–68.
8. Gar Hildenbrand et al., "Five-Year Survival Rates of Melanoma Patients Treated by Diet Therapy After the Manner of Gerson: A Retrospective Review," *Alternative Therapies*, Sept. 1995, p. 29.
9. American Cancer Society Cancer Response System #8254, printed May 24, 1995.
10. Michael Lerner, *Choices in Healing: Integrating the Best of Conventional and Complementary Approaches to Cancer* (Cambridge, MA: MIT Press, 1994), p. 261.

11. Anthony Sattillaro, *Recalled by Life* (New York: Avon Books, 1982). Neil Barnard, "Surviving Cancer," *Good Medicine*, Summer 1993, p. 14.
12. Vivien Newbold, "Complete Remission of Advanced Medically Incurable Cancer in Six Patients Following a Macrobiotic Approach to Healing," *Townsend Letter for Doctors*, Oct. 1990, p. 638.
13. Ibid., p. 642. Vivien Newbold, letter to Helen Sheehan, director of Professional Education Programs, American Cancer Society, Mar. 4, 1988. M. Lerner, as per note 10, pp. 306–7.
14. James Carter et al., "Hypothesis: Dietary Management May Improve Survival From Nutrionally Linked Cancers . . ." *Journal of the American College of Nutrition*, 12(3), 1993, pp. 209–26. James Carter et al., "Cancers With Suspected Nutritional Links: Dietary Management?" Tulane University School of Public Health and Tropical Medicine, Feb. 1990.
15. Harold Foster, "Lifestyle Changes and the 'Spontaneous' Regression of Cancer . . ." *International Journal of Biosocial Research*, 10(1), 1988, pp. 17–33.
16. American Cancer Society Cancer Response System #8679, printed May 24, 1995.
17. Murray Smith, "The Burzynski Controversy: A Comparative Case Study in the Sociology of Alternative Medicine in the U.S. and Canada," *Canadian Journal of Sociology*, 17(2), 1992; reprinted in *Townsend Letter for Doctors*, Apr. 1994, pp. 352–63.
18. R. Walters, as per note 6, pp. 17–18.
19. M. Lerner, as per note 10, p. 410.
20. Ibid., p. 412.
21. M. Smith, as per note 17.
22. American Cancer Society Cancer Response System #8015, "Anti-neoplastons," printed May 24, 1995.
23. "A Patient's Son Speaks Out," *The Cancer Chronicles*, Jan.–Feb. 1993, p. 4.
24. Ralph Moss, *The Cancer Industry* (New York: Paragon House, 1991), p. 331.
25. R. Walters, as per note 6, p. 21.
26. Ibid.
27. "You Might Like to Hear Some Good News," *The Cancer Chronicles*, Summer 1991, p. 7.
28. "Alternative Medicine and the Law," *Townsend Letter for Doctors*, May 1995, p. 136.
29. "Judge Restores Burzynski's License, Chastises Texas Board," *The Cancer Chronicles*, Feb. 1995, p. 4.
30. Ibid.
31. As per note 28.
32. "FDA and Postal Agents Raid Burzynski Clinic," *The Cancer Chronicles*, May 1995, p. 4.
33. "Congress Launches Probe of Burzynski Connection," *The Cancer Chronicles*, Oct. 1995, p. 3.
34. "Burzynski vs. Grand Jury, Round Five," *Townsend Letter for Doctors*, July 1995, p. 19.
35. As per note 32.
36. Ibid., p. 5.
37. Ibid.
38. Ibid.
39. American Cancer Society, as per note 22.
40. "General Information on Questionable Methods of Cancer Treatment Risks and Dangers," American Cancer Society Cancer Response System, #8249, printed May 24, 1995.
41. David Eisenberg and Thomas Wright, *Encounters With Qi: Exploring Chinese Medicine* (New York: Penguin, 1987), pp. 68–74.
42. Bernie Siegel, *Peace, Love, and Healing* (New York: Harper, 1989), p. 95.
43. Janny Scott, "Study Says Cancer Survival Rises With Group Therapy," *Los Angeles Times*, May 11, 1989. David Spiegel, "A Psychosocial Intervention and Survival Time of Patients With Metastatic Breast Cancer," *Advances*, 7(3), Summer 1991, pp. 10–19.
44. D. Lamm et al., "Megadose Vitamins in Bladder Cancer: A Double-Blind Clinical Trial," *Journal of Urology*, 151, 1994, pp. 21–26.
45. V. Vinciguerra et al., "Inhalation Marijuana as an Anti-emetic for Cancer Chemotherapy," *New York State Journal of Medicine*, 88, Oct. 1988, pp. 525–27.
46. Lester Grinspoon and James Bakalar, *Marijuana, The Forbidden Medicine* (New Haven, CT: Yale University Press, 1993), pp. 28–31.
47. Ibid., p. 32.
48. Ibid., pp. 37–38.
49. Ibid., p. 38.
50. Ibid., pp. 1–175.
51. Lester Grinspoon et al., "Marijuana as Medicine: A Plea for Reconsideration," *Journal of the American Medical Association*, June 21, 1995, pp. 1875–76.

52. Peter Gwynne, "Trials of Marijuana's Potential Languish as Government Just Says No," *The Scientist* Nov. 27, 1995, p. 7.
53. "Springer's New Test," *The Cancer Chronicles*, July 1994, p. 5
54. Claudia Dowling, "Fighting Back," *Life*, May 1994, p. 82.
55. "Chicago Immunologist Uses 'T/Tn Antigen' Treatment," *The Cancer Chronicles*, July 1994, p. 5
56. Ibid., p. 2
57. Ibid.
58. Ibid.
59. C. Dowling, as per note 54, p. 81
60. Ibid., p. 00.
61. Nathaniel Mead, "Breakthroughs in Cancer Research," *Natural Health*, Jan.–Feb. 1996, p. 138
62. Ibid.
63. Keith Block, "Block Nutrition Program," in *New Clinical Care Model: Applications to Cancer Patient Care*; prepared for Office of Technology Assessment, U.S. Congress.
64. N. Mead, as per note 61, p. 82.
65. Keith Block, personal communication with author.
66. "Dr. Warner's Battle With Disciplinary Board," *Townsend Letter for Doctors*, June 1994, p. 595
67. Lois Berry, personal communication with author, July 1995
68. Personal communication with author, July 1995.
69. Ibid.
70. L. Berry, as per note 67.
71. Cited in "Washington Oncologist Raided and Shut Down," *The Cancer Chronicles*, Oct 1995
72. J. T. Quigg, personal communication with author, July 1995
73. As per note 66, p. 596

Chapter 15: Toward Partnership: Integrating the Best of Alternative and Orthodox Medicine
1. Riane Eisler, *The Chalice and the Blade* (San Francisco: Harper and Row, 1987)
2. Laurie Garrett, *The Coming Plague* (New York: Penguin, 1994), p. 209
3. Ibid.
4. F. Bennett, "A Comparison of Community Health in Uganda With Its Two East African Neighbors in the Period 1970–1979," in C. Dodge and P. Wiebe, eds., *Crisis in Uganda* (Oxford, England· Pergamon Press, 1985), pp. 43–52.
5. A. Enns, "The Clocks Have Stopped in Uganda," in C. Dodge, as per note 4, pp. 53–54.
6. Book in progress by Stuart A. Schlegel, *The Gracious Vision: Spiritual Wisdom From a Rainforest People.*
7. Personal communication with author, 1996.
8. Ruth Sivard, *World Military and Social Expenditures* (Washington, DC: World Priorities, 1983), pp. 5, 26
9. Ibid.
10. "Citings," *WorldWatch*, May–June 1993, p. 8.
11. Rene Dubos, *Mirage of Health* (New York: Harper, 1959), pp. 110–11.
12. Andrew Weil, *Spontaneous Healing: How to Discover and Enhance Your Body's Natural Ability to Maintain and Heal Itself* (New York: Alfred Knopf, 1995), pp. 4–7.
13. Robert Duggan, "Complementary Medicine: Transforming Influence or Footnote to History?" *Alternative Therapies*, May 1995, p. 29.
14. Thomas McKeown, *The Role of Medicine* (Princeton, NJ: Princeton University Press, 1979). Thomas McKeown, *The Origins of Human Disease* (Oxford, England: Blackwell, 1988)
15. Christiaan Barnard, "Medicine Negated," in Robert Lanza, ed., *One World: The Health and Survival of the Human Species in the 21st Century* (Santa Fe: Health Press, 1996), p. 105
16. Ibid., p. 106.
17. Ibid., p. 109.
18. D. Barua and W. Greenough, *Current Topics in Infectious Disease: Cholera* (New York: Plenum, 1992). J. Duffy, "Social Impact of Disease in the late 19th Century," in J. Leavitt et al., eds., *Sickness and Health in America* (Madison: University of Wisconsin Press, 1985).
19. Paul Ewald, "On Darwin, Snow, and Deadly Diseases," *Natural History*, June 1994, pp. 42–45
20. Ibid.
21. Thomas McKeown, *The Origins of Human Disease*, as per note 14, p. 83.
22. Jeffrey Fisher, *The Plague Makers* (New York: Simon and Schuster, 1994), p. 12.
23. J. Najera, "Malaria and the Work of WHO," *Bulletin of the World Health Organization*, 1989 pp. 229–43

24. J. Fisher, as per note 22, p. 17.
25. W. Stewart, "A Mandate for Action," presented at the Association of State and Territorial Health Officers, Washington, DC, Dec. 4, 1967
26. L. Garrett, as per note 2, p. 40.
27. Ibid., p. 47.
28. Institute of Medicine, *Malaria: Obstacles and Opportunities* (Washington, DC: National Academy Press, 1991).
29. Meri McCoy-Thompson, "Brazil Enlists DDT Against Malaria Outbreak," *WorldWatch*, July–Aug. 1990, p. 10.
30. Institute of Medicine, as per note 28.
31. L. Garrett, as per note 2, p. 49.
32. Rachel Carson, *Silent Spring* (Boston: Houghton Mifflin, 1962), p. 8.
33. Institute of Medicine, as per note 28.
34. G. Coatney, "Pitfalls in a Discovery: The Chronicle of Chloroquine," *American Journal of Tropical Medicine and Hygiene*, 12, 1963, pp. 121–28. D. Wyler, "The Ascent and Decline of Chloroquine," *Journal of the American Medical Association*, 251, 1984, pp. 2420–22.
35. J. Najera, as per note 23.
36. American Association for the Advancement of Science, *Malaria and Development in Africa*, AFR-0481-A-00-0037-00, U.S. Agency for International Development, Africa Bureau, Washington, DC, 1991.
37. D. Brothwell and A. Sandison, *Diseases in Antiquity* (Springfield, IL: Charles Thomas, 1967), pp. 238–46. W. McNeill, *Plagues and People* (New York: Doubleday, 1976), p. 103.
38. Ibid. F. Fenner et al., *Smallpox and Its Eradication* (Geneva: World Health Organization, 1988). W. Denevan, *The Native Populations of the Americas in 1492* (Madison: University of Wisconsin Press, 1992).
39. Ibid.
40. Ibid.
41. L. Garrett, as per note 2, p. 41. Larry Brilliant, "The Health of Humanity," *Whole Earth Review*, Fall 1993, p. 66.
42. F. Fenner, as per note 38. June Goodfield, *Quest for Killers* (Boston: Birkhauser, 1985), pp. 191–244. Horace Ogden, *CDC and the Smallpox Crusade*, HHS Publication No. 87-8400 (Washington, DC: U.S. Govt. Printing Office, 1987).
43. Larry Brilliant, *The Health of Humanity: A Progress Report*, presented at Symposium on Human and Environmental Health, March 22, 1991, sponsored by Presbyterian Hospital/Pacific Medical Center Program in Medicine and Philosophy.
44. L. Garrett, as per note 2, p. 42.
45. Thirty-third World Health Assembly, *Declaration of Global Eradication of Smallpox*, Geneva, May 8, 1980.
46. L. Brilliant, as per note 43.
47. Harris Coulter, *Vaccination, Social Violence, and Criminality* (Berkeley, CA: North Atlantic Books, 1990). Harris Coulter and Barbara Fisher, *A Shot in the Dark* (New York: Avery, 1991). Viera Scheibner, *Vaccination* (Maryborough, Victoria, Australia: Aust. Print Group, 1993). Neil Miller, *Vaccines: Are They Really Safe and Effective?* (Santa Fe, NM: New Atlantean Press, 1992). Peggy O'Mara, ed., *Vaccinations: The Rest of the Story* (Santa Fe, NM: Mothering, 1992). Walene James, *Immunization: The Reality Behind the Myth* (Westport, CT: Bergin and Garvey, 1995).
48. "Pertussis Returns With a Vengeance," *Patient Care*, Feb. 15, 1994; noted in *Birth Gazette*, Spring 1994, p. 36.
49. Anne Platt, "Epidemics in the Former Soviet Union," *WorldWatch*, Nov.–Dec. 1995, p. 6. Centers for Disease Control and Prevention, *Diphtheria Outbreak, Russian Federation*.
50. Anne Platt, "The Resurgence of Infectious Diseases," *WorldWatch*, July–Aug. 1995, p. 29.
51. P. O'Mara, as per note 47, p. 9.
52. H. Buttram and J. Hoffman, "Vaccinations and Immune Malfunction," in J. Pizzorno et al., *A Textbook of Natural Medicine* (Seattle: Bastyr College Publications, 1986).
53. J. Froom et al., "Diagnosis and Antibiotic Treatment of Acute Otitis Media: Report From International Primary Care Network," *British Medical Journal*, 300, 1990, pp. 582–86.
54. F. Buchem, "Therapy of Acute Otitis Media: Myringotomy, Antibiotics, or Neither? A Double-Blind Study in Children," *Lancet*, 8252, Oct. 24, 1981, pp. 883–87.
55. M. Diamant et al., "Abuse and Timing of Antibiotics in Acute Otitis Media," *Archives of Otolaryngology*, 1974, pp. 226–32. E. Cantekin et al., "Antimicrobial Therapy for Otitis Media," *Journal of the American Medical Association*, 266(23), 1991, pp. 3309–17.

56. Michael Schmidt, "Response to Ear Infections," *Mothering*, Fall 1991, p. 21.
57. S. Solovitch, "Certain Foods May Bring on Ear Infections," *San Jose Mercury News*, Jan. 31, 1996, p. 5E
58. Michael Schmidt, "Ear Infections in Children," *Mothering*, Spring 1991, pp. 41–42.
59. J. Fisher, as per note 22, p. 15.
60. Ibid., p. 22.
61. H. Neu, "The Crisis in Antibiotic Resistance," *Science*, 257, 1992, pp. 1064–73. M. Cohen, "Epidemiology of Drug Resistance . . . " *Science*, 257, 1992, pp. 1050–55. S. Finegold, "Antimicrobial Therapy of Anaerobic Infections. A Status Report," *Hospital Practice*, Oct. 1979, pp. 71–81. L. Gentry, "Bacterial Resistance," *Orthopedic Clinics of North America*, 22, 1991, pp. 379–88. A. Gibbons, "Exploring New Strategies to Fight Drug-Resistant Microbes," *Science*, 257, 1992. Marc Lappe, *Germs That Won't Die* (Garden City, NY: Anchor Press, 1982). Stuart Levy, *The Antibiotic Paradox* (New York: Plenum, 1992).
62. J. Fisher, as per note 22, p. 30.
63. L. Garrett, as per note 2, p. 437.
64. J. Fisher, as per note 22, p. 31.
65. Ibid.
66. Ibid., p. 40.
67. J. Lederberg, speech before Irvington Trust, New York City, Feb. 8, 1994
68. M. Cohen, as per note 61.
69. A. Weil, as per note 12, pp. 225–26.
70. "The Tobacco-Health Insurance Connection," *Lancet*, July 8, 1995. "Health Care Giants Invest Their Juicy Profits in Tobacco Stock," *Public Citizen Health Letter*, Aug. 1995, p. 12.
71. "Civil Suits Awards a Pittance Compared to CEO Salaries, Study Shows," *Public Citizen*, 1995, p. 7
72. Joan Claybrook, *Public Citizen Member Letter*, 1995.
73. Robert Pear, "Hospitals Say HMOs Often Refuse Emergencies," New York Times, *San Francisco Chronicle*, July 9, 1995, p. A-1.
74. George Anders, "HMOs Pile Up Billions in Cash," *Wall Street Journal*, Dec. 21, 1994. Mitt Freudenheim, "Penny-Pinching HMOs Showed Their Generosity in Executive Paychecks," *New York Times*, April 11, 1995.
75. Allen Meyerson, "Final Stats: Mantle's Last Medical Bills," *New York Times*, Aug. 20, 1995

Chapter 16: The Health of Humanity

1. "Vital Signs," *WorldWatch*, Sept.–Oct. 1991, p. 6.
2. Laurie Garrett, *The Coming Plague* (New York: Penguin, 1994), p. 250.
3. Ibid.
4. *Global Marine Biological Diversity* (Washington, DC: Center for Marine Conservation, 1993).
5. Paul Epstein, "Marine Ecosystem Health: Implications for Public Health," annals of the *New York Academy of Science*, vol. 740, "Diseases in Evolution," pp. 14–23. Paul Epstein, "Cholera and the Environment," *Lancet*, 339, 1992, pp. 1167–68. Paul Epstein et al., "Marine Ecosystems," *Lancet*, 342, Nov. 13, 1993, pp. 1216–19. L. Garrett, as per note 2, p. 562.
6. Ibid., p. 564.
7. A. Lockwood, "Aliens and Interlopers at Sea," *Lancet*, 342, 1993, pp. 942–43. C. Anderson, "Cholera Epidemic Traced to Risk Miscalculation," *Nature*, 354, 1992, p. 255. E. Rice et al., "Cholera in Peru," *Lancet*, 338, 1991, p. 455. V. Witt et al., "Environmental Health Conditions and Cholera Vulnerability in Latin America . . ." *Journal of Public Health Policy*, Winter 1991, pp. 450–63. R. Tauxe et al., "Cholera Epidemic in Latin America," *Journal of the American Medical Association*, 267, 1992, pp. 1388–90.
8. Nancy Chege, "Pasteurizing Water," *WorldWatch*, Sept.–Oct. 1995, p. 8.
9. W. McNeill, Appendix, "Epidemics in China" in *Plagues and People* (New York: Doubleday, 1976).
10. J. Heckler, *The Epidemics of the Middle Ages*; cited in L. Garrett, as per note 2, p. 643.
11. Ibid.
12. L. Garrett, as per note 2, p. 238.
13. Ibid., p. 28.
14. Ibid., pp. 13–29.
15. Ibid., p. 28.
16. Nick Chiles, "In Rat's Realm," *New York Newsday*, May 9, 1994, p. A-8.
17. "Plague! India, Africa Confront the Ultimate Nightmare," *Animal People*, Nov. 1994, p. 15.
18. Robert Pinner et al., "Trends in Infectious Disease Mortality in the United States," *Journal of the American Medical Association*, 275(3), Jan. 17, 1996, pp. 189–93.
19. Richard Preston, *The Hot Zone* (New York: Anchor Books Doubleday, 1994), pp. 407–9.

20. L. Garrett, as per note 2, p. 319.
21. Jonathan Mann, "AIDS," in Robert Lanza, ed., *One World: The Health and Survival of the Human Species in the 21st Century* (Santa Fe, NM: Health Press, 1996), p. 76.
22. Ibid., p. 77.
23. "Needle Exchanges Slow AIDS Spread," New York Times, *San Francisco Chronicle*, Nov. 26, 1994, p. A-10.
24. L. Garrett, as per note 2, p. 464.
25. J. Mann, as per note 21, p. 79.
26. L. Garrett, as per note 2, p. 491.
27. "India: Prostitutes and the Spread of AIDS," *Lancet*, 335, 1990, p. 1332.
28. L. Garrett, as per note 2, pp. 692–93.
29. J. Mann, as per note 21, p. 79.
30. Ibid.
31. C. Everett Koop, *Koop: The Memories of a Family Physician* (New York: Random House, 1991)
32. C. Decker, "Robertson Tailors His Message to Audiences," *Los Angeles Times*, Nov. 23, 1987.
33. L. Garrett, as per note 2, p. 466.
34. Ibid., p. 469.
35. A. Kumar, "AIDS in India: Fear and Ignorance Are Combining to Produce the Public Health Crisis of the Century," *India Currents*, Aug. 1991, pp. 17–18.
36. Ibid.
37. M. Ellis, "AMA Denounces WHO," *World Health*, Jan. 1948.
38. "Clinton Intensifies Support for AIDS," Washington Post, *San Jose Mercury News*, Dec. 7, 1995.
39. Patricia Holt, "Doctor Says He Keeps AIDS Patients Healthy," *San Francisco Chronicle*, 1994, p. C-4
40. Jon Kaiser, *Immune Power: A Comprehensive Treatment for HIV* (New York: St. Martin's Press, 1993)
41. Leon Chaitow and James Strohecker, *You Don't Have to Die: Unraveling the AIDS Myth* (Puyallup, WA: Future Medicine, 1994), p. 198.
42. Personal communication with author.
43. Jonathan Patz et al., "Global Climate Change and Emerging Infectious Diseases," *Journal of the American Medical Association*, 275(3), Jan. 17, 1996, pp. 217–23. "Health Implications of Climate Variability and Change," Climate Research Committee, *National Academy of Sciences, National Research Council*, May 8, 1995, Washington, DC. Richard Stone, "If the Mercury Soars, So May Health Hazards," *Science*, 267, Feb. 1995. Michael Loevinsohn, "Climate Warming and Increased Malaria Incidence," *Lancet*, 343, Mar. 19, 1994. Paul Epstein, "Emerging Diseases and Ecosystem Instability New Threats to Public Health," *American Journal of Public Health*, 85(2), Feb. 1995, pp. 168–71
44. L. Garrett, as per note 2, p. 536.
45. Ibid., p. 530.
46. L. Altman, "Virus That Caused Deaths in New Mexico Is Isolated," *New York Times*, Nov. 21, 1993, p. A21. L. Garrett, "Medical Gumshoes Confront a Mystery," *Newsday*, Sept. 28, 1993, pp. 69–72. J. Horgan, "Were Four Corners Victims Biowar Casualties?," *Scientific American*, Nov. 1993. J. Hughes et al., "Hantavirus Pulmonary Syndrome: An Emerging Infectious Disease," *Science*, 262, 1993, pp. 850–51. B. Le Guenno, "Identifying a Hantavirus . . ." *Lancet*, 342, 1993, pp. 1438–39 R. Levins et al., "Hantavirus Disease Emerging," *Lancet*, 342, 1993, p. 1292.
47. "Biologists Fear Hantavirus Outbreak," Associated Press, *Santa Cruz Sentinel*, July 5, 1995, p. A5
48. Lester Brown, "Facing Food Scarcity," *WorldWatch*, Nov.–Dec. 1995, pp. 10–11.
49. Lester Brown, "The Cairo Plan," *WorldWatch*, Nov.–Dec. 1994, p. 2.
50. Riane Eisler, *The Chalice and the Blade* (San Francisco: Harper and Row, 1987), p. 176.
51. Richard Franke and Barbara Chasin, *Kerala: Radical Reform as Development in an Indian State*, Institute for Food and Development Policy, 1994.
52. Ann Austin, "State of Grace," *Earthwatch*, Mar.–Apr. 1993, p. 21.
53. Ibid.
54. Nicholas Kristof, "China Sets Example in Health Care," New York Times, *Ann Arbor News*, April 14, 1991 p. A-6. Jane Lii, "China Booms, The World Holds Its Breath," *New York Times Magazine*, Feb. 18, 1996 p. 27.
55. Ibid.
56. Bill Caradonna and Mazair Emadi, "Antibiotic Update," *Journal of Naturopathic Medicine*, 5(1) 1994, pp. 62–67 "Making Medicine, Making Money," *Seattle Times*, Jan. 3 1993, A-3

Index

Abel, Ulrich, 237
Abortion, 95–99
Access to Medical Treatment Act, 222
Acupuncture, 262–63, 293–94
ADHD, 159–81
Aetna Insurance Co., 346
Agency for Health Care Policy and Research, 194
A Good Birth, A Safe Birth, 24
AIDS, 354–61; alternative treatments for, 358–61
Alaska State Medical Association, 221
Allen, Woody, 295
American Academy of Pediatrics, 180
American Cancer Society: alternative cancer treatments and, 9, 220, 252–55, 263, 270, 278, 281, 283–87, 291–92; Keith Block and, 302, 304; chemotherapy and, 244; chemotherapy drug patents and, 270; dominator medicine and, 322; Hubert Humphrey and, 245; Betsy Lehman and, 242; Look Good, Feel Better and, 248–49; medical marijuana and, 300; radiation and, 231, 245; Reach to Recovery and, 247–49; tobacco and, 207, 208, 247; toxicity of wealth of, 246
American College of Obstetricians and Gynecologists: cesareans and, 38; changes in sexual response due to hysterectomy and, 133, 135;

dominator medicine and, 322; fetal monitors and, 49; gender balance in board of, 103; home births and, 30–31; midwife-attended births and, 79; out-of-hospital births and, 20; women's right to medical self-determination and, 79–80
American College of Orthopedic Surgeons, 191
American College of Physicians, 191
American College of Radiology, 191
American College of Surgeons, 191
American Dietetic Association, 179–80
American Hospital Association, 191
American International Group Insurance Co., 346
American Lung Association, 213
American Medical Association: abortion and, 95–99; acupuncture and, 8–9; alternative cancer treatments and, 220, 255, 273–76, 279–80, 282; alternative medicine and, 8–9; 185–96, 220, 255, 273–76, 279–80, 282; biofeedback and, 8–9; birth control and, 97, 99–101, 119, 198; chiropractic and, 185–96; choice of name of, 96; dominant medical paradigm and, 227; estrogen and, 138; extent of influence of, 182–84, 219; FEC and, 183–84; Ben Feingold and, 170; homeopathy